Kennedy Boulevard • Suite 1800 • Philadelphia, Pennsylvania 19103-2899

eclinics.com

CLINICS OF NORTH AMERICA Volume 97, Number 1
13 ISSN 0025-7125, ISBN-13: 978-1-4557-7116-5

mela Hetherington

Medical Clinics of North America (ISSN 0025-7125) is published bimonthly by Elsevier Inc., 360 Park Avenue
South, New York, NY 10010-1710. Months of issue are January, March, May, July, September, and November.
Periodicals postage paid at New York, NY, and additional mailing offices. Subscription prices are USD 232 per
year for US individuals, USD 424 per year for US institutions, USD 117 per year for US students, USD 295 per
year for Canadian individuals, USD 551 per year for Canadian institutions, USD 184 per year for Canadian students, USD 358 per year for international individuals, USD 551 per year for international institutions and USD
184 per year for international students. To receive student/resident rate, orders must be accompanied by
name of affiliated institution, date of term, and the signature of program/residency coordinator on institution
letterhead. Orders will be billed at individual rate until proof of status is received. Foreign air speed delivery
is included in all Clinics subscription prices. All prices are subject to change without notice. POSTMASTER:
Send address changes to Medical Clinics of North America, Elsevier Health Sciences Division, Subscription
Customer Service, 3251 Riverport Lane, Maryland Heights, MO 63043. Customer Service: Telephone:
1-800-654-2452 (U.S. and Canada); 1-314-447-8871 (outside U.S. and Canada). Fax: 1-314-447-8029.
E-mail: journalscustomerservice-usa@elsevier.com (for print support); journalsonlinesupport-usa@
elsevier.com (for online support).

Reprints. For copies of 100 or more of articles in this publication, please contact the Commercial Reprints
Department, Elsevier Inc., 360 Park Avenue South, New York, NY 10010-1710. Tel.: 212-633-3812; Fax:
212-462-1935; E-mail: reprints@elsevier.com.

Medical Clinics of North America is also published in Spanish by McGraw-Hill Interamericana Editores S. A.,
P.O. Box 5-237, 06500 Mexico, D.F., Mexico.

Medical Clinics of North America is covered in MEDLINE/PubMed (Index Medicus), Current Contents, ASCA,
Excerpta Medica, Science Citation Index, and ISI/BIOMED.

Printed in the United States of America.

Diabetic Chronic Kidney Disease

Editor

MARK E. WILLIAMS

MEDICAL CLINICS
OF NORTH AMERICA

www.medical.theclinics.com

January 2013 • Volume 97 • Number 1

PROGRAM OBJECTIVE:

The goal of *Medical Clinics of North America* is to keep practicing physicians up to date with current clinical practice by providing timely articles reviewing the state of the art in patient care.

TARGET AUDIENCE

All practicing physicians and other healthcare professionals.

ACCREDITATION

The Elsevier Office of Continuing Medical Education (EOCME) is accredited by the Accreditation Council for Continuing Medical Education (ACCME) to provide continuing medical education for physicians.

The EOCME designates this journal-based CME activity for a maximum of 11 *AMA PRA Category 1 Credit*(s)™. Physicians should claim only the credit commensurate with the extent of their participation in the activity.

All other health care professionals completing continuing education credit for this activity will be issued a certificate of participation.

DISCLOSURE OF CONFLICTS OF INTEREST

The EOCME assesses conflict of interest with its instructors, faculty, planners, and other individuals who are in a position to control the content of CME activities. All relevant conflicts of interest that are identified are thoroughly vetted by EOCME for fair balance, scientific objectivity, and patient care recommendations. EOCME is committed to providing its learners with CME activities that promote improvements or quality in healthcare and not a specific proprietary business or a commercial interest.

The planning committee, staff, authors and editors listed below have identified no financial relationships or relationships to products or devices they or their spouse/life partner have with commercial interest related to the content of this CME activity:

Andrea Bittner, PharmD Candidate; W. Kline Bolton, MD; Santha Priya Boorasamy; Brendan T. Bowman, MD; Paola Fioretto, MD, PhD; Jeannette Forcina; Rajesh Garg, MD; Jasmine D. Gonzalvo, PharmD; Deanna S. Kania, PharmD; Amanda J. Kleiner, MD; Andrezj S. Korlewski, MD, PhD; Jill McNair; Christy L. Nash, PharmD; Marcus G. Pezzolesi, PhD, MPH; Anne T. Reutens, MBBS, PhD; Eberhard Ritz, MD; Brian M. Shepler, PharmD; Cory T. Smith, PharmD; Katelynn Steck; Peter N. Van Buren, MD; and Mark E. Williams, MD.

The planning committee, staff, authors and editors listed below have identified financial relationships or relationships to products or devices they or their spouse/life partner have with commercial interest related to the content of this CME activity:

Jamie P. Dwyer, MD has received a research grant from Eli Lilly, Keryx Biopharmaceuticals and Nyphrogenex; and is a consultant/advisor for Boehringer Ingelheim.
Julie Lewis, MD and spouse have received research grants from Keryx, Lilly and Nephrogenix.
Christine Maric-Bilkan, PhD has received a research grant from NIH/NIDDK.
Michael Mauer, MD is a consultant/advisor for Sanofi, Noxxon, and Merck.
Robert D. Toto, MD is a consultant/advisor for Reata Pharmaceuticals, Amgen, Abbott, Mitsubishi and Otsukam; is on the speaker's bureau for Merck & Co. and Amgen; and has received a research grant from Reata Pharmaceuticals, Merck & Co. and Novartis.

UNAPPROVED / OFF-LABEL USE DISCLOSURE

The EOCME requires CME faculty to disclose to the participants:

1. When products or procedures being discussed are off-label, unlabelled, experimental, and/or investigational (not US Food and Drug Administration (FDA) approved; and
2. Any limitations on the information presented, such as data that are preliminary or that represent ongoing research, interim analyses, and/or unsupported opinions. Faculty may discuss information about pharmaceutical agents that is outside of DA-approved labelling. This information is intended solely for CME and is not intended to promote off-label use of these medications. If you have any questions, contact the medical affairs department of the manufacturer for the most recent prescribing information.

TO ENROLL

To enroll in the *Medical Clinics of North America* Continuing Medical Education program, call customer service at 1-800-654-2452 or sign up online at http://www.theclinics.com/home/cme. The CME program is available to subscribers for an additional annual fee of USD $267.

METHOD OF PARTICIPATION

In order to claim credit, participants must complete the following:

1. Complete enrolment as indicated above.
2. Read the activity.
3. Complete the CME Test and Evaluation. Participants must achieve a score of 70% on the test. All CME Tests and Evaluations must be completed online.

CME INQUIRIES/SPECIAL NEEDS

For all CME inquiries or special needs, please contact elsevierCME@elsevier.com.

MEDICAL CLINICS OF NORTH AMERICA

FORTHCOMING ISSUES

March 2013
Management of Acute & Chronic Headache Pain
Steven D. Waldman, *Editor*

May 2013
Early Diagnosis and Intervention in Predementia Alzheimer's Disease
Jose Molinuevo, Jeffrey Cummings, Bruno Dubois, and Philip Scheltens, *Editors*

July 2013
The Diabetic Foot
Andrew Boulton, *Editor*

RECENT ISSUES

November 2012
Interventions in Infectious Disease Emergencies
Nancy Misri Khardori, MD, PhD, FACP, FIDSA, *Editor*

July 2012
Chronic Obstructive Pulmonary Disease
Stephen I. Rennard, MD, and Bartolome R. Celli, MD, *Editors*

May 2012
Immunotherapy in Clinical Medicine
Nancy Misri Khardori, MD, PhD, FACP, FIDSA, and Romesh Khardori, MD, PhD, FACP, FACE, *Editors*

RELATED INTEREST

Geriatric Clinics, August 2009
Renal Disease
E.V. Lerma, *Editor*

NOW AVAILABLE FOR YOUR iPhone and iPad

Contributors

EDITOR

MARK E. WILLIAMS, MD, FACP, FASN
Harvard Medical School, Joslin Diabetes Center, Boston, Massachusetts

AUTHORS

ANDREA BITTNER
Candidate, Purdue University College of Pharmacy, West Lafayette, Indiana

W. KLINE BOLTON, MD
Division of Nephrology, Department of Medicine, University of Virginia Health System, Charlottesville, Virginia

BRENDAN T. BOWMAN, MD
Division of Nephrology, Department of Medicine, University of Virginia Health System, Charlottesville, Virginia

JAMIE P. DWYER, MD
Assistant Professor of Medicine, Division of Nephrology and Hypertension, and Nephrology Clinical Trials Center, Vanderbilt University Medical Center, Nashville, Tennessee

PAOLA FIORETTO, MD, PhD
Associate Professor of Medicine (Endocrinology), University of Padova, Padova, Italy

RAJESH GARG, MD
Division of Endocrinology, Diabetes and Hypertension, Brigham and Women's Hospital, Boston, Massachusetts

JASMINE D. GONZALVO, PharmD, BCPS, BC-ADM, CDE
Clinical Assistant Professor of Pharmacy Practice, Clinical Pharmacy Specialist, Primary Care, Purdue University College of Pharmacy and Pharmaceutical Sciences, West Lafayette, Indiana

DEANNA S. KANIA, PharmD, BCPS
Clinical Associate Professor of Pharmacy Practice, Purdue University College of Pharmacy and Pharmaceutical Sciences, West Lafayette, Indiana; R.L. Roudebush VA Medical Center

AMANDA J. KLEINER, MD
Division of Endocrinology, Department of Medicine, University of Virginia Health System, Charlottesville, Virginia

ANDRZEJ S. KROLEWSKI, MD, PhD
Section Head, Section on Genetics and Epidemiology, Research Division, Joslin Diabetes Center; Associate Professor, Department of Medicine, Harvard Medical School, Boston, Massachusetts

JULIA B. LEWIS, MD
Professor of Medicine, Division of Nephrology and Hypertension, and Nephrology Clinical Trials Center, Vanderbilt University Medical Center, Nashville, Tennessee

CHRISTINE MARIC-BILKAN, PhD, FASN, FAHA
Associate Professor, Department of Physiology and Biophysics, University of Mississippi Medical Center, Jackson, Mississippi

MICHAEL MAUER, MD
Professor of Pediatrics and Medicine, University of Minnesota, Minneapolis, Minnesota

CHRISTY L. NASH, PharmD, CDE
Clinical Assistant Professor of Pharmacy Practice, Associate Director of Advanced Pharmacy Practice Experiences, Purdue University College of Pharmacy and Pharmaceutical Sciences and Mathes Pharmacy, West Lafayette, Indiana

MARCUS G. PEZZOLESI, PhD, MPH
Research Associate, Section on Genetics and Epidemiology, Research Division, Joslin Diabetes Center; Instructor, Department of Medicine, Harvard Medical School, Boston, Massachusetts

ANNE T. REUTENS, MBBS, PhD, FRACP
Department of Epidemiology and Preventive Medicine, Alfred Centre, Monash University; Department of Clinical Diabetes and Epidemiology, Baker IDI Heart and Diabetes Institute, Melbourne, Victoria, Australia

EBERHARD RITZ, MD
Professor, University of Heidelberg, Nierenzentrum, Heidelberg, Germany

BRIAN M. SHEPLER, PharmD
Clinical Associate Professor of Pharmacy Practice, Director Advanced Pharmacy Practice Experiences, Purdue University College of Pharmacy, West Lafayette, Indiana

CORY T. SMITH, PharmD
Visiting Clinical Assistant Professor of Pharmacy Practice, Purdue University College of Pharmacy and Pharmaceutical Sciences, West Lafayette, Indiana; Floyd Memorial Hospital

ROBERT D. TOTO, MD
Professor, Associate Dean of Translational Science, Mary M. Conroy Professorship in Kidney Disease, Division of Nephrology, Department of Internal Medicine, University of Texas Southwestern Medical Center, Dallas, Texas

PETER N. VAN BUREN, MD
Instructor, Dedman Family Scholar in Clinical Care, Division of Nephrology, Department of Internal Medicine, University of Texas Southwestern Medical Center at Dallas, Dallas, Texas

MARK E. WILLIAMS, MD, FACP, FASN
Renal Division, Joslin Diabetes Center, Boston, Massachusetts

Contents

Preface: Diabetic Chronic Kidney Disease: When the Other Shoe Drops   xi

Mark E. Williams

Epidemiology of Diabetic Kidney Disease   1

Anne T. Reutens

Diabetes currently affects 8.3% of the world's adults and will increase in prevalence in future decades. Diabetic kidney disease is a leading cause of end stage renal disease (ESRD) and health care expenditure. Diabetic kidney disease can develop along an albuminuric or non-albuminuric pathway. The risks of death from all causes and from cardiovascular disease increase with lower glomerular filtration rates. For those with albuminuria, the risks of ESRD and of all-cause mortality and cardiovascular mortality increase with higher levels of albumin excretion. Survival has improved compared to outcomes from the 1980s, and progression to ESRD is now more common than premature death. This chapter reviews the epidemiology of diabetic kidney disease in type 1 and type 2 diabetes.

Clinical Manifestations and Natural History of Diabetic Kidney Disease   19

Eberhard Ritz

Renal failure in type 2 diabetes has been termed "a medical catastrophe of worldwide dimension". In 2001, we found in our unit that 49% of incident patients requiring maintenance hemodialysis had diabetes (i.e. 98/million population/year), 6% of whom had type 1 and most (94%) had type 2 diabetes, i.e. more than the than reported frequency in Germany (approximately 35% of incident patients). The frequency is underestimated because hyperglycemia is often lost in the preterminal phase when diabetic patients lose weight and fasting hyperglycemia.

The Pathogenesis and Management of Hypertension in Diabetic Kidney Disease   31

Peter N. Van Buren and Robert D. Toto

Hypertension is one of the hallmark features of diabetic kidney disease. It contributes to both the progression of kidney disease and the risk for cardiovascular events in these patients. Although lowering blood pressure is critical in managing diabetic kidney disease, the ability to achieve this goal is complicated by the complexity of blood pressure regulation in these patients related to both extracellular volume expansion and increased vasoconstriction. This review includes a discussion of our current understanding of the etiology of hypertension in patients with diabetic kidney disease and an update of the most current clinical trials investigating antihypertensive interventions.

Nonproteinuric Diabetic Nephropathy: When Diabetics Don't Read the Textbook   53

Jamie P. Dwyer and Julia B. Lewis

Diabetic nephropathy (DN) refers to the structural and functional changes in the kidneys of patients with diabetes mellitus (type 1 or 2). A subset of patients with presumed DN may not have overt proteinuria as a prerequisite to renal failure, contrary to the classical paradigm. No animal model fully recapitulates the human subset. All studies on this subject are observational and most lack biopsy data. Many mechanisms have been postulated, including use of renin-angiotensin system agents, recurrent bouts of acute kidney injury, genetic predisposition, and renal lesions other than DN. A well-designed biopsy study and a series of intervention trials are needed to fully understand this entity.

Obesity and Diabetic Kidney Disease   59

Christine Maric-Bilkan

Obesity and diabetes are major health concerns worldwide. Along with other elements of the metabolic syndrome, including hypertension, they contribute to the development and progression of renal disease, which, if not treated, may lead to end-stage renal disease (ESRD). Although early intervention and management of body weight, hyperglycemia, and hypertension are imperative, novel therapeutic approaches are also necessary to reduce the high morbidity and mortality associated with renal disease. This review provides perspectives regarding the mechanisms by which obesity may lead to ESRD and discusses prevention strategies and treatment of obesity-related renal disease.

Diabetic Kidney Disease in Elderly Individuals   75

Mark E. Williams

Chronic kidney disease (CKD) complicates diabetes and also has an increased prevalence in elderly individuals. Particularly in those older than 60 years, the most common cause of CKD and end-stage renal disease in the United States is diabetic kidney disease. This growing population represents unique challenges in multidisciplinary medical management. Elderly diabetic patients with CKD may be underserved with regard to fundamental standards of care like the role of glucose control, hypertension management, and the use of renin-angiotensin blocking agents. Current management therefore needs to be reassessed in terms of the special needs of this growing population.

The Genetic Risk of Kidney Disease in Type 2 Diabetes   91

Marcus G. Pezzolesi and Andrzej S. Krolewski

In this review, the authors discuss the major approaches being used to identify diabetic nephropathy (DN) susceptibility genes in type 2 diabetes (T2D) and highlight the salient findings from studies whereby these approaches have been implemented. The recent advent of next-generation sequencing technology is beginning to impact DN gene mapping strategies. As the field moves forward, family based approaches should greatly facilitate efforts to identify variants in genes that have a major effect on the risk of DN in T2D. To be successful, the ascertainment and comprehensive study of families with multiple affected members is critical.

Pancreas Transplantation and Reversal of Diabetic Nephropathy Lesions   109

Michael Mauer and Paola Fioretto

Pancreas transplantation is the only available treatment that has restored long-term (10 or more years) normoglycemia without the risks of severe hypoglycemia, allowing testing of the reversibility of diabetic nephropathy lesions. The authors studied renal structure before and 5 and 10 years after pancreas transplantation in nonuremic patients with long-term type 1 diabetes, with established diabetic nephropathy lesions at baseline. Diabetic glomerular lesions were not significantly changed at 5 years but were dramatically improved after 10 years, with most patients' glomerular structure returning to normal at the 10-year follow-up. These studies also showed that tubulointerstitial remodeling was also possible.

Potential New Treatments for Diabetic Kidney Disease   115

Deanna S. Kania, Cory T. Smith, Christy L. Nash, Jasmine D. Gonzalvo, Andrea Bittner, and Brian M. Shepler

Diabetic kidney disease is a complex pathologic process that involves many biochemical associations. As our understanding of this processes deepens, potential new targets for drug therapy become apparent. There are several mechanisms by which medications may be able to inhibit or slow the progression of kidney disease. Existing medications and entirely new compounds have been studied in human subjects that have antifibrotic and antioxidant effects as well as the ability to bind with and antagonize specific receptors known to contribute to the deleterious effects observed in diabetic kidney disease patients. While most potential new drug therapies remain highly experimental, there is a growing body of data from clinical trials show that many new drugs may eventually lead to new standards for drug treatment in diabetic kidney disease. Potential new drug therapies discussed include antifibrotic agents, antioxidant agents, ET-a receptor antagonists and other compounds with non-specific or multi-faceted mechanisms of action such as paricalcitol, ruboxistaurin, palosuran, allopurinol, and fasudil.

Diabetes Management in the Kidney Patient   135

Rajesh Garg and Mark E. Williams

Hyperglycemia management in chronic kidney disease (CKD) patients presents difficult challenges, partly due to the complexity involved in treating these patients, and partly due to lack of data supporting benefits of tight glycemic control. While hyperglycemia is central to the pathogenesis and management of diabetes, hypoglycemia and glucose variability also contribute to outcomes. Multiple agents with different mechanisms of action are now available; some can lower glucose levels without the risk of hypoglycemia. This article reviews metabolic changes present in kidney impairment/failure, current views about glycemic goals, and treatment options for the diabetic patient with CKD.

Comanagement of Diabetic Kidney Disease by the Primary Care Provider and Nephrologist   157

Brendan T. Bowman, Amanda Kleiner, and W. Kline Bolton

Diabetic kidney disease (DKD) is a common disorder, and few patients achieve current therapeutic targets. Careful collaboration between all health care providers and the creation of disorder-specific health care systems seem to offer the best opportunity for improving the management and clinical outcomes of these patients. This article explores the barriers to effective collaboration between physicians in the management of patients with DKD, attitudes and perceptions of physicians toward collaborative management, and the physiologic challenges in patients with DKD that would warrant specialist involvement in their care. A model for collaborative DKD care delivery is also proposed.

Index   **175**

Preface

Diabetic Chronic Kidney Disease: When the Other Shoe Drops

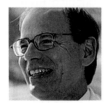

Mark E. Williams, MD, FACP, FASN
Editor

Diabetes mellitus currently affects over 8% of the world's adult population. When chronic kidney disease complicates diabetes, as a patient recently confessed to me as her physician, it is like the other shoe has dropped. In the aggregate, the increasing prevalence of diagnosed diabetes mellitus in the United States and elsewhere over the past 2 decades has significantly affected practice within the medical clinics of North America and throughout the world. It is also associated with poorer outcomes and higher medical costs for patients with diabetes and kidney disease. The epidemic of chronic kidney disease complicating this systemic illness thus becomes a topic of current interest for a physician audience outside as well as inside of nephrology.

The prevalence of both diabetes and prediabetes has reached new levels. The most recent data from the Centers for Disease Control and Prevention (CDC)[1] document the substantial increase in the prevalence of diagnosed diabetes throughout the 50 states, Washington DC, and Puerto Rico from 1995 to 2010. Although the rate of increase was not uniform, the age-adjusted prevalence of diabetes increased by more than 50% in most states. Even more remarkable was the fact that the rate increased by at least 100% in 18 states! In 1995 the age-adjusted prevalence of diabetes was ≥6% in only 3 states, but by 2010 it was present in all states within the United States. The epidemic of diabetes that has emerged has been attributed to population aging, urbanization, physical inactivity, poor nutrition, and greater problems with obesity. The increase in diabetes prevalence has coincided with the increase in obesity rates across the United States. Increasing diabetes prevalence, not unexpectedly, is being reflected in greater numbers of patients with diabetic chronic kidney disease.

Effective and efficient care is required if the patient with diabetes and chronic kidney disease is to have optimal health. Referral and comanagement of the patient with diabetes and chronic kidney disease is a necessity. For example, a lesser but notable factor causing the current epidemic of diabetes (and, by inference, diabetic chronic kidney disease) described above has been improved survival of persons already

Med Clin N Am 97 (2013) xi–xii
http://dx.doi.org/10.1016/j.mcna.2012.11.005
0025-7125/13/$ – see front matter © 2013 Published by Elsevier Inc.

diagnosed with diabetes. Mortality rates among US adults with diabetes declined substantially between 1997 and 2006, at an even faster rate than for those adults without diabetes. The trend, highlighted in the latest CDC report, may be related to improvements in health for patients with diabetes, improved quality of care and medical treatments, and decreased rates of complications. A separate analysis from the CDC[2] recently determined that an important decline in diabetes-related end-stage renal disease (ESRD) incidence occurred starting in the late 1990s and has included all age groups, including those who were older than 75 years of age. Although the absolute number of patients with diabetes-attributed ESRD almost tripled between 1990 and 2006, therefore, the age-adjusted incidence rates fell. The authors cited widespread use of renin-angiotensin-aldosterone blockers for the improvements in rates of patients with diabetes and chronic kidney disease reaching ESRD.

Nonetheless, diabetic nephropathy remains by far the most common cause of ESRD in Western societies. It accounts for 40% to 45% of ESRD cases, and for greater than 20% of kidney transplant recipients transplanted in the United States. The prognosis for patients with diabetes and kidney disease thus remains grim, with fewer than 50% of those with ESRD surviving 5 years after diagnosis.

It has been predicted that the coming global increase in diabetes mellitus will be 2.7%, a level 1.7 times the anticipated annual growth in the world's population. The care of patients with diabetes poses significant challenges to the clinician. Interventions to prevent kidney disease, delay its progression, and decrease the comorbidity associated with it are now an important part of chronic kidney disease care for the nonnephrologist. Diabetic kidney disease can be detected by screening for persistent abnormal urine albumin excretion and by determining the estimated glomerular filtration rate. The main evidence-based strategies for preventing or delaying loss of kidney function in diabetic patients include blood pressure control, blockade of the renin-angiotensin system, and glycemic control. Controlling these factors and reducing proteinuria are now the main focus of diabetic kidney disease management. Through a multidisciplinary approach of implementing guidelines and timely referral, care of the diabetic kidney disease patient can be improved. The key is preventing and slowing the progression of this complication, to keep the other shoe from dropping.

Mark E. Williams, MD, FACP, FASN
Harvard Medical School
Joslin Diabetes Center
One Joslin Place
Boston, MA 02215, USA

E-mail address:
mark.williams@joslin.harvard.edu

REFERENCES

1. Geiss LS, Li Y, Kirtland K, et al. Increasing prevalence of diagnosed diabetes— United States and Puerto Rico, 1995–2010. Morb Mortal Wkly Rep (MMWR) November 16, 2012;61(45):918.
2. Burrows NR. Incidence of treatment for end-stage renal disease among individuals with diabetes in the U.S. continues to decline. Diabetes Care 2010;33:73–7.

Epidemiology of Diabetic Kidney Disease

Anne T. Reutens, MBBS, PhD, FRACP[a,b,*]

KEYWORDS

- Diabetes • Prevalence • Incidence • Microalbuminuria • Macroalbuminuria
- End-stage renal disease

KEY POINTS

- Diabetic kidney disease is a leading cause of chronic kidney disease. This reflects the increasing prevalence of type 2 diabetes globally.
- In type 1 and type 2 diabetes, the presence of microalbuminuria and macroalbuminuria or decreased glomerular filtration rate confers increased risk of developing ESRD and of death.
- Increased risk of albuminuria has been identified in certain non-European ethnic groups.
- Renal impairment in diabetic kidney disease may occur in the absence of albuminuria.

DEFINITION OF DIABETIC KIDNEY DISEASE

Diabetic kidney disease (DKD) refers to chronic kidney disease (CKD) presumed to be caused by diabetes.[1] DKD is detected clinically by screening for persistent abnormal urine albumin excretion (defined as at least two abnormal specimens within a 3- to 6-month period) and by screening for a decreased estimated glomerular filtration rate (eGFR). In most cases, kidney biopsies are not used to establish the presence of diabetic glomerulopathy. Albuminuria has traditionally been divided into microalbuminuria (urine albumin creatinine ratio [ACR] of 30–300 mg/g, equivalent to timed collections of 20–200 µg/min or 30–300 mg/24 hours) or macroalbuminuria (ACR >300 mg/d, timed albumin excretion >200 µg/min or >300 mg/24 hours) (**Table 1**). Serum creatinine-derived estimates of GFR (previously calculated from the Modification of Diet in Renal Disease Study equation and now estimated using the Chronic Kidney Disease Epidemiology Collaboration formula) can be used to stage DKD, but eGFR alone can only accurately detect stages 3 or higher of CKD (eGFR <60 mL/min/1.73 m^2) (**Table 2**).

The author has no conflict of interest with regard to this manuscript.

[a] Department of Epidemiology and Preventive Medicine, Alfred Centre, Monash University, Level 5, 99 Commercial Road, Melbourne, Victoria 3004, Australia; [b] Department of Clinical Diabetes and Epidemiology, Baker IDI Heart and Diabetes Institute, Level 4, Alfred Centre, 99 Commercial Road, Melbourne, Victoria 3004, Australia

* Baker IDI Heart and Diabetes Institute, Level 4, Alfred Centre, 99 Commercial Road, Melbourne, Victoria 3004, Australia.

E-mail addresses: anne.reutens@bakeridi.edu.au; anne.reutens@monash.edu

Table 1
Definitions of abnormalities in albumin excretion

Category	Spot Collection (mg/g creatinine)	24-Hour Collection (mg/24 hours)	Timed Collection (μg/min)
Normoalbuminuria	<30	<30	<20
Microalbuminuria	30–300	30–300	20–200
Macroalbuminuria	>300	>300	>200

Data from National Kidney Foundation. KDOQI clinical practice guidelines and clinical practice recommendations for diabetes and chronic kidney disease. Am J Kidney Dis 2007;49:S1–180.

WORLDWIDE BURDEN OF DIABETES AND DKD

The International Diabetes Federation Diabetes Atlas estimated that in 2011, there were 366 million patients with diabetes worldwide (8.3% of adults), and by 2030, this will increase to 552 million people.[2] Forty-eight percent of this increase is predicted to occur in China and India. The increased diabetes prevalence will disproportionately affect low- and middle-income countries compared with high-income countries. To put the global increase in diabetes in perspective, the average annual growth in diabetes prevalence will be 2.7%, which is 1.7 times the anticipated annual growth in the world's population. In the United States, 11.3% of people aged 20 years or older had diabetes in 2011 (25.6 million people), with prevalence increasing in older age groups (26.9% of people aged ≥65 years).[3]

Increasing diabetes prevalence is already being reflected in high DKD prevalence. In 2006, the DEMAND study evaluated the presence of DKD in 32,308 patients with type 2 diabetes drawn from medical clinics in 33 countries.[4] The global prevalence of microalbuminuria and macroalbuminuria was 39% and 10% respectively, with Asian and Hispanic patients having the highest prevalence of albuminuria. Twenty-two percent of patients had impaired renal function (eGFR <60 mL/min/1.73 m^2). The results from the 2007 to 2010 nationally representative China National Survey of Chronic Kidney Disease give a glimpse of the magnitude of future challenges.[5] The overall prevalence of CKD was 10.7%, affecting an estimated 119.5 million people in China. There was a low prevalence of people with renal impairment (1.7%) compared with albuminuria prevalence (9.4%). Zhang and colleagues[5] noted that this may be because renal impairment from diabetes and other chronic diseases may take another 10 years to be reflected at the population level. A total of 19.1% of those with eGFR less than 60

Table 2
Stages of CKD

Stage	Description	GFR (mL/min/1.73 m^2)
1	Kidney damage with normal or increased GFR	≥90
2	Kidney damage with mild decreased GFR	60–89
3	Moderately decreased GFR	30–59
4	Severely decreased GFR	15–29
5	Kidney failure	<15 or dialysis

Data from National Kidney Foundation. K/DOQI clinical practice guidelines for chronic kidney disease: evaluation, classification and stratification. Am J Kidney Dis 2002;39:S1–266.

mL/min/1.73 m^2 had diabetes, and 17.3% of those with albuminuria had diabetes. The adjusted prevalence of diabetes in the total Chinese population was 4.9%, based on abnormal fasting plasma glucose or a history of diabetes. This prevalence may be an underestimate, because another recent Chinese representative survey that used an oral glucose tolerance test for diabetes diagnosis reported a prevalence of 9.7%.[6] From India, the other country with an expected large increase in diabetes prevalence, a population-based examination of DKD in urban Chennai reported a prevalence of 2.2% for macroalbuminuria and 26.9% for microalbuminuria.[7] These figures estimate that more than 850,000 people in India had overt DKD in 2007. Unfortunately, most would not be able to afford the cost of renal replacement therapy (RRT) after disease progressed to end-stage renal disease (ESRD).

The US Renal Data System reported high incidence rates of ESRD caused by diabetes in 2009 in certain countries: 58% to 60% in Malaysia and Mexico, and more than 40% in Thailand, New Zealand, Hong Kong, Republic of Korea, Japan, Taiwan, the United States, Israel, and the Philippines.[8] In the United States in 2009, diabetes accounted for most incident cases of ESRD (154 per million patients with ESRD) and also caused most of the prevalent cases (647 per million patients).[8] Since 1996, there has been a 35% decline in the age-adjusted incidence rate for ESRD caused by diabetes,[9] a decline of 3.9% per year.[10] This means that although the total number of ESRD cases caused by diabetes is increasing because of the increasing number of patients with diabetes, the likelihood of developing ESRD if a person is diabetic is decreasing. In the renal registry data from Australia and New Zealand (ANZDATA), the proportion of patients with DKD requiring RRT rose from 17% in 1980 to 35% of new ESRD cases in 2009, but the rate of increase seems to be leveling off since 2005.[11]

The cost of DKD is considerable. The annual treatment cost in 2009 to 2010 for people with ESRD caused by diabetes in Australia was estimated to be $73,527 per person for RRT and $12,174 for conservative treatment.[12] The total cost of DKD in Australia in 2009 to 2010 was $20.5 million for people with diabetes in CKD stages 1 to 4 and $446.3 million for people with ESRD and diabetes. This total cost is projected to double by 2020.[12] In the United States in 2009, Medicare expenditure was $18 billion for people with CKD caused by diabetes.[8] The cost of DKD progression was recently analyzed using information from the Kaiser Permanente Northwest health maintenance organization.[13] Annualized cost increase was calculated for transition to higher stages of DKD. The costs of progression were $2764 from normoalbuminuria, $3618 from microalbuminuria, and $56,745 from macroalbuminuria. This demonstrated clearly that most of the increased cost is caused by development of ESRD. If the rate of GFR decline could be slowed by 10%, the saving to the US health budget would be approximately $9.06 billion.[14]

In summary, the diabetes epidemic has led to substantial increases in numbers of people with DKD and ESRD. The costs for health care are immense. Unfortunately, increased diabetes prevalence will affect regions and populations that may be unable to bear these costs. Urgent attention is therefore needed to prevent DKD and to prevent progression of DKD. The following section will analyze the current epidemiology of diabetic kidney disease in greater detail.

NEPHROPATHY IN TYPE 1 DIABETES
Early Studies

The clinical significance of microalbuminuria in DKD
The concept of microalbuminuria arose with the development of a sensitive radioactive iodine assay for albumin[15] and demonstration that increased albumin excretion

could be detected in people with diabetes without proteinuria.[16,17] Several small studies in the early 1980s established that microalbuminuria was important for DKD prognosis in type 1 diabetes.[18-20] A 14-year follow-up of a cohort from Guy's Hospital, London (United Kingdom), showed that proteinuria and death occurred in 87.5% and 37.5%, respectively, of those with microalbuminuria compared with 3.6% and 9.1% of those with normal albumin excretion.[19] When this cohort was followed for a further 23 years, 62.5% of those with initial microalbuminuria had died (50% from cardiovascular disease) and 25% had progressed to ESRD.[20] The relative risk (in those with microalbuminuria compared with those with normoalbuminuria) was 9.3 for progression to proteinuria and 2.9 for cardiovascular death.

Mogensen and Christensen[21] published a study of 44 patients with type 1 diabetes and no proteinuria, initially tested in 1969 to 1976 and restudied in 1983. In those who were initially normoalbuminuric, none developed proteinuria and 14% developed microalbuminuria, whereas 86% of those with microalbuminuria progressed to proteinuria. Similar results from Mathiesen and colleagues[22] confirmed that that those with albumin excretion at the higher end of the microalbuminuric range had the highest risk of developing proteinuria. Retinopathy, neuropathy, and hypertension were highly prevalent in those with microalbuminuria.[22,23]

Incidence of proteinuria in DKD

Epidemiologic studies published in the mid 1980s showed a high incidence of ESRD, cardiovascular disease, and death in people with kidney disease caused by type 1 diabetes. For 25 years, Andersen and colleagues[24] at the Steno Memorial Hospital followed 1475 people with type 1 diabetes diagnosed before 1953. A total of 41% developed persistent proteinuria. The cumulative incidence of DKD was 45% after 40 years of diabetes. Maximum DKD prevalence (21%) occurred after 20 years duration of diabetes and declined to 10% by 40 years. A total of 83% of those with proteinuria died (66% from uremia, 19% from cardiovascular disease), compared with 28% of the nonproteinuric patients. Those who developed proteinuria relatively early (<20 years from diagnosis of diabetes) were more likely to die from uremia and survived for approximately 7 years from onset of uremia. Those with later-onset kidney disease died more frequently from ischemic heart disease than uremia.

A study of 1134 patients with type 1 diabetes published 2 years later from the same hospital by Borch-Johnsen and colleagues[25] showed that 40% of patients developed persistent proteinuria, with maximal incidence between 13 and 18 years of diabetes duration. This cohort of patients differed from the cohort in the previous study because the date of diagnosis of type 1 diabetes was limited to 1933 to 1952. Mortality increased after 3 years of proteinuria to 17% per year at 10 to 20 years after onset of proteinuria, after which it declined. Life expectancy was longer for those who were diagnosed later in 1950 compared with 1935. Those without proteinuria maintained a low relative mortality throughout the study.

At the Joslin Clinic, Krolewski and colleagues[26] followed three cohorts of people with type 1 diabetes diagnosed in 1939, 1949, and 1959 for 20 to 40 years to determine if the natural history of nephropathy was changing. The cohorts were limited to whites from eastern Massachusetts who had diabetes less than 1 year before the first visit. The cumulative incidence of persistent proteinuria was 35% after 40 years of diabetes (67 patients), and 42 of these people developed ESRD. The median interval between appearance of persistent proteinuria and ESRD was 10 years. In this study, those who had been diagnosed with diabetes in 1939 had twice the risk of developing proteinuria compared with those in later cohorts.

Summary of early studies

These early studies set the historical context of type 1 DKD. By the 1980s, microalbuminuria had been identified as an early stage of renal damage, and as a predictor of the risk of death or DKD progression. A total of 80% to 90% of those with microalbuminuria progressed to proteinuria. Incident proteinuria occurred in 30% to 40% of patients with type 1 diabetes. Most patients developed ESRD within 10 years of proteinuria onset, and there was high mortality from uremia and cardiovascular disease.

Later Studies

The path from microalbuminuria to proteinuria is not inexorable

From the early studies, it seemed that after a patient developed microalbuminuria, he or she was committed to a path of proteinuria and premature death. However, recent observational studies have shown that microalbuminuria frequently remits. At the Steno Diabetes Center, 10-year follow-up of adult patients with microalbuminuria recruited in 1994 showed that 33% progressed to persistent proteinuria and 16% regressed to persistent normoalbuminuria. Of those who showed regression of microalbuminuria, in 55% it occurred after starting hypertension treatment.[27] The Joslin Study of the Natural History of Microalbuminuria followed 386 patients recruited in 1991 to 1992. The 6-year cumulative incidence of persistent proteinuria was 19%. The cumulative proportion of people who regressed in their urine albumin excretion was approximately 60%. Factors independently associated with regression were shorter duration of microalbuminuria and better glycemic, lipid, and blood pressure control.[28] These figures are similar to those obtained by Steinke and colleagues[29] who followed patients from North America and France over a 5-year period. A total of 64% of patients with persistent microalbuminuria reverted spontaneously to normal albumin excretion during follow-up. In the Diabetes Control and Complications Trial (DCCT), an intensive glycemic treatment group of patients with recently diagnosed type 1 diabetes was compared with a standard diabetes care control group.[30] Patients were enrolled from 1983 to 1989 and the trial terminated in 1993 after 6.5 years of treatment. The Epidemiology of Diabetes Interventions and Complications (EDIC) study continued observation of the participants after the end of the DCCT study. Reports from year 16 of the EDIC study (2008–2010) showed that in those who had developed persistent microalbuminuria, 40% regressed to normoalbuminuria.[31] Of these, only 24.6% were using renin angiotensin system (RAS) inhibitors at the time of regression. Some patients regressed after more than 10 years of persistent microalbuminuria.

In summary, modern studies demonstrated that in DKD caused by type 1 diabetes, regression of microalbuminuria was more common than progression to proteinuria or ESRD.

Prevalence of DKD caused by type 1 diabetes

A cross-sectional study of people with type 1 diabetes from North Wales from 1999 showed a prevalence of 27.2% for microalbuminuria and 9.6% for overt DKD.[32] Renal disease was reported for a large German and Austrian cohort of 27,805 children, adolescents, and adults with type 1 diabetes followed until 2007.[33] After 40 years of diabetes, the calculated prevalence of microalbuminuria was 25.4% and calculated prevalence of macroalbuminuria and ESRD combined was 9.4%. Risk factors for development of microalbuminuria were diabetes duration, HbA_{1c}, dyslipidemia, and blood pressure; and for macroalbuminuria, the risk factors were diabetes duration, HbA_{1c}, dyslipidemia, and male gender. Onset of diabetes in childhood protected against development of microalbuminuria.

Incidence of proteinuria in DKD

In 2003, Hovind and colleagues[34] from the Steno Diabetes Center published data from at least 20 years of follow-up of Danish patients with type 1 diabetes. The patients were divided into 5-year cohorts depending on year of diagnosis (Group A 1965–1969, through to Group D 1979–1984). Cumulative incidence of proteinuria was significantly reduced as the calendar year of diagnosis became more recent: 31.1% in Group A compared with 13.7% in Group D. In the later cohort, antihypertensive medications were started earlier after diagnosis, HbA_{1c} and blood pressure were lower, and smokers were less prevalent. Similar results came from the Swedish Linköping study, which studied cohorts of patients diagnosed with childhood type 1 diabetes between 1961 and 1985.[35] The cumulative proportion of persistent proteinuria occurring after 30 years of follow-up was 32% in those diagnosed between 1961 and 1965 compared with 10.8% in the next oldest cohort from 1966 to 1970. Prevalence of microalbuminuria was not statistically significantly different between the cohorts. Those with nephropathy had the highest mortality (33.3%) compared with 5.7% in those without nephropathy. In contrast to these promising Scandinavian results, in the Pittsburgh Epidemiology of Diabetes Complications Study, there was no decline in proteinuria incidence with calendar year.[36] This study stratified participants into five cohorts according to year of diagnosis, ranging from 1950 to 1959, to 1975 to 1980. By 25 years, the cumulative incidence of persistent proteinuria was similar in all the cohorts, with a pooled incidence of 25%. However, there was a dramatic decline in 30-year incidence of ESRD, from the cohort diagnosed in the 1950s (31%) to the cohort from 1965 to 1969 (18%). Mortality also fell from 39% to 23% in the respective cohorts. A recent review of type 1 diabetes studies has proposed that the changing pattern of proteinuria may reflect a 5- to 15-year delay in onset of albuminuria due to improved management of glucose, blood pressure and cholesterol, reduced rates of cigarette smoking and increased use of RAS inhibitors, rather than a decrease in cumulative incidence of proteinuria.[37]

Incidence of ESRD and death

A recent Swedish study showed a 3.3% cumulative 30-year incidence of ESRD in patients with type 1 diabetes.[38] Onset of ESRD was delayed if the person was prepubertal when diabetes was diagnosed, or if female and 20 years and older at diabetes diagnosis. The Finnish Diabetes Register study of patients with type 1 diabetes diagnosed between 1965 and 1999 had a cumulative 30-year ESRD incidence of 7.8%, with declining risk in those diagnosed after 1969 compared with those diagnosed between 1965 and 1969.[39] Those diagnosed with diabetes before 5 years of age had the lowest incidence of ESRD. The risk of dying with ESRD was 3.3% after 30 years. The prospective Finnish Diabetic Nephropathy (FinnDiane) study followed adults with type 1 diabetes recruited between 1997 and 2006 for 7 years.[40] Mortality was compared with that of the age- and gender-matched general Finnish population to obtain a standardized mortality ratio. The standardized mortality ratio was 2.8 for people with microalbuminuria, 9.2 for those with macroalbuminuria, and 18.3 if people had ESRD. An eGFR less than 60 mL/min/1.73 m^2 was also associated with increased mortality (adjusted hazard ratio, 1.7). Twenty-year outcomes were reported in Austrian patients with type 1 diabetes followed from 1983 to 1984.[41] ESRD occurred in 5.6% (incidence rate 311 per 100,000 person-years) and mortality was 13% (mortality rate 708 per 100,000 person-years). Mortality risk was twofold higher in patients who originally had microalbuminuria and fourfold higher in those with macroalbuminuria compared with those who had normoalbuminuria.

After 23 years of follow-up in the DCCT/EDIC study, the cumulative incidence of sustained eGFR less than 60 mL/min/1.73 m^2 was 11.4%.[42] Of these people, 16%

had microalbuminuria and 61% had macroalbuminuria before developing a reduced eGFR. The rate of decline of eGFR was significantly greater in people with current macroalbuminuria (5.7% per year) or who previously had macroalbuminuria (5.1% per year) compared with those with a current or a previous history of microalbuminuria (1.8% and 1.4%, respectively). The rate of eGFR decline in those with normoalbuminuria was 1.2% per year. Renal outcomes were separately assessed for the 325 participants who developed incident microalbuminuria during the DCCT/EDIC study.[31] Ten-year cumulative incidences were 28% for progression to macroalbuminuria, 15% for development of eGFR less than 60 mL/min/1.73 m^2, and 4% for ESRD.

A prospective study from the Steno Diabetes Center published in 2005 followed two groups of people with type 1 diabetes over 10 years, one group with persistent macroalbuminuria, the other with persistent normoalbuminuria.[43] Median survival in the group with DKD was 21.7 years. A total of 30% in this group died, compared with 8% in the group with normoalbuminuria. In those with DKD, 42% died of cardiovascular disease and 50% of ESRD. The risk of ESRD in this study was 1.6 per 100 person-years. This low figure contrasts with higher figures from the FinnDiane study[44] and the Joslin Clinic.[45] In the competing-risk analysis of the FinnDiane study,[44] 35.5% of patients with proteinuria developed ESRD and 9.5% died during the median follow-up time of 9.9 years. The incidence of ESRD was 5.1 per 100 person-years. From the Joslin Clinic, Rosolowsky and colleagues[45] reported 15-year cumulative risks of 52% for ESRD and 11% for death before developing ESRD. The incidence rate for ESRD was 5.8 per 100 person-years and mortality rate was 1 per 100 person-years. The disparity between the Steno Diabetes Center results and the other two studies is puzzling, because all the studies were conducted after it became routine clinical practice to use RAS blockade and to treat hypertension and lipids aggressively.

In summary, recent studies have confirmed the older findings relating the risk of eGFR decline, ESRD, and mortality with the level of urinary albumin excretion. In several studies, childhood onset of diabetes was associated with a lower risk of developing advanced DKD. The incidence of proteinuria, ESRD, and death varies considerably among centers. The reported 30-year cumulative incidence of proteinuria is 11% to 32%. The 30-year incidence of ESRD is 3.3% to 7.8%, which is considerably lower than previous reports. Patients with proteinuria are now more likely to proceed to ESRD than to die prematurely. However, cardiovascular disease remains an important cause of mortality.

Renal impairment can occur without albuminuria or without progression from microalbuminuria to proteinuria

From the DCCT/EDIC study, 24% of the patients who developed persistent GFR less than 60 mL/min/1.73 m^2 did not have any preceding microalbuminuria or macroalbuminuria.[42] This uncoupling of renal impairment from albuminuria was found in previous biopsy studies. The eight renal biopsies reported by Lane and colleagues[46] from women with type 1 diabetes and renal impairment but normal albumin excretion showed similar glomerular pathology to biopsies taken from diabetic women with microalbuminuria, or with microalbuminuria and low GFR. In the study by Caramori and colleagues[47] of normoalbuminuric patients with type 1 diabetes, those with a reduced eGFR had more advanced glomerular lesions on electron microscopic examination. These subjects were more likely to be female, a finding confirmed in the study by Tsalamandris and colleagues.[48]

A study from the Joslin Clinic tracked GFR and urinary albumin excretion in patients with type 1 diabetes and newly diagnosed microalbuminuria for 12 years.[49] A total of 29% developed advanced renal disease (ESRD or stage 3–4 CKD) and these cases had a 50% to 75% decline in GFR over 12 years compared with a 20% decline in those who did not develop severe renal disease. With regard to the urinary albumin excretion of the advanced renal cases, in those who developed stage 3 to 4 CKD, microalbuminuria had regressed in 18%, persisted in 47%, and 35% progressed to proteinuria. All the patients with ESRD had proteinuria, which developed only after or at the time that GFR began to decline (i.e. proteinuria did not usually precede the onset of GFR decline). In the other patients who did not develop advanced DKD, 50% regressed to normoalbuminuria, 34% had persistent microalbuminuria, and 16% had proteinuria.

In summary, these findings indicate that loss of renal function does not depend on prior development of proteinuria but can occur without any development of microalbuminuria or soon after microalbuminuria onset.

NEPHROPATHY IN TYPE 2 DIABETES
Prevalence of Albuminuria

The understanding of DKD associated with type 2 diabetes has evolved in parallel with the advances made in understanding DKD caused by type 1 diabetes. Cross-sectional studies of diabetes clinic patients from the 1980s showed a wide range of microalbuminuria prevalence. A Swiss study from 1982 reported a prevalence of 48%; 8.7% of these clinic patients had a GFR less than 60 mL/min.[50] By contrast, Parving and colleagues[51] from Denmark reported the prevalence of albuminuria in 1987 was 13.8% in adult patients with type 2 diabetes of approximately 10 years duration.

This paragraph presents prevalence of albuminuria from population-based studies. In the Wisconsin Epidemiologic Study of Diabetic Retinopathy, participants were selected from southern Wisconsin and serially evaluated.[52] From the 1984 to 1986 examination, there were 840 participants with type 2 diabetes and in these people, the prevalence of microalbuminuria was 24.8% and 20.5% had proteinuria. In the 1988 Italian prevalence survey conducted in Casale Monferrato, 80% (1574) of the total population with type 2 diabetes was examined.[53] The prevalence of microalbuminuria was 32.1% and prevalence of macroalbuminuria was 17.6%. Population-based cross-sectional analysis of adults with type 2 diabetes aged 40 years and older was done in the US Third National Health and Nutrition Examination Survey (NHANES III), which sampled the entire adult US civilian population between 1988 and 1994.[54] Albuminuria was defined according to the study procedure of single assessment of urinary ACR. Prevalence of microalbuminuria was 35% and prevalence of macroalbuminuria was 6%. The Shanghai Diabetic Complications Study was a community-based sample of 3714 subjects, of which 930 people had type 2 diabetes.[55] In those with diabetes, the prevalence of microalbuminuria was 22.8% and the prevalence of macroalbuminuria was 3.4%. A total of 29.6% had an eGFR less than 60 mL/min/1.73 m^2. The Australian Diabetes, Obesity, and Lifestyle Study (AusDiab study) was a population-based survey of 11,247 adults 25 years and older initially conducted in 1999 to 2000.[56] Overall, the prevalence of microalbuminuria in participants known to have diabetes (with type 1 or type 2 diabetes) and participants newly diagnosed with diabetes was 25.3% (21% with microalbuminuria and 4.3% with macroalbuminuria). The prevalence of albuminuria increased with increasing glycemia, so that for the participants newly diagnosed with diabetes (of which most had type 2 diabetes) the prevalence was 17.8% and for participants known to have type 2 diabetes, the prevalence was 32.6%. Longer duration of diabetes increased the prevalence of albuminuria, from 20.9% if duration of diabetes was less than 4 years, to 54.1% if the duration was greater than or equal to 20 years.

In summary, population-based cross-sectional studies show that the prevalence of microalbuminuria in type 2 diabetes is 25% to 35%. The prevalence of macroalbuminuria is 3.5% to 20.5%.

Incidence and Progression of Albuminuric DKD

In 1984, Mogensen[57] published 10-year follow-up results of a group of adult patients with type 2 diabetes and found that 22% of those with microalbuminuria had developed proteinuria. Mortality was significantly associated with elevated albumin excretion and if proteinuria was present, mortality was 148% higher compared with normal control subjects. Two studies published in 1988, a 10-year follow-up of Danish patients with type 2 diabetes[58] and the study by Nelson and colleagues[59] in Pima Indians with type 2 diabetes, confirmed that mortality, particularly cardiovascular mortality, was significantly increased in those with increased urine albumin excretion. The Pima Indians with proteinuria had a relative mortality rate of 3.5 compared with those without proteinuria.[59] The cumulative incidence of overt proteinuria in Pima Indians after 20 years of type 2 diabetes was 50%.[60] Gall and colleagues[61] from the Steno Diabetes Center followed patients who initially had normoalbuminuria for a median of 5.8 years, starting from 1987. A total of 20% developed persistent microalbuminuria and 3% developed persistent macroalbuminuria. Compared with those who remained normoalbuminuric, the patients with DKD tended to be older, male, with higher blood pressure, poor glycemic control, and associated retinopathy.

Results of the United Kingdom Prospective Diabetes Study (UKPDS) have helped to define the natural history of DKD caused by type 2 diabetes. In the UKPDS, 5102 patients with early type 2 diabetes were recruited between 1977 and 1991. These patients were mainly white, normoalbuminuric, and with normal serum creatinine. After a median of 15 years diabetes duration, 38% developed albuminuria (microalbuminuria or macroalbuminuria); 28% had renal impairment (eGFR $\leq$60 mL/min/1.73 m^2); and 14% had both albuminuria and renal impairment.[62] Annual transition rates were 2% per year from no kidney disease to microalbuminuria, 2.8% per year from microalbuminuria to macroalbuminuria, and 2.3% from macroalbuminuria to elevated plasma creatinine ($\geq$175 μmol/L) or RRT.[63] Mortality was high in those who were in this last stage, at 19.2% per year. Similar transition rates were seen in a prospective Swedish National Register study of 3667 adult patients with type 2 diabetes and no baseline renal disease, followed from 2002 to 2007. The rate of transition to albuminuria (mainly to microalbuminuria) was 4% per year, and this occurred in 20% of patients. Of the patients who developed microalbuminuria, 16% developed renal impairment. The rate of development of an eGFR less than 60 mL/min/1.73 m^2 was 2.2% per year (11% of all patients).[64]

The prospective Casale Monferrato study followed a community-based sample of 1253 people with type 2 diabetes and normoalbuminuria or microalbuminuria who were recruited in 1991 to 1992.[65] Median follow-up was 5.33 years, during which time 3.7% per year progressed to proteinuria (2.5% per year if normoalbuminuric and 5.4% per year if initially microalbuminuric). Microalbuminuria therefore conferred a 42% increased risk of developing overt DKD. Recent evaluation of the DIAMETRIC database derived from two large clinical trials of patients with type 2 diabetes and overt proteinuria at baseline found that over 2.8 years of follow-up, 19.5% developed ESRD.[66] The incidence of developing ESRD was 2.5 times the incidence of dying from cardiovascular causes, and 1.5 times the incidence of all-cause mortality. Recently, a meta-analysis was published by the Chronic Kidney Disease Prognosis Consortium in which data were analyzed from 1,024,977 participants, of which 128,505 had diabetes.[67] These participants came from cohorts followed for an average of 8.5 years (general population cohorts) or 9.2 years (high-risk cardiovascular cohorts). Across the ranges of eGFR and ACR, the hazard ratios for all-cause mortality and cardiovascular mortality were 1.2–1.9 times higher in those who had diabetes, compared to those without diabetes. When mortality was analyzed for fixed ACR and eGFR categories and compared to reference ranges of ACR <10 mg/g or eGFR 90–104 ml/min/1.73 m^2, the hazard ratios for all-cause mortality and cardiovascular mortality increased with lower eGFR or higher ACR in individuals with diabetes.

The recent large glycemic control studies in type 2 diabetes have provided more information about predictors of renal events and cardiovascular outcomes. The Action in Diabetes and Vascular Disease: Preterax and Diamicron-MR Controlled Evaluation study enrolled 10,640 patients.[68] At baseline, 69%, 27%, and 4% were normoalbuminuric, microalbuminuric, and macroalbuminuric, respectively. After 4.3 years of follow-up, 1% developed a renal event (defined as death from kidney disease, RRT, or doubling of serum creatinine >200 μmol/L). After adjusting for regression dilution, for each 10-fold increase in baseline albumin/creatinine ratio, the increase in risks for cardiovascular events, cardiovascular death, and renal events were 2.5-fold, 3.9-fold, and 10.5-fold, respectively. For every halving of baseline eGFR, the risks increased 2.2-fold, 3.6-fold, and 63.6-fold for cardiovascular events, cardiovascular death, and renal events. These data have allowed further refinement of predictors for onset of microalbuminuria (eGFR, urine ACR, systolic blood pressure, HbA$_{1c}$, retinopathy, baseline antihypertensive medication, Asian ethnicity, and waist circumference) and of major renal events (eGFR, urine ACR, systolic blood pressure, HbA$_{1c}$, retinopathy, gender, and level of education).[69]

Ethnic Background and DKD

The effect of ethnic background was explored in a cohort of type 2 patients with diabetes of general practitioners in the United Kingdom.[70] This study found that South Asian patients, when compared with white patients, had a higher prevalence of overt proteinuria and a lower prevalence of microalbuminuria. When duration of diabetes was taken into account, the South Asians had a lower risk of microalbuminuria early in the course of their diabetes, but also had an odds ratio (OR) of 2.17 versus whites for overt proteinuria. This suggested that DKD in South Asians, once it starts, more rapidly progresses to proteinuria. Ethnic differences in the prevalence of albuminuria in type 2 diabetes have also been documented in a New Zealand study of 65,171 patients with type 2 diabetes attending primary care doctors between 2000 and 2006.[71] After controlling for multiple risk factor variables, compared with Europeans, the ORs for albuminuria were 3.9 for Maori, 4.7 for Pacific Islanders, 2 in Indo-Asians, and 4.1 for East-Asians. Ethnic differences in DKD incidence may reflect genetic predisposition and different access to care. To eliminate the effect of disparity of access, the Pathways Study in the United States was conducted in a setting of uniform access to good quality primary health care (in a large health maintenance organization in Washington state).[72] In this cross-sectional study of 2969 patients with diabetes, ethnic differences in prevalence of albuminuria were found. In patients without hypertension, Asians had ORs of 2.01 for microalbuminuria and 3.17 for macroalbuminuria compared with whites. If patients had hypertension, Hispanics had greater odds of microalbuminuria (OR, 3.82) and blacks had greater odds of macroalbuminuria (OR, 3.32) compared with whites. From the 2009 ANZDATA renal registry data, examination of the incidence rate of RRT for DKD in Australia and New Zealand revealed that 35% of new patients had DKD, of which 92% was caused by type 2 diabetes.[11] Australian indigenous people had a significantly higher incidence rate for RRT compared with nonindigenous Australians (particularly in the age group ≥60 years). Indigenous Australians made up 16.7% of the patients with DKD commencing RRT but only 2.5% of the Australian population in 2009.[11]

In summary, in DKD caused by type 2 diabetes, there is a gradation of risk of ESRD and mortality depending on the level of urine albumin excretion, similar to what is seen with type 1 diabetes. The range of annual transition rates from normoalbuminuria to microalbuminuria is 2% to 4%, from microalbuminuria to macroalbuminuria 2.8% to 5.4%, and from macroalbuminuria to RRT or high serum creatinine 2.3%. People from Hispanic, black, Asian, Indian, indigenous, Maori, and Pacific Island ethnic backgrounds have increased prevalence of albuminuric DKD compared with Europeans.

The Nonalbuminuric Pathway of DKD

As in type 1 diabetes, renal impairment often develops in those with type 2 diabetes without preceding abnormalities in urine albumin excretion. MacIsaac and colleagues[73] determined the prevalence of impaired GFR in 301 people with type 2 diabetes attending a hospital clinic by using the gold standard of plasma isotopic marker disappearance. In this study, after excluding those taking RAS inhibitors because of their effect on urinary albumin excretion, 23% of the people with renal impairment of CKD stage 3 or worse had preceding persistent normoalbuminuria. In the UKPDS, after a median follow-up of 15 years, 28% of the people with type 2 diabetes developed renal impairment, defined as eGFR less than or equal to 60 mL/min/1.73 m^2.[62] Of these, 51% had never had microalbuminuria or macroalbuminuria during the study and 16% developed albuminuria only after reaching an impaired eGFR. A total of 33% had albuminuria before onset of renal insufficiency. These results are similar to those obtained by the United States NHANES III.[54] In those with type 2 diabetes and eGFR less than 60 mL/min/1.73 m^2, 30% had no retinopathy or microalbuminuria or macroalbuminuria. In the Swedish National Diabetes Register cohort studied by Afghahi and colleagues,[64] 6% to 7% developed nonalbuminuric renal impairment within the 5 years of follow-up. Only one-third of those who developed renal failure had developed albuminuria.

A contemporary Australian study of patients attending general practitioners for type 2 diabetes management showed that 55% of those with stage 3 or lower CKD had persistent normoalbuminuria.[74] The clinic-based, cross-sectional, global DEMAND study examined the prevalence of normoalbuminuric renal dysfunction in 11,573 adults with type 2 diabetes.[75] The overall prevalence of normoalbuminuria was 51%. For CKD stages 3 to 5, those with normoalbuminuria formed 41%, 26% and 29% respectively of the total number of patients within each stage. A cross-sectional Italian study (The Renal Insufficiency and Cardiovascular Events [RIACE] study) of 15,773 adult patients with type 2 diabetes attending public hospital clinics in 2007 to 2008 showed that 56.6% of those with eGFR less than 60 mL/min/1.73 m^2 were normoalbuminuric.[76] In this population, when those with nonalbuminuric renal impairment were compared with those with albuminuric renal impairment, the two groups had different clinical associations. The nonalbuminuric pathway had weaker associations with retinopathy, HbA$_{1c}$, and hypertension, but significant associations with female gender, nonsmoker status, and cardiovascular complications. The patients tended to have shorter duration of diabetes and were less likely to be on an angiotensin-converting enzyme inhibitor or on angiotensin receptor blocker treatment compared with those who had progressed down the albuminuric pathway. The two pathways had a similar association with age of the patient.[76] Logistic regression analysis showed the OR of cardiovascular events was 1.52 for nonalbuminuric CKD and 1.90 for albuminuric CKD. For cardiovascular events, there was a stronger relationship between nonalbuminuric CKD and coronary events (OR, 1.514) than for cerebrovascular or peripheral events, and conversely, the association with cerebrovascular and peripheral events (OR, 1.69 and 1.88, respectively) was stronger for albuminuric CKD than for nonalbuminuric CKD.[77]

In summary, renal impairment without albuminuria has become the most common presentation of renal disease in type 2 diabetes. The recent RIACE Italian study does not support previous conjecture that this change in presentation was caused by age-related GFR classification as stage 3 or higher CKD or because of widespread use of RAS inhibitors. The two pathways of developing DKD (albuminuric vs nonalbuminuric) have different risks of associated cardiovascular disease.

KIDNEY FUNCTION IN PREDIABETIC STATES

Changes in kidney function can be detected in the stages of impaired glucose tolerance (IGT) or impaired fasting glucose (IFG), collectively termed "prediabetes." Prediabetes affects 35% of US adults.[3] A total of 280 million adults worldwide were estimated to have IGT in 2011 (6.4%) and this is projected to reach 398 million (7.1%) by 2030.[78] Even in these prediabetic stages, abnormalities are evident in pathways leading to kidney damage; for example, young adult African Americans with IGT had elevated urinary transforming growth factor-β levels compared with those with normal glucose tolerance.[79] There has been a body of work examining the significance of abnormal GFR in people with prediabetes. Definition of an abnormal GFR, such as hyperfiltration, depends in part on identification of the age-appropriate GFR within a control healthy population.[80] So far, there has been no consensus on the definition of hyperfiltration. A carefully conducted Japanese study by Okada and colleagues[81] recently found that the prevalence of hyperfiltration increased as prediabetes worsened. In this study, hyperfiltration was defined as an eGFR greater than the 95th percentile of the age- and gender-specific eGFR, determined in 99,140 people in the Aichi prefecture. Prediabetes was diagnosed if the person had IFG.[81] The ORs of hyperfiltration were 1.29 for stage 1 prediabetes (fasting plasma glucose 100–109 mg/dL) and 1.58 for stage 2 prediabetes (fasting plasma glucose 110–125 mg/dL). However, in this study, there was no association between prediabetes and decreased GFR. Similar results were found in a Norwegian study, the Renal Iohexol Clearance Survey.[82] The OR for hyperfiltration in those with IFG compared with those with normal fasting glucose was 1.56. Decreased GFR has also been associated with prediabetes. In the 1999 to 2006 US NHANES, the prevalence of CKD stage 3 to 4 in people with IFG was 8.5%.[83] Overall prevalence of CKD (defined by low eGFR or albuminuria) in prediabetes was 16.6%.

In summary, studies in people with prediabetes have shown evidence of early renal damage, demonstrated by albuminuria or abnormal GFR.

SUBCLINICAL CHANGES IN KIDNEY FUNCTION THAT OCCUR EARLY IN DIABETES

Nelson and colleagues[84] assessed serial GFR changes in Pima Indians with normal glucose tolerance and IGT. Although at baseline there was no statistically significant difference in GFR between those with normal glucose tolerance and IGT, people who progressed to type 2 diabetes showed a 30% increase in GFR at onset of diabetes. A recent longitudinal study of people with type 2 diabetes and GFR greater than or equal to 120 mL/min/1.73 m^2 showed that those with persistent hyperfiltration had a hazard ratio of 2.16 for progression to albuminuria compared with those in whom hyperfiltration resolved or who did not have baseline hyperfiltration.[85] Over 4 years, GFR decline was relatively rapid at 3.37 mL/min/1.73 m^2 per year. A meta-analysis of 10 studies in people with type 1 diabetes concluded that those with hyperfiltration had increased risk of progressing to DKD.[86]

Measurement of serum cystatin C can improve detection of mild degrees of renal dysfunction.[87] In a landmark study, Perkins and colleagues[88] demonstrated that serial cystatin C measurements done over 4 years, when compared with iothalamate clearance in Pima Indians with type 2 diabetes and GFR greater than 120 mL/min/1.73 m^2, could be used to detect early trends in renal function. Directly measured GFR declined at 4.4% per year. This technique was used to detect early renal function decline in people with type 1 diabetes from the Joslin Clinic, followed for 8 to 12 years.[89] Early renal function decline was detected in 9% of people with normoalbuminuria and 31% with microalbuminuria. Skupien and colleagues[90] have recently demonstrated that the slope of the early eGFR decline observed over 5 years predicted the risk of developing ESRD in people with type 1 diabetes.

In summary, subtle changes in GFR (hyperfiltration and rate of GFR decline) occurring early in the course of diabetes have been associated with DKD prognosis but these associations need to be confirmed.

SUMMARY

The increasing prevalence of diabetes has led to DKD becoming the leading cause of ESRD in many regions. The economic cost of DKD will grow to prohibitive amounts unless strategies to prevent its onset or progression are urgently implemented. In type 1 and type 2 diabetes, the presence of microalbuminuria and macroalbuminuria confers increased risk of developing ESRD and of death. Comparison of recent studies with earlier historical studies shows that the incidence of ESRD and death has decreased in DKD. Increased risk of albuminuria has been identified in certain non-European ethnic groups. However, the initial concept of progression of DKD as an albuminuric phenotype involving development of microalbuminuria, macroalbuminuria, and then ESRD has had to be modified. Albumin excretion frequently regresses, and GFR can decline without abnormality in albumin excretion. There is emerging evidence that changes in renal function occurring early in the course of diabetes predict future outcomes. The major challenges are to prevent DKD onset, to detect it early, and to improve DKD outcomes globally.

REFERENCES

1. National Kidney Foundation. KDOQI clinical practice guidelines and clinical practice recommendations for diabetes and chronic kidney disease. Am J Kidney Dis 2007;49:S1–180.
2. Whiting D, Guariguata L, Weil C, et al. IDF diabetes atlas: global estimates of the prevalence of diabetes for 2011 and 2030. Diabetes Res Clin Pract 2011;94: 311–21.
3. Centers for Disease Control and Prevention. National diabetes fact sheet: national estimates and general information on diabetes and prediabetes in the United States, 2011. US Department of Health and Human Services. Atlanta (GA): Centers for Disease Control and Prevention; 2011.
4. Parving H, Lewis J, Ravid M, et al. Prevalence and risk factors for microalbuminuria in a referred cohort of type II diabetic patients: a global perspective. Kidney Int 2006;69:2057–63.
5. Zhang L, Wang F, Wang L, et al. Prevalence of chronic kidney disease in China: a cross-sectional survey. Lancet 2012;379:815–22.
6. Yang W, Lu J, Weng J, et al. Prevalence of diabetes among men and women in China. N Engl J Med 2010;362:1090–101.
7. Unnikrishnan R, Rema M, Pradeepa R, et al. Prevalence and risk factors of diabetic nephropathy in an urban South Indian population: the Chennai Urban Rural Epidemiology Study (CURES 45). Diabetes Care 2007;30:2019–24.
8. United States Renal Data System. USRDS 2011 annual data report: atlas of chronic kidney disease and end-stage renal disease in the United States.

Bethesda (MD): National Institutes of Health. National Institute of Diabetes and Digestive and Kidney Diseases; 2011.

9. Centers for Disease Control and Prevention. Incidence of end-stage renal disease attributed to diabetes among persons with diagnosed diabetes—United States and Puerto Rico, 1996–2007. MMWR Morb Mortal Wkly Rep 2010;59:1361–6.

10. Burrows N, Li Y, Geiss L. Incidence of treatment for end-stage renal disease among individuals with diabetes in the U.S. continues to decline. Diabetes Care 2010;33:73–7.

11. Grace B, Clayton P, McDonald S. Increases in renal replacement therapy in Australia and New Zealand: understanding trends in diabetic nephropathy. Nephrology (Carlton) 2012;17:76–84.

12. Deloitte Access Economics. Two of a KinD (Kidneys in Diabetes): the burden of diabetic kidney disease and the cost effectiveness of screening people with type 2 diabetes for chronic kidney disease. Kidney Health Australia. Melbourne (Victoria): Kidney Health Australia; 2011.

13. Nichols G, Vupputuri S, Lau H. Medical care costs associated with progression of diabetic nephropathy. Diabetes Care 2011;34:2374–8.

14. Trivedi H, Pang M, Campbell A, et al. Slowing the progression of chronic renal failure: economic benefits and patients' perspectives. Am J Kidney Dis 2002; 39:721–9.

15. Keen H, Chlouverakis C. An immunoassay for urinary albumin at low concentrations. Lancet 1963;2:913–4.

16. Keen H, Chlouverakis C, Fuller J, et al. The concomitants of raised blood sugar: studies in newly-detected hyperglycaemics. II. Urinary albumin excretion, blood pressure and their relation to blood sugar levels. Guys Hosp Rep 1969;118: 247–54.

17. Mogensen C. Urinary albumin excretion in early and long-term juvenile diabetes. Scand J Clin Lab Invest 1971;28:183–93.

18. Parving H, Oxenboll B, Svendsen P, et al. Early detection of patients at risk of developing diabetic nephropathy: a longitudinal study of urinary albumin excretion. Acta Endocrinol (Copenh) 1982;100:550–5.

19. Viberti G, Hill R, Jarrett R, et al. Microalbuminuria as a predictor of clinical nephropathy in insulin-dependent diabetes mellitus. Lancet 1982;1:1430–2.

20. Messent J, Elliott T, Hill R, et al. Prognostic significance of microalbuminuria in insulin-dependent diabetes mellitus: a twenty-three year follow-up study. Kidney Int 1992;41:836–9.

21. Mogensen C, Christensen C. Predicting diabetic nephropathy in insulin-dependent patients. N Engl J Med 1984;311:89–93.

22. Mathiesen E, Oxenbøll B, Johansen K, et al. Incipient nephropathy in type 1 (insulin-dependent) diabetes. Diabetologia 1984;26:406–10.

23. Parving H, Hommel E, Mathiesen E, et al. Prevalence of microalbuminuria, arterial hypertension, retinopathy and neuropathy in patients with insulin dependent diabetes. Br Med J 1988;296:156–60.

24. Andersen A, Christiansen J, Andersen J, et al. Diabetic nephropathy in type 1 (insulin-dependent) diabetes: an epidemiological study. Diabetologia 1983;25: 496–501.

25. Borch-Johnsen K, Andersen P, Deckert T. The effect of proteinuria on relative mortality in type 1 (insulin-dependent) diabetes mellitus. Diabetologia 1985;28: 590–6.

26. Krolewski A, Warram J, Christlieb A, et al. The changing natural history of nephropathy in type 1 diabetes. Am J Med 1985;78:785–94.

27. Rossing P, Houggaard P, Parving H- H. Progression of microalbuminuria in type 1 diabetes: ten-year prospective observational study. Kidney Int 2005;68:1446–50.
28. Perkins B, Ficociello L, Silva K, et al. Regression of microalbuminuria in type 1 diabetes. N Engl J Med 2003;348:2285–93.
29. Steinke J, Sinaiko A, Kramer M, et al. The early natural history of nephropathy in type 1 diabetes: III. Predictors of 5-year urinary albumin excretion rate patterns in initially normoalbuminuric patients. Diabetes 2005;54:2164–71.
30. The Diabetes Control, Complications Trial Research Group. The effect of intensive treatment of diabetes on the development and progression of long-term complications in insulin-dependent diabetes mellitus. N Engl J Med 1993;329: 977–86.
31. de Boer I, Rue T, Cleary P, et al. Long-term renal outcomes of patients with type 1 diabetes mellitus and microalbuminuria: an analysis of the diabetes control and complications trial/epidemiology of diabetes interventions and complications cohort. Arch Intern Med 2011;171:412–20.
32. Harvey J, Rizvi K, Craney L, et al. Population-based survey and analysis of trends in the prevalence of diabetic nephropathy in type 1 diabetes. Diabet Med 2001; 18:998–1002.
33. Raile K, Galler A, Hofer S, et al. Diabetic nephropathy in 27,805 children, adolescents, and adults with type 1 diabetes: effect of diabetes duration, A1C, hypertension, dyslipidemia, diabetes onset, and sex. Diabetes Care 2007;30:2523–8.
34. Hovind P, Tarnow L, Rossing K, et al. Decreasing incidence of severe diabetic microangiopathy in type 1 diabetes. Diabetes Care 2003;26:1258–64.
35. Nordwall M, Bojestig M, Arnqvist H, et al. Declining incidence of severe retinopathy and persisting decrease of nephropathy in an unselected population of type 1 diabetes: the Linkoping Diabetes Complications Study. Diabetologia 2004;47: 1266–72.
36. Pambianco G, Costacou T, Ellis D, et al. The 30-year natural history of type 1 diabetes complications. The Pittsburgh Epidemiology of Diabetes Complications Study experience. Diabetes 2006;55:1463–9.
37. Marshall S. Diabetic nephropathy in type 1 diabetes: has the outlook improved since the 1980s? Diabetologia 2012;55:2301–6.
38. Möllsten A, Svensson M, Waernbaum I, et al. Cumulative risk, age at onset, and sex-specific differences for developing end-stage renal disease in young patients with type 1 diabetes. A nationwide population-based cohort study. Diabetes 2010;59:1803–8.
39. Finne P, Reunanen A, Stenman S, et al. Incidence of end-stage renal disease in patients with type 1 diabetes. JAMA 2005;294:1782–7.
40. Groop P, Thomas M, Moran J, et al. The presence and severity of chronic kidney disease predicts all-cause mortality in type 1 diabetes. Diabetes 2009;58: 1651–8.
41. Stadler M, Auinger M, Anderwald C, et al. Long-term mortality and incidence of renal dialysis and transplantation in type 1 diabetes mellitus. J Clin Endocrinal Metab 2006;91:3814–20.
42. Molitch M, Steffes M, Sun W, et al. Development and progression of renal insufficiency with and without albuminuria in adults with type 1 diabetes in the diabetes control and complications trial and the epidemiology of diabetes interventions and complications study. Diabetes Care 2010;33:1536–43.
43. Astrup A, Tarnow L, Rossing P, et al. Improved prognosis in type 1 diabetic patients with nephropathy: a prospective follow-up study. Kidney Int 2005;68: 1250–7.

44. Forsblom C, Harjutsalo V, Thorn L, et al. Competing-risk analysis of ESRD and death among patients with type 1 diabetes and macroalbuminuria. J Am Soc Nephrol 2011;22:537–44.
45. Rosolowsky E, Skupien J, Smiles A, et al. Risk for ESRD in type 1 diabetes remains high despite renoprotection. J Am Soc Nephrol 2011;22:545–53.
46. Lane P, Steffes M, Mauer S. Glomerular structure in IDDM women with low glomerular filtration rate and normal urinary albumin excretion. Diabetes 1992;41:581–6.
47. Caramori M, Fioretto P, Mauer M. Low glomerular filtration rate in normoalbuminuric type 1 diabetic patients. Diabetes 2003;52:1036–40.
48. Tsalamandris C, Allen T, Gilbert R, et al. Progressive decline in renal function in diabetic patients with and without albuminuria. Diabetes 1994;43:649–55.
49. Perkins B, Ficociello L, Roshan B, et al. In patients with type 1 diabetes and new-onset microalbuminuria the development of advanced chronic kidney disease may not require progression to proteinuria. Kidney Int 2010;77:57–64.
50. Fabre J, Balant L, Dayer P, et al. The kidney in maturity onset diabetes mellitus: a clinical study of 510 patients. Kidney Int 1982;21:730–8.
51. Parving H, Gall M, Skott P, et al. Prevalence and causes of albuminuria in non-insulin-dependent diabetic patients. Kidney Int 1992;41:758–62.
52. Valmadrid C, Klein R, Moss S, et al. The risk of cardiovascular disease mortality associated with microalbuminuria and gross proteinuria in persons with older-onset diabetes mellitus. Arch Intern Med 2000;160:1093–100.
53. Bruno G, Cavallo-Perin P, Bargero G, et al. Prevalence and risk factors for micro- and macroalbuminuria in an Italian population-based cohort of NIDDM subjects. Diabetes Care 1996;19:43–7.
54. Kramer H, Nguyen Q, Curhan G, et al. Renal insufficiency in the absence of albuminuria and retinopathy among adults with type 2 diabetes mellitus. JAMA 2003; 289:3273–7.
55. Jia W, Gao X, Pang C, et al. Prevalence and risk factors of albuminuria and chronic kidney disease in Chinese population with type 2 diabetes and impaired glucose regulation: Shanghai Diabetic Complications Study (SHDCS). Nephrol Dial Transplant 2009;24:3724–31.
56. Tapp R, Shaw J, Zimmet P, et al. Albuminuria is evident in the early stages of diabetes onset: results from the Australian Diabetes, Obesity, and Lifestyle Study (AusDiab). Am J Kidney Dis 2004;44:792–8.
57. Mogensen C. Microalbuminuria predicts clinical proteinuria and early mortality in maturity onset diabetes. N Engl J Med 1984;310:356–60.
58. Schmitz A, Vaeth M. Microalbuminuria: a major risk factor in non-insulin-dependent diabetes. A 10-year follow-up study of 503 patients. Diabet Med 1988;5:126–34.
59. Nelson R, Pettitt D, Carraher M, et al. Effect of proteinuria on mortality in NIDDM. Diabetes 1988;37:1499–504.
60. Kunzelman C, Knowler W, Pettitt D, et al. Incidence of proteinuria in type2 diabetes mellitus in the Pima Indians. Kidney Int 1989;35:681–7.
61. Gall M, Hougaard P, Borch-Johnsen K, et al. Risk factors for development of incipient and overt diabetic nephropathy in patients with non-insulin dependent diabetes mellitus: prospective, observational study. Br Med J 1997;314:783–8.
62. Retnakaran R, Cull C, Thorne K, et al. Risk factors for renal dysfunction in type 2 diabetes: U.K. Prospective Diabetes Study 74. Diabetes 2006;55:1832–9.
63. Adler A, Stevens R, Manley S, et al. Development and progression of nephropathy in type 2 diabetes: the United Kingdom Prospective Diabetes Study (UKPDS 64). Kidney Int 2003;63:225–32.

64. Afghahi H, Cederholm J, Eliasson B, et al. Risk factors for the development of albuminuria and renal impairment in type 2 diabetes: the Swedish National Diabetes Register (NDR). Nephrol Dial Transplant 2011;26:1236–43.
65. Bruno G, Merletti F, Biggeri A, et al. Progression to overt nephropathy in type 2 diabetes: the Casale Monferrato Study. Diabetes Care 2003;26:2150–5.
66. Packham D, Alves T, Dwyer J, et al. Relative incidence of ESRD versus cardiovascular mortality in proteinuric type 2 diabetes and nephropathy: results from the DIAMETRIC (Diabetes Mellitus Treatment for Renal Insufficiency Consortium) database. Am J Kidney Dis 2012;59:75–83.
67. Fox C, Matsushita K, Woodward M, et al. Associations of kidney disease measures with mortality and end-stage renal disease in individuals with and without diabetes: a meta-analysis. In: Lancet 2012.
68. Ninomiya T, Perkovic V, de Galan B, et al. Albuminuria and kidney function independently predict cardiovascular and renal outcomes in diabetes. J Am Soc Nephrol 2009;20:1813–21.
69. Jardine M, Hata J, Woodward M, et al. Prediction of kidney-related outcomes in patients with type 2 diabetes. Am J Kidney Dis 2012;60:770–8.
70. Raymond N, O'Hare J, Bellary S, et al. Comparative risk of microalbuminuria and proteinuria in UK residents of south Asian and white European ethnic background with type 2 diabetes: a report from UKADS. Curr Med Res Opin 2011;27:47–55.
71. Kenealy T, Elley C, Collins J, et al. Increased prevalence of albuminuria among non-European peoples with type 2 diabetes. Nephrol Dial Transplant 2012;27: 1840–6.
72. Young B, Katon W, Von Korff M, et al. Racial and ethnic differences in microalbuminuria prevalence in a diabetes population: the pathways study. J Am Soc Nephrol 2005;16:219–28.
73. MacIsaac R, Tsalamandris C, Panagiotopoulos S, et al. Nonalbuminuric renal insufficiency in type 2 diabetes. Diabetes Care 2004;27:195–200.
74. Thomas M, Macisaac R, Jerums G, et al. Nonalbuminuric renal impairment in type 2 diabetic patients and in the general population (national evaluation of the frequency of renal impairment cO-existing with NIDDM [NEFRON] 11). Diabetes Care 2009;32:1497–502.
75. Dwyer J, Parving H, Hunsicker L, et al. Renal dysfunction in the presence of normoalbuminuria in type 2 diabetes: results from the DEMAND study. Cardiorenal Med 2012;2:1–10.
76. Penno G, Solini A, Bonora E, et al. Clinical significance of non albuminuric renal impairment in type 2 diabetes. J Hypertens 2011;29:1802–9.
77. Solini A, Penno G, Bonora E, et al. Diverging association of reduced glomerular filtration rate and albuminuria with coronary and noncoronary events in patients with type 2 diabetes. Diabetes Care 2012;35:143–9.
78. International Diabetes Federation. International Diabetes Federation diabetes atlas. 5th edition. Brussels (Belgium): International Diabetes Federation; 2011.
79. Huan Y, DeLoach S, Daskalakis C, et al. Regulation of transforming growth factor-b1 by insulin in prediabetic African Americans. Kidney Int 2010;78:318–24.
80. Jerums G, Premaratne E, Panagiotopoulos S, et al. The clinical significance of hyperfiltration in diabetes. Diabetologia 2010;53:2093–104.
81. Okada R, Yasuda Y, Tsushita K, et al. Glomerular hyperfiltration in prediabetes and prehypertension. Nephrol Dial Transplant 2012;27:1821–5.
82. Melsom T, Mathisen U, Ingebretsen O, et al. Impaired fasting glucose is associated with renal hyperfiltration in the general population. Diabetes Care 2011;34: 1546–51.

83. Plantinga L, Crews D, Coresh J, et al. Prevalence of chronic kidney disease in US adults with undiagnosed diabetes or prediabetes. Clin J Am Soc Nephrol 2010;5: 673–82.

84. Nelson R, Tan M, Beck G, et al. Changing glomerular filtration with progression from impaired glucose tolerance to type II diabetes mellitus. Diabetologia 1999;42:90–3.

85. Ruggenenti P, Porrini E, Gaspari F, et al. Glomerular hyperfiltration and renal disease progression in type 2 diabetes. Diabetes Care 2012;35(10):2061–8.

86. Magee G, Bilous R, Cardwell C, et al. Is hyperfiltration associated with the future risk of developing diabetic nephropathy? A meta-analysis. Diabetologia 2009;52: 691–7.

87. Macisaac R, Tsalamandris C, Thomas M, et al. The accuracy of cystatin C and commonly used creatinine-based methods for detecting moderate and mild chronic kidney disease in diabetes. Diabet Med 2007;24:443–8.

88. Perkins B, Nelson R, Ostrander B, et al. Detection of renal function decline in patients with diabetes and normal or elevated GFR by serial measurements of serum cystatin C concentration: results of a 4-year follow-up study. J Am Soc Nephrol 2005;16:1404–12.

89. Perkins B, Ficociello L, Ostrander B, et al. Microalbuminuria and the risk for early progressive renal function decline in type 1 diabetes. J Am Soc Nephrol 2007;18: 1353–61.

90. Skupien J, Warram J, Smiles A, et al. The early decline in renal function in patients with type 1 diabetes and proteinuria predicts the risk of end-stage renal disease. Kidney Int 2012;82:589–97.

Clinical Manifestations and Natural History of Diabetic Kidney Disease

Eberhard Ritz, MD

KEYWORDS

- Diabetes • Kidney disease • Natural history • Clinical manifestations

KEY POINTS

- Diabetes mellitus, mostly type 2, has become the single most frequent cause of dialysis dependency.
- There are two key interventions to prevent, or at least retard, progression of diabetic kidney disease are blood pressure lowering and blockade of the renin-angiotensin-system.
- Beyond the classical presentation with nephromegaly and proteinuria, an increasing proportion of diabetic patients with CKD presents with minor (or no) proteinuria.

In order to be a competent nephrologist, one has to be a knowledgeable diabetologist.

—*Eli Friedman (New York)*

EPIDEMIOLOGY OF CHRONIC KIDNEY DISEASE AND END-STAGE KIDNEY DISEASE IN DIABETES

Renal failure in type 2 diabetes has been termed a medical catastrophe of worldwide dimension.[1] In 2001, at the author's unit in Heidelberg, it was found that 49% of incident patients requiring maintenance hemodialysis had diabetes (ie, 98 per million population [pmp] per year), 6% of whom had type 1 diabetes and most of the 94% had type 2 diabetes.[2] This frequency was much higher than the then reported frequency in Germany of approximately 35% of incident patients. The main cause for this underestimate was that the diagnosis of type 2 diabetes is often missed if an oral glucose tolerance test is not performed. Patients with diabetes with chronic kidney disease (CKD) tend to lose weight in the preterminal phase of renal failure.[3] This factor also explains why several reports stated that 10% to 15% of patients undergoing dialysis develop apparent de novo type 2 diabetes (presumably reappearance of type 2

University of Heidelberg, Nierenzentrum, Im Neuenheimer Feld 162, Heidelberg 69120, Germany
E-mail address: bueroritz@gmx.de

Med Clin N Am 97 (2013) 19–29
http://dx.doi.org/10.1016/j.mcna.2012.10.008
0025-7125/13/$ – see front matter © 2013 Elsevier Inc. All rights reserved.

diabetes after hyperglycemia had disappeared in the preterminal stage of CKD). In patients with CKD, the prevalence of undiagnosed diabetes or prediabetes is high.[4] Importantly, presumed new-onset diabetes after the initiation of hemodialysis is associated with a similarly poor prognosis and survival rate as in patients with known pre-existing type 2 diabetes.[5]

In the 1990s, a continuous increase of the incident rates of end-stage renal disease (ESRD) in patients with diabetes was noted both in Europe and in the United States.[6] In proteinuric patients with diabetes, it is only in relatively advanced stages of estimated glomerular filtration rate (eGFR) loss that the risk to develop ESRD exceeds the risk to die of cardiovascular causes. This point was recently confirmed by the Diabetes Mellitus Treatment for Renal Insufficiency Consortium in a meta-analysis of controlled intervention trials.[7] The progressive increase of ESRD in patients with diabetes in the past might have also been, at least in part, the result of improved cardiac care. Interestingly, the rate of patients with diabetes with ESRD per million population has recently stabilized in Europe as well as in the United States. According to the last report of the United States Renal Data System, the annual rate (per million population) of patients with diabetes reaching end-stage kidney disease was 160 pmp and the prevalence of patients with diabetes on dialysis is currently 650 pmp.

Patients with type 2 diabetes with CKD may have classic Kimmelstiel-Wilson disease or alternatively from a type of more nonspecific nephropathy.[8] In the author's clinical series,[2] 70% of the patients had the classic clinical features of Kimmelstiel-Wilson nephropathy (ie, renomegaly, heavy proteinuria with or without retinopathy); varying from year to year, up to 20% had small kidneys, little or no proteinuria, presumably ischemic nephropathy, and between 10% and 20% had primary kidney disease with superimposed type 2 diabetes.

One further mode of presentation of impaired renal function in patients with type 2 diabetes is acute kidney injury (AKI), usually in the form of AKI superimposed on CKD. Patients may or may not recover from AKI, and in the latter case remain dialysis dependent. If the patients recover, accelerated progression and increased risk of ESRD are common.[9,10] If patients with preexisting diabetic nephropathy survive an episode of AKI, the predictors of subsequent fast progression are high baseline serum creatinine, high blood pressure, and high proteinuria; any given level of serum creatinine proteinuria is a risk factor for more rapid development of end-stage kidney disease.[11]

In juvenile patients with type 1 diabetes, the diabetes control an complication trial/epidemiology of diabetes interventions and complications (DCCT/EDIC) trial showed that it takes decades until ESRD is reached.[12] In contrast, juvenile patients with type 2 diabetes have a substantially higher renal risk of early renal failure,[13] a point of considerable concern in view of the increasing frequency of obesity and type 2 diabetes in juveniles.

At what clinical stage can pathologic changes be documented in the kidney? Caramori and colleagues[14] found even advanced glomerular lesions in patients with type 1 diabetes who had normoalbuminuria but lower glomerular filtration rates. Numerous observational studies documented that patients with type 1 or 2 diabetes and advanced loss of GFR might have no proteinuria at all. This finding is presumably not, or at least not fully, explained as the result of the antiproteinuric effect of renin-angiotensin system (RAS) blockade.[15] The underlying renal histology in this subpopulation is not well known.

One specific form of nonproteinuric progressive renal failure has been identified in a prospective study in Japan.[16] In patients with type 2 diabetes with small vessel disease documented by cerebral magnetic resonance imaging, a high risk was found to develop dialysis-dependent renal failure within 10 years' time despite the absence of microalbuminuria, suggesting a form of progressive nonproteinuric vascular kidney disease.

The threshold for an adverse effect of glycemia on renal function may be lower than conventionally thought. Succurro and colleagues[17] documented kidney dysfunction in patients with a high risk of type 2 diabetes, but not overt diabetes, who had 1-hour postload plasma glucose levels more than 155 mg/dL.

A special form of type 2 diabetes is onset of type 2 diabetes after kidney transplantation.[18] In some series, up to 24% of patients developed type 2 diabetes 3 years after renal transplantation; this was more frequent in males, in patients with hepatitis C, in patients with a high body mass index, and in patients undergoing tacrolimus treatment. Posttransplant diabetes is also associated with a higher risk of cardiovascular events[19] and a higher risk of more rapid deterioration of renal function.

It is important to consider that not all kidney disease in patients with type 2 diabetes is diabetic nephropathy. One example is postinfectious glomerulonephritis and impaired renal function, which may be seen particularly in elderly patients with diabetes,[20] even in the absence of diabetic glomerulosclerosis.

Of concern are also reports of diffuse diabetic glomerulosclerosis[21] and even nodular diabetic glomerulosclerosis[22] in patients with metabolic syndrome and abnormal glucose tolerance but not with overt type 2 diabetes. These observations raise the issue of whether renal lesions may exist in prediabetic individuals before the criteria of type 2 diabetes have been met or whether patients may have had overt type 2 diabetes in the past.

It is also of note that even nodular glomerulosclerosis is not absolutely specific for diabetic nephropathy; it may be found in nondiabetic smokers[23] or, even more confusing, in smokers with metabolic syndrome.[24] In this context, it is of interest that active and passive exposure to cigarette smoke does not only increase the risk of type 2 diabetes[25] but also increases the risk of albuminuria[26] and progressive loss of GFR.

In the natural history of diabetes, at what stage are renal abnormalities demonstrable? In prediabetic patients with slightly elevated postprandial glycemia, but not yet overt type 2 diabetes, lower eGFR was found in a notable proportion of individuals.[17] In individuals with type 1 diabetes, Caramori and colleagues[14] found that thickening of the basement membrane and increased mesangial volume preceded the onset of microalbuminuria. This finding is in agreement with their finding[27] that in a rhesus monkey diabetes model, glomerular hypertrophy begins in the prediabetic hyperinsulinemic phase; aging rhesus monkeys are frequently obese and exhibit spontaneous type 2 diabetes and may, thus, provide a model for the evolution of diabetic nephropathy. Early on, they develop increased glomerular volume, increased width of glomerular basement membrane, and increased glomerular tuft volume, which are features that were correlated to the degree of glucose tolerance. Mouse models also present some features of diabetic nephropathy, but they do not reproduce features of advanced nephropathy (eg, glomerular nodules); a recent murine model, the PPARϒ2 knockout mouse in a genetic ob/ob background may, therefore, be of interest.[28]

STRATEGIES TO DELAY PROGRESSION AND COMPLICATIONS OF DIABETIC NEPHROPATHY

The main strategies with proven evidence to prevent or, in later stages, delay progressive loss of renal function in patients with diabetes include (1) blood pressure control, (2) blockade of the RAS, and (3) glycemic control. Some further interventions have, so far, provided only incomplete evidence of benefit.

Blood Pressure Control

One of the most important treatment targets in diabetic nephropathy is hypertension. In type 1 diabetes, hypertension usually starts with the onset of nephropathy; but in type 2 diabetes, matters are more complex. In the general population, higher blood pressure values predict a higher risk of future end-stage kidney disease, even in individuals without renal disease at baseline; this risk is much more pronounced in individuals with diabeties.[29]

In the 1970s, early studies of Mogensen[30] and Parving[31] documented the frequency of hypertension in patients with diabetes with nephropathy; they documented the efficacy of blood pressure lowering by antihypertensive agents even before RAS blockers had become available. When RAS blockade became available, a great number of studies documented the specific effect of RAS blockade to interfere with the progressive loss of GFR in addition to blood pressure lowering.

What has recently been added to the issue of blood pressure control? Some recently discussed major blood pressure–related issues include the target for blood pressure lowering and the technique of blood pressure measurement. Since the classic study by Mogensen,[30] it is beyond doubt that elevated office blood pressure per se has an adverse effect on the progression of diabetic nephropathy. Recent studies documented that taking albuminuria in type 2 diabetes as a renal damage indicator, nocturnal blood pressure is the most important predictor.[32,33] In a 9.2-year follow-up study, nighttime dipping was also associated with less mortality.[34] It is, therefore, of interest that taking additional antihypertensive medication in the evening provides better nighttime blood pressure control.[35] The predictive value of clinic blood pressure is grossly inferior to morning blood pressure.[36] Therefore, blood pressure measurements in the morning by patients or caregivers is preferable.

Whether there is one optimal target blood pressure for all patients with diabetes is debatable and the answer is presumably negative. The UKPDS study had shown that the higher the systolic blood pressure, the higher the frequency of death and of end points, including renal endpoints[37]; this was true even for relatively low systolic blood pressures. Substantial lowering is presumably correct for early stages of diabetic nephropathy, but aggressive blood pressure lowering is presumably hazardous in individuals with longstanding diabetes and latent or overt cardiovascular damage. It seems more appropriate to go for lower blood pressure values in younger patients in early stages of diabetes, and it may be prudent to be less aggressive in elderly patients, in patients with diabetes of long duration, and particularly in patients with documented cardiovascular complications. Current advise is not based on controlled evidence, because, as pointed out by Mancia and colleagues,[38] one is confronted with the dilemma that none of the controlled trials on blood pressure lowering in diabetes had actually achieved a systolic blood pressure less than 130 mm Hg. They gave the wise advice that the cardiovascular risk profile should determine the aggressiveness of blood pressure lowering. In the Irbesartan Diabetic Nephropathy Trial (IDNT) study, Pohl[39] noted that in patients with type 2 diabetes with advanced diabetic nephropathy, lowering systolic blood pressure to levels less than 120 mm Hg systolic caused less renal end points but at the expense of higher mortality. Particular attention should also be given to avoid excessive lowering of the diastolic blood pressure; in the same study, Berl and colleagues[40] reported that the risk of myocardial infarction was progressively higher with lower diastolic blood pressures. Findings in the recent Randomized Olmesartan And Diabetes MicroAlbuminuria Prevention (ROADMAP) also pointed to the potential risk of blood pressure lowering and cardiac events or death,[41] and this is particularly relevant in advanced diabetic nephropathy with a high risk of concomitant cardiovascular damage.

In patients with longstanding diabetes and advanced CKD, a point of particular concern is orthostatic hypotension,[42] particularly after bed rest,[43] increasing cardiovascular risk.[44]

Blockade of the RAS

In prediabetic patients, RAS blockade reduces new-onset diabetes.[45] Furthermore, in the prediabetic stage, RAS blockade causes less renal damage after the onset of diabetes in animal studies.[46] In patients with diabetes, blockade of the RAS provides blood pressure–independent renal benefit. In the early stages of type 2 diabetes, the angiotensin-converting enzyme (ACE) inhibitor trandolapril reduced the onset of microalbuminuria in the Bergamo Nephrologic Diabetes Complications Trial (BENEDICT).[47] More recently, the ROADMAP study[41] provided similar evidence for the angiotensin receptor blocker olmesartan. It must be admitted, however, that the reduction of albuminuria and attenuation of GFR loss may not always go in parallel. In relatively early stages of overt diabetic nephropathy, Barnett and colleagues[48] had documented the beneficial effect of RAS blockade to retard the progressive loss of GFR and to stabilize GFR after 4 to 5 years. This was achieved with angiotensin receptor blockers as well as with ACE inhibitors.

In advanced nephropathy, the 2 major studies in patients with type 2 diabetes and relatively advanced CKD (ie, RENAAL[49] and IDNT[50]), using the angiotensin receptor blockers losartan and irbesartan, respectively, documented that both drugs reduced the risk of ESRD blood pressure independently. Blockade of the RAS was beneficial across a broad spectrum of serum creatinine concentrations.[51] Furthermore, in the IDNT study, Pohl and colleagues[39] could document that the effects of blood pressure control and RAS blockade are independent and additive (ie, even when patients were on RAS blockade with the angiotensin receptor blocker irbesartan, blood pressure control was still relevant); doubling serum creatinine was progressively more frequent at progressively higher achieved systolic blood pressure values.[39] This observation illustrates that both blood pressure lowering and RAS blockade are important targets. The ON TARGET study included a substantial number of patients with diabetes; the findings documented that no additional benefit could be achieved with the combination of ACE inhibitors and angiotensin receptor blocker (ARB).

An important issue is the dose of ACE inhibitors or angiotensin receptor blockers. The licensed doses of either drug class are based on blood pressure–lowering studies; in patients with diabetes, the reduction of albuminuria requires dose escalation of angiotensin receptor blockers more than the doses licensed for blood pressure lowering,[52] and higher doses are necessary to retard progressive loss of GFR in patients with CKD.[53]

When assessing the literature, one must be cautious not to extrapolate too liberally from the reduction of albuminuria to the reduction of renal outcomes; the ON TARGET study included many patients with diabetes and showed that the 2 outcomes do not always go in parallel.[54]

Another difficulty is the interpretation of loss of GFR as an end point. In diabetes, glomerular filtration is initially increased and presumably even in patients with reduced GFR still inappropriately high. The reduction of hyperfiltration might be beneficial as recently documented in a study on ACE inhibition on 600 patients with type 2 diabetes in an early stage[55]; after RAS blockade, the subsequent evolution of renal end points was more benign in patients with an initial GFR decrease (ie, reversal of hyperfiltration).

An important issue is the choice of salt intake. In a controlled study in nondiabetic patients with CKD on angiotensin receptor blockers, Vogt and colleagues[56] found that salt restriction was associated with significantly greater reduction of proteinuria. To what extent salt intake lowering is also adequate in patients who have diabetes is currently uncertain because recent observational, but not fully conclusive, evidence indicates that low salt intake in type 1 diabetes is associated with worse outcomes.[57]

Great hopes had been connected with the renin inhibitor aliskiren, which had significantly reduced albuminuria in patients with type 2 diabetes blood pressure independently.

Glycemia Control

It is important to differentiate between glycemic control in (1) prediabetes, (2) early diabetes, and (3) late diabetes with complications.

In a 14-year observational study, the hazard ratio (HR) to develop diabetic kidney disease was strongly correlated to the hemoglobin A_{1c} (HbA_{1c}) at baseline in a cohort with no diabetes at baseline.[58]

In patients with juvenile type 1 diabetes (DCCT, EDIC trial), intensified glycemic control attenuated the rate of impairment of eGFR[12]; onset of nephropathy was reduced from 25% to 9%.

In patients with type 2 diabetes of considerable duration (eg, in the ADVANCE study),[59] patients with an HbA_{1c} target of 6.5% compared with 7.3% had 21% less renal end points (new or worsening of nephropathy); in the VA-Diabetes trial,[60] however, no significant reduction of renal events was seen in elderly type 2 diabetics with long-standing diabetes.

The interpretation is rendered difficult because it takes a long time to develop kidney malfunction (ie, GFR loss) as shown in the EDIC trial[12]; conversely after pancreas transplantation, the benefit of normoglycemia on renal function is seen only after more than a decade.[61] Cardiovascular mortality is particularly high in patients at a high renal risk[62] so that many may have died before advanced renal end points had time to develop.

The most meaningful information on renal function comes from the UKPDS study whereby patients were observed starting at early stages of diabetes[62]; the prespecified outcomes were similar to the ones in the type 1 diabetes EDIC trial.[12] Two percent of patients yearly progressed from normoalbuminuria to microalbuminuria and from microalbuminuria to macroalbuminuria; increased albuminuria was associated with higher mortality. During 12 years of observation, more intensive glycemic control reduced the onset of microalbuminuria and proteinuria by 33%.

Multifactorial Treatment

The aforementioned interventions document significant benefit with several modes of intervention, but the net effect for most interventions is rather modest. This state of affairs led to the hypothesis that combining several different interventions might amplify the therapeutic benefit. In a relatively small but well-executed study, 160 patients with type 2 diabetes were allocated either to standard treatment (according to the then valid guidelines) or intensive treatment, including behavior modification and intense treatment of hyperglycemia, hypertension, dyslipidemia, and microalbuminuria; such intensified intervention slowed progression of diabetic nephropathy.[63] It took many years to see the definite long-term benefit. After 7.8 years, the risk of nephropathy was significantly lower in the group with intensified treatment (HR 0.39)[64]; and only when the study had ended, rates of death (HR 0.54) and cardiovascular death (HR 0.43) were found to be reduced after further follow-up, yielding a total of 13.3 years observation. Late renal outcome was different, although of course not statistically significant; only 1 patient in the group with intensified treatment versus 6 patients in the control group had developed terminal renal failure.[65]

A recent Asian study complemented this finding by documenting that not only progression of diabetic nephropathy but even onset of diabetic nephropathy can be improved by intensified treatment in patients with normoalbuminuric type 2 diabetes. In 1290 Chinese patients with type 2 diabetes, new onset of microalbuminuria could be significantly delayed in a 4.5-year prospective trial comprising tight simultaneous control of multiple targets (ie, HbA$_{1c}$, blood pressure control, and lipid control versus no intensified intervention).[66]

PATIENTS WITH DIABETIC NEPHROPATHY: ADDITIONAL INTERVENTIONS

Unfortunately in many diabetic patients with renal disease, the aforementioned established interventions (blood pressure lowering, RAS blockade, glycemic control) fail to satisfactorily reduce proteinuria and to arrest the progressive loss of GFR. Recent studies assessed complementary interventions on top of blood pressure lowering and RAS blockade. The investigators comment briefly on mineralocorticoid receptor blockade, endothelin receptor blockade, uric acid lowering, and the terpenoid bardoxolone.

Sato and colleagues[67] found that patients with type 2 diabetes with a secondary increase in albuminuria despite continued RAS blockade (escape) responded to 25 mg/d spironolactone with 40% reduction in albuminuria despite no significant change in blood pressure. Escape is caused by a secondary increase in plasma aldosterone concentration. A correlation exists between p-aldosterone and GFR loss.[68] Recently, controlled evidence has been provided that aldosterone receptor blockade, in addition to standard renoprotective treatment, lowers albuminuria in patients with microalbuminuric type 1 diabetes.[69] Novel intestinal potassium binders reduce the potential risk of hyperkalemia.[70]

In patients who failed to respond satisfactorily to standard therapy, the endothelin receptor blocker avosentan caused significant further reduction of albuminuria[71]; but in patients with impaired renal function, unacceptable sodium/fluid retention was observed.[72] More Endothelin A (ET-A) receptor–specific blockers are still promising, however.[73]

Uric acid might become a potential therapeutic target in diabetic nephropathy. Serum uric acid concentration predicts future onset of type 2 diabetes[74] and is a predictor of nephropathy.[75] A meta-analysis documented a relation between lowering uricemia and attenuated GFR loss in diabetic nephropathy.[76] In a controlled study of patients with CKD, including patients with diabetes, allopurinol attenuated the progressive loss of GFR.[77]

Bardoxolone, a terpenoid with antiinflammatory action, interacts with the Nrf 2/Keap system and caused an increase of estimated GFR in patients with type 2 diabetes.[78] A large controlled study is currently underway. It is still undecided whether the increase of GFR is beneficial or adverse; this issue is currently assessed in a prospective trial.

REFERENCES

1. Ritz E, Rychlik I, Locatelli F, et al. End-stage renal failure in type 2 diabetes: a medical catastrophe of worldwide dimensions. Am J Kidney Dis 1999;34(5):795–808.
2. Schwenger V, Müssig C, Hergesell O, et al. Incidence and clinical characteristics of renal insufficiency in diabetic patients. Dtsch Med Wochenschr 2001;126(47):1322–6 [in German].
3. Kalantar-Zadeh K, Derose SF, Nicholas S, et al. Burnt-out diabetes: impact of chronic kidney disease progression on the natural course of diabetes mellitus. J Ren Nutr 2009;19(1):33–7.

4. Plantinga LC, Crews DC, Coresh J, et al. Prevalence of chronic kidney disease in US adults with undiagnosed diabetes or prediabetes. Clin J Am Soc Nephrol 2010;5(4):673–82.
5. Salifu MO, Abbott KC, Aytug S, et al. New-onset diabetes after hemodialysis initiation: impact on survival. Am J Nephrol 2010;31(3):239–46.
6. Van Dijk PC, Jager KJ, Stengel B, et al. Renal replacement therapy for diabetic end-stage renal disease: data from 10 registries in Europe (1991–2000). Kidney Int 2005;67(4):1489–99.
7. Packham DK, Alves TP, Dwyer JP, et al. Relative incidence of ESRD versus cardiovascular mortality in proteinuric type 2 diabetes and nephropathy: results from the DIAMETRIC (Diabetes Mellitus Treatment for Renal Insufficiency Consortium) database. Am J Kidney Dis 2012;59(1):75–83.
8. Fioretto P, Caramori ML, Mauer M. The kidney in diabetes: dynamic pathways of injury and repair. The Camillo Golgi Lecture 2007. Diabetologia 2008;51(8):1347–55.
9. Ishani A, Xue JL, Himmelfarb J, et al. Acute kidney injury increases risk of ESRD among elderly. J Am Soc Nephrol 2009;20(1):223–8.
10. Liangos O, Wald R, O'Bell JW, et al. Epidemiology and outcomes of acute renal failure in hospitalized patients: a national survey. Clin J Am Soc Nephrol 2006; 1(1):43–51.
11. Shahinfar S, Dickson T, Zhang Z, et al. Baseline predictors of end-stage renal disease risk in patients with type 2 diabetes and nephropathy: new lessons from the RENAAL study. Kidney Int Suppl 2005;(93):S48–51.
12. de Boer IH, Sun W, Cleary PA, et al. Intensive diabetes therapy and glomerular filtration rate in type 1 diabetes. N Engl J Med 2011;365(25):2366–76.
13. Dart AB, Sellers EA, Martens PJ, et al. High burden of kidney disease in youth-onset type 2 diabetes. Diabetes Care 2012;35(6):1265–71.
14. Caramori ML, Fioretto P, Mauer M. Low glomerular filtration rate in normoalbuminuric type 1 diabetic patients: an indicator of more advanced glomerular lesions. Diabetes 2003;52(4):1036–40.
15. MacIsaac RJ, Tsalamandris C, Panagiotopoulos S, et al. Nonalbuminuric renal insufficiency in type 2 diabetes. Diabetes Care 2004;27(1):195–200.
16. Uzu T, Kida Y, Shirahashi N, et al. Cerebral microvascular disease predicts renal failure in type 2 diabetes. J Am Soc Nephrol 2010;21(3):520–6.
17. Succurro E, Arturi F, Lugarà M, et al. One-hour postload plasma glucose levels are associated with kidney dysfunction. Clin J Am Soc Nephrol 2010;5(11):1922–7.
18. Kasiske BL, Snyder JJ, Gilbertson D, et al. Diabetes mellitus after kidney transplantation in the United States. Am J Transplant 2003;3(2):178–85.
19. Cosio FG, Kudva Y, van der Velde M, et al. New onset hyperglycemia and diabetes are associated with increased cardiovascular risk after kidney transplantation. Kidney Int 2005;67(6):2415–21.
20. Nasr SH, Fidler ME, Valeri AM, et al. Postinfectious glomerulonephritis in the elderly. J Am Soc Nephrol 2011;22(1):187–95.
21. Altiparmak MR, Pamuk ON, Pamuk GE, et al. Diffuse diabetic glomerulosclerosis in a patient with impaired glucose tolerance: report on a patient who later develops diabetes mellitus. Neth J Med 2002;60(6):260–2.
22. Souraty P, Nast CC, Mehrotra R, et al. Nodular glomerulosclerosis in a patient with metabolic syndrome without diabetes. Nat Clin Pract Nephrol 2008;4(11):639–42.
23. Nasr SH, D'Agati VD. Nodular glomerulosclerosis in the nondiabetic smoker. J Am Soc Nephrol 2007;18(7):2032–6.
24. Li W, Verani RR. Idiopathic nodular glomerulosclerosis: a clinicopathologic study of 15 cases. Hum Pathol 2008;39(12):1771–6.

25. Zhang L, Curhan GC, Hu FB, et al. Association between passive and active smoking and incident type 2 diabetes in women. Diabetes Care 2011;34(4):892–7.
26. Phisitkul K, Hegazy K, Chuahirun T, et al. Continued smoking exacerbates but cessation ameliorates progression of early type 2 diabetic nephropathy. Am J Med Sci 2008;335(4):284–91.
27. Cusumano AM, Bodkin NL, Hansen BC, et al. Glomerular hypertrophy is associated with hyperinsulinemia and precedes overt diabetes in aging rhesus monkeys. Am J Kidney Dis 2002;40(5):1075–85.
28. Martinez-Garcia C, Izquierdo A, Velagapudi V, et al. Accelerated renal disease is associated with the development of metabolic syndrome in a glucolipotoxic mouse model. Dis Model Mech 2012;5(5):636–48.
29. Hsu CY, McCulloch CE, Darbinian J, et al. Elevated blood pressure and risk of end-stage renal disease in subjects without baseline kidney disease. Arch Intern Med 2005;165(8):923–8.
30. Mogensen CE. Progression of nephropathy in long-term diabetics with proteinuria and effect of initial anti-hypertensive treatment. Scand J Clin Lab Invest 1976; 36(4):383–8.
31. Parving HH, Persson F, Lewis JB, et al. Aliskiren combined with losartan in type 2 diabetes and nephropathy. N Engl J Med 2008;358(23):2433–46.
32. Palmas W, Pickering T, Teresi J, et al. Nocturnal blood pressure elevation predicts progression of albuminuria in elderly people with type 2 diabetes. J Clin Hypertens (Greenwich) 2008;10(1):12–20.
33. Knudsen ST, Laugesen E, Hansen KW, et al. Ambulatory pulse pressure, decreased nocturnal blood pressure reduction and progression of nephropathy in type 2 diabetic patients. Diabetologia 2009;52(4):698–704.
34. Astrup AS, Nielsen FS, Rossing P, et al. Predictors of mortality in patients with type 2 diabetes with or without diabetic nephropathy: a follow-up study. J Hypertens 2007;25(12):2479–85.
35. Hermida RC, Ayala DE, Mojón A, et al. Bedtime dosing of antihypertensive medications reduces cardiovascular risk in CKD. J Am Soc Nephrol 2011;22(12): 2313–21.
36. Kamoi K, Miyakoshi M, Soda S, et al. Usefulness of home blood pressure measurement in the morning in type 2 diabetic patients. Diabetes Care 2002; 25(12):2218–23.
37. Adler AI, Stratton IM, Neil HA, et al. Association of systolic blood pressure with macrovascular and microvascular complications of type 2 diabetes (UKPDS 36): prospective observational study. BMJ 2000;321(7258):412–9.
38. Mancia G, Laurent S, Agabiti-Rosei E, et al. Reappraisal of European guidelines on hypertension management: a European Society of Hypertension Task Force document. J Hypertens 2009;27(11):2121–58.
39. Pohl MA, Blumenthal S, Cordonnier DJ, et al. Independent and additive impact of blood pressure control and angiotensin II receptor blockade on renal outcomes in the irbesartan diabetic nephropathy trial: clinical implications and limitations. J Am Soc Nephrol 2005;16(10):3027–37.
40. Berl T, Blumenthal S, Cordonnier DJ, et al. Impact of achieved blood pressure on cardiovascular outcomes in the Irbesartan Diabetic Nephropathy Trial. J Am Soc Nephrol 2005;16(7):2170–9.
41. Haller H, Ito S, Izzo JL Jr, et al. Olmesartan for the delay or prevention of microalbuminuria in type 2 diabetes. N Engl J Med 2011;364(10):907–17.
42. Spallone V, Morganti R, Fedele T, et al. Reappraisal of the diagnostic role of orthostatic hypotension in diabetes. Clin Auton Res 2009;19(1):58–64.

43. Schneider SM, Robergs RA, Amorim FT, et al. Impaired orthostatic response in patients with type 2 diabetes mellitus after 48 hours of bed rest. Endocr Pract 2009;15(2):104–10.
44. Fedorowski A, Hedblad B, Melander O. Early postural blood pressure response and cause-specific mortality among middle-aged adults. Eur J Epidemiol 2011; 26(7):537–46.
45. Jandeleit-Dahm KA, Tikellis C, Reid CM, et al. Why blockade of the renin-angiotensin system reduces the incidence of new-onset diabetes. J Hypertens 2005;23(3):463–73.
46. Nagai Y, Yao L, Kobori H, et al. Temporary angiotensin II blockade at the prediabetic stage attenuates the development of renal injury in type 2 diabetic rats. J Am Soc Nephrol 2005;16(3):703–11.
47. Ruggenenti P, Fassi A, Ilieva AP, et al. Preventing microalbuminuria in type 2 diabetes. N Engl J Med 2004;351(19):1941–51.
48. Barnett AH, Bain SC, Bouter P, et al. Angiotensin-receptor blockade versus converting-enzyme inhibition in type 2 diabetes and nephropathy. N Engl J Med 2004;351(19):1952–61.
49. Brenner BM, Cooper ME, de Zeeuw D, et al. Effects of losartan on renal and cardiovascular outcomes in patients with type 2 diabetes and nephropathy. N Engl J Med 2001;345(12):861–9.
50. Lewis EJ, Hunsicker LG, Clarke WR, et al. Renoprotective effect of the angiotensin-receptor antagonist irbesartan in patients with nephropathy due to type 2 diabetes. N Engl J Med 2001;345(12):851–60.
51. Remuzzi G, Ruggenenti P, Perna A, et al. Continuum of renoprotection with losartan at all stages of type 2 diabetic nephropathy: a post hoc analysis of the RENAAL trial results. J Am Soc Nephrol 2004;15(12):3117–25.
52. Krimholtz MJ, Karalliedde J, Thomas S, et al. Targeting albumin excretion rate in the treatment of the hypertensive diabetic patient with renal disease. J Am Soc Nephrol 2005;16(Suppl 1):S42–7.
53. Hou FF, Zhang X, Zhang GH, et al. Efficacy and safety of benazepril for advanced chronic renal insufficiency. N Engl J Med 2006;354(2):131–40.
54. Mann JF, Schmieder RE, McQueen M, et al. Renal outcomes with telmisartan, ramipril, or both, in people at high vascular risk (the ONTARGET study): a multicentre, randomised, double-blind, controlled trial. Lancet 2008;372(9638): 547–53.
55. Ruggenenti P, Porrini EL, Gaspari F, et al. Glomerular hyperfiltration and renal disease progression in type 2 diabetes. Diabetes Care 2012;35:2061–8.
56. Vogt L, Waanders F, Boomsma F, et al. Effects of dietary sodium and hydrochlorothiazide on the antiproteinuric efficacy of losartan. J Am Soc Nephrol 2008; 19(5):999–1007.
57. Thomas MC, Moran J, Forsblom C, et al. The association between dietary sodium intake, ESRD, and all-cause mortality in patients with type 1 diabetes. Diabetes Care 2011;34(4): 861–6.
58. Selvin E, Ning Y, Steffes MW, et al. Glycated hemoglobin and the risk of kidney disease and retinopathy in adults with and without diabetes. Diabetes 2011; 60(1):298–305.
59. Patel A, MacMahon S, Chalmers J, et al. Effects of a fixed combination of perindopril and indapamide on macrovascular and microvascular outcomes in patients with type 2 diabetes mellitus (the ADVANCE trial): a randomised controlled trial. Lancet 2007;370(9590):829–40.

60. Duckworth W, Abraira C, Moritz T, et al. Glucose control and vascular complications in veterans with type 2 diabetes. N Engl J Med 2009;360(2):129–39.
61. Morath C, Zeier M, Döhler B, et al. Metabolic control improves long-term renal allograft and patient survival in type 1 diabetes. J Am Soc Nephrol 2008;19(8): 1557–63.
62. Bilous R. Microvascular disease: what does the UKPDS tell us about diabetic nephropathy? Diabet Med 2008;25(Suppl 2):25–9.
63. Gaede P, Vedel P, Parving HH, et al. Intensified multifactorial intervention in patients with type 2 diabetes mellitus and microalbuminuria: the Steno type 2 randomised study. Lancet 1999;353(9153):617–22.
64. Gaede P, Vedel P, Larsen N, et al. Multifactorial intervention and cardiovascular disease in patients with type 2 diabetes. N Engl J Med 2003;348(5):383–93.
65. Gaede P, Lund-Andersen H, Parving HH, et al. Effect of a multifactorial intervention on mortality in type 2 diabetes. N Engl J Med 2008;358(6):580–91.
66. Tu ST, Chang SJ, Chen JF, et al. Prevention of diabetic nephropathy by tight target control in an Asian population with type 2 diabetes mellitus: a 4-year prospective analysis. Arch Intern Med 2010;170(2):155–61.
67. Sato A, Hayashi K, Naruse M, et al. Effectiveness of aldosterone blockade in patients with diabetic nephropathy. Hypertension 2003;41(1):64–8.
68. Schjoedt KJ, Andersen S, Rossing P, et al. Aldosterone escape during blockade of the renin-angiotensin-aldosterone system in diabetic nephropathy is associated with enhanced decline in glomerular filtration rate. Diabetologia 2004; 47(11):1936–9.
69. Nielsen SE, Persson F, Frandsen E, et al. Spironolactone diminishes urinary albumin excretion in patients with type 1 diabetes and microalbuminuria: a randomized placebo-controlled crossover study. Diabet Med 2012;29(8):e184–90.
70. Pitt B, Anker SD, Bushinsky DA, et al. Evaluation of the efficacy and safety of RLY5016, a polymeric potassium binder, in a double-blind, placebo-controlled study in patients with chronic heart failure (the PEARL-HF) trial. Eur Heart J 2011;32(7):820–8.
71. Wenzel RR, Littke T, Kuranoff S, et al. Avosentan reduces albumin excretion in diabetics with macroalbuminuria. J Am Soc Nephrol 2009;20(3):655–64.
72. Mann JF, Green D, Jamerson K, et al. Avosentan for overt diabetic nephropathy. J Am Soc Nephrol 2010;21(3):527–35.
73. Kohan DE, Pritchett Y, Molitch M, et al. Addition of atrasentan to renin-angiotensin system blockade reduces albuminuria in diabetic nephropathy. J Am Soc Nephrol 2011;22(4):763–72.
74. Bhole V, Choi JW, Kim SW, et al. Serum uric acid levels and the risk of type 2 diabetes: a prospective study. Am J Med 2010;123(10):957–61.
75. Hovind P, Rossing P, Tarnow L, et al. Serum uric acid as a predictor for development of diabetic nephropathy in type 1 diabetes: an inception cohort study. Diabetes 2009;58(7):1668–71.
76. Miao Y, Ottenbros SA, Laverman GD, et al. Effect of a reduction in uric acid on renal outcomes during losartan treatment: a post hoc analysis of the reduction of endpoints in non-insulin-dependent diabetes mellitus with the Angiotensin II Antagonist Losartan Trial. Hypertension 2011;58(1):2–7.
77. Goicoechea M, de Vinuesa SG, Verdalles U, et al. Effect of allopurinol in chronic kidney disease progression and cardiovascular risk. Clin J Am Soc Nephrol 2010; 5(8):1388–93.
78. Pergola PE, Raskin P, Toto RD, et al. Bardoxolone methyl and kidney function in CKD with type 2 diabetes. N Engl J Med 2011;365(4):327–36.

The Pathogenesis and Management of Hypertension in Diabetic Kidney Disease

Peter N. Van Buren, MD*, Robert D. Toto, MD

KEYWORDS

• Hypertension • Vasoconstriction • ACE inhibitor • RAAS therapy • Hyperkalemia

KEY POINTS

- Hypertension commonly coexists with diabetes, and its prevalence is even higher in the presence of diabetic kidney disease.
- The pathogenesis of hypertension in this population stems from increased extracellular volume and increased vasoconstriction that result from mechanisms that may be attributed to both diabetes and the eventual impairment of renal function.
- Antihypertensive therapy aimed at reducing blood pressure remains a primary goal in preventing the incidence of diabetic kidney and slowing its progression. Initial therapy should consist of an ACE inhibitor or ARB titrated to the maximally tolerated dose.
- Using combination RAAS therapy further reduces proteinuria, but the benefits of this strategy compared with the potential risks of hyperkalemia and acute deterioration of renal function are still unknown.
- Endothelin receptor antagonists also lower proteinuria, but these can be associated with volume overload and edema with no clear long-term benefit on renal function yet identified.

INTRODUCTION

Diabetic kidney disease is one of the potential microvascular complications that can occur in diabetic patients. It is the leading cause of end-stage renal disease (ESRD) in the United States that also carries an augmented risk for cardiovascular morbidity

This work was supported by funding from the American Heart Association Fellow to Faculty Transition Award (PVB) and the UT Southwestern O'Brien Center (NIH P30DK079328). This work was also conducted with support from UT-STAR, NIH/NCATS Grant Number KL2RR024983. The conduct is solely the responsibility of the authors and does not necessarily represent the official views of the UT-STAR, The University of Texas Southwestern Medical Center at Dallas and its affiliated academic and health care centers, the National Center for Advancing Translational Sciences, or the National Institutes of Health.
The authors have no further disclosures to report.
Division of Nephrology, Department of Internal Medicine, University of Texas Southwestern Medical Center at Dallas, 5939 Harry Hines Boulevard, Dallas, TX 75390-8516, USA
* Corresponding author.
E-mail address: Peter.vanburen@utsouthwestern.edu

and mortality in patients who still have some preservation of renal function. Blood pressure control, along with glycemic control and inhibition of the renin-angiotensin-aldosterone system (RAAS), has been established as a primary goal to reduce the incidence of and slow the progression of diabetic kidney disease. As hypertension is a common comorbidity associated with diabetes that has a multifactorial origin, this task remains difficult to achieve in many diabetic patients. Furthermore, the specific blood pressure targets that offer optimal benefit from both a renal and cardiovascular standpoint remain uncertain. This review article focuses on some of the predominant mechanisms responsible for increased blood pressure in diabetic kidney disease and the current clinical evidence on the antihypertensive agents that are used to manage diabetic kidney disease.

DIABETIC KIDNEY DISEASE

When kidney disease presents in diabetic patients as albuminuria and/or renal impairment, specific clinical cues may further guide the determination of whether or not diabetes is the underlying cause. The presence of extrarenal microvascular disease (diabetic retinopathy, diabetic neuropathy) and a long duration of diabetes before the onset of albuminuria support the diagnosis of diabetic kidney disease.[1] The lack of these findings, the presence of hematuria, or evidence of another systemic disease warrant consideration of a renal biopsy to establish the diagnosis. As diabetic kidney disease may take many years to develop and progress in patients with either type 1 or type 2 diabetes, a diagnosis will often be made late in the course of the disease at a time when the disease is progressing at a faster rate. The first phase, hyperfiltration, has usually already passed even when the diagnosis is made early. During the hyperfiltration phase, which is marked by an increase in glomerular filtration rate, clinical symptoms of albuminuria and hypertension are typically absent. Subsequent phases of diabetic kidney disease involve microalbuminuria and then macroalbuminuria with progressive decreases in the glomerular filtration rate and increases in blood pressure. Once overt diabetic nephropathy is present, there is increased risk for both ESRD and cardiovascular mortality. Hypertension is a critical comorbidity that further increases the risk of these outcomes at this stage of the disease.

Hypertension in Diabetic Kidney Disease

For individuals in the general population, a blood pressure of 140/90 mm Hg marks the threshold of stage I hypertension and the point at which antihypertensive therapy is indicated.[2] For individuals with diabetes or kidney disease (regardless of the underlying etiology), the recommended treatment target is a blood pressure lower than 130/80 mm Hg.[3,4] As these recommendations reflect relatively recent guidelines for blood pressure targets, the reported prevalence of hypertension among patients with diabetes may vary depending on when a study was conducted and the specific definition for hypertension that was used.

The clinical context in which hypertension presents will differ between patients with type 1 and type 2 diabetes. In type 1 diabetic patients, hypertension most frequently presents after microalbuminuria develops. One large epidemiologic study showed the prevalence of hypertension among patients with type 1 diabetes without microalbuminuria to be 4% (similar to the age-matched control population),[5] whereas another study showed its prevalence in this population to be 19%.[6] Both studies defined hypertension at values higher than the currently recommended blood pressure targets, but they were consistent in showing that the prevalence of hypertension increases as the amount of proteinuria increases. This association between hypertension and albuminuria in patients with type 1 diabetes has been further defined by evidence that the failure of blood pressure to decrease during the nighttime on ambulatory blood pressure monitoring occurs before the development of microalbuminuria.[7] In patients with type 2 diabetes, hypertension may be present well before any manifestation of microalbuminuria or renal disease, indicating that insulin resistance is associated with increased blood pressure.[8] In fact, the prevalence of hypertension has been estimated to be as high as 58% to 70% in patients with type 2 diabetes without microalbuminuria.[9,10] Similar to type 1 diabetic patients, hypertension becomes even more prevalent as renal disease progresses in patients with type 2 diabetes and further augments the risk for cardiovascular events in these patients.[11]

PATHOPHYSIOLOGY

The underlying mechanisms responsible for hypertension in diabetic kidney disease involve increased extracellular volume, increased vasoconstriction, and the general inability of these components to appropriately balance out each other. Increased renal reabsorption of sodium and/or impaired renal excretion of sodium mediate the increase in extracellular volume, whereas increased vasoconstriction is mediated by numerous systems including the RAAS, endothelin system, and sympathetic nervous system. Some of the mediators from these systems are directly involved in promoting local renal damage, but the overall increase in systemic blood pressure these mediators induce and the inherent hemodynamic autoregulatory impairment in the renal microvasculature of diabetics facilitate further renal injury if hypertension is inadequately treated.

Hyperfiltration and Sodium Reabsorption

One of the first changes in renal function that may occur in diabetes is an increase in the glomerular filtration rate, referred to as hyperfiltration.[12] Because serum creatinine will be low and blood pressure will be normal in this context, overall renal function may be inappropriately perceived as normal. However, both the underlying cause and subsequent consequences of hyperfiltration are associated with the development of an unfavorable hemodynamic state that permits the eventual deterioration of renal function.

Increased proximal tubular reabsorption of sodium may coexist with hyperfiltration in patients with insulin-dependent diabetes.[13] In fact, it is hypothesized that hyperfiltration is an appropriate response of the tubuloglomerular feedback reacting to an inappropriate increase in sodium reabsorption. An animal study showed lower concentrations of tubular sodium and chloride measured proximal to the macula densa in diabetic rats compared with control animals.[13] With pharmacologic inhibition of proximal tubule sodium/glucose transporters, there were increased concentrations of sodium and chloride downstream to these transporters, which subsequently resulted in a decreased single-nephron glomerular filtration rate (GFR). There is experimental evidence that hyperfiltration is nitric oxide dependent and that this process also prevents increases in blood pressure early in the course of diabetes.[14,15] Although the primary mechanisms contributing to the increase in sodium reabsorption remain incompletely understood, the ultimate consequence is an expansion of extracellular volume. Furthermore, patients with diabetes respond to salt loading with an inadequate inhibition of RAAS activity.[16] As RAAS activity promotes renal sodium reabsorption throughout the nephron, achieving euvolemia can become even more difficult if this system is not adequately suppressed in volume-overloaded individuals.

The implications of various interventions related to either dietary salt ingestion or the use of diuretics in the context of pharmacologic RAAS inhibition are discussed later in the management section.

In patients who develop diabetic kidney disease, hyperfiltration ceases and reductions in GFR take place as there is progression through the phases of microalbuminuria and macroalbuminuria. Renal excretion of sodium and water becomes more difficult with reduction in GFR, and this further contributes to the increased prevalence of extracellular volume expansion and hypertension at these later stages.

RAAS

The RAAS has the potential to influence diabetic kidney disease through several mechanisms. One of the systemic functions of this system is to restore euvolemia and maintain sufficient blood pressure in the context of volume depletion. Both angiotensin II (Ang II) and aldosterone have functions that (1) promote increased reabsorption of sodium by binding to various receptors on renal tubules and (2) increase vascular tone by binding to receptors on vascular smooth muscle cells in the peripheral circulation. Local tissue levels of the angiotensin-converting enzyme (ACE) and Ang II have been shown to be increased in the glomeruli and renal tubules of streptozocin-induced diabetic rats and diabetic patients with or without nephropathy.[17–20] On the systemic level, the plasma renin activity of diabetic patients and patients with diabetic nephropathy is frequently the same as or lower than that of healthy individuals.[21,22] However, these levels seen in diabetic patients are still higher than would be expected given the degree of extracellular volume overload that is present.[22] Thus, deregulation of this axis may contribute to increased blood pressure by creating a persistent state of volume overload and increased vasoconstriction.

Beyond the traditional RAAS mediators (Ang II and aldosterone), there is emerging evidence that other novel components of this system may be important mediators of hypertension and diabetic kidney disease (**Fig. 1**). ACE 2 is responsible for the enzymatic conversion of Ang II to Ang-(1–7), as well as the conversion of Ang I to Ang-(1–9). In Zucker diabetic rats, independent of Ang II levels, infusion of Ang-(1–7) (1) lowered blood pressure, (2) reduced oxidative stress and inflammation in the kidney, (3) reduced renal extracellular matrix expansion, (4) reduced proteinuria, and (5) increased GFR compared with saline infusion.[23] Conversely, in diabetic mice, pharmacologic inhibition of ACE 2 promoted an increase in extracellular matrix production and proteinuria.[24] The significance of these findings has yet to be confirmed in humans. Current studies in patients with diabetes or CKD are limited by variability in research methods and consequently variable results regarding the renal expression of ACE 2 or ACE 2 activity.[25–27] The full implications of how the ACE 2 fits into the management of hypertension and diabetic nephropathy remains yet to be determined. The use of pharmacologic agents to inhibit the traditional components of the RAAS is discussed in significant detail in the management section.

Endothelial Cell Dysfunction

Endothelial cells are involved in important interactions with vascular smooth muscle cells to facilitate the regulation of vasodilation and vasoconstriction. In CKD, blood pressure correlates with the severity of endothelial cell dysfunction.[28] Furthermore, diabetes is independently associated with a greater degree of endothelial cell dysfunction compared with healthy individuals, and the amount of proteinuria correlates with the severity of this dysfunction.[29,30] A unifying abnormality among CKD and diabetes is the potential disruption of the balance of vasoconstrictors and vasodilators that modify vascular tone and function. Under physiologic conditions, nitric

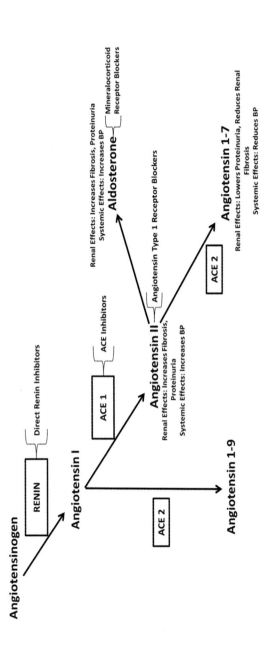

Fig. 1. The RAAS pathway is depicted along with the effects and potential therapeutic options for the individual mediators. Renin enzymatically converts angiotensinogen to angiotensin I. Direct renin inhibitors have been explored as an option to reduce renin activity, but the current clinical trial evidence does not support its use in combination with other RAAS inhibiting agents. ACE 1 converts Ang I to Ang II. ACE inhibitors are considered first-line antihypertensive therapies for patients with diabetic kidney disease. Ang II promotes renal fibrosis and proteinuria and also increases blood pressure systemically. Accordingly, ARBs are another consideration as first-line therapy. Ang II also promotes release of aldosterone, which can further promote fibrosis, proteinuria, and increased blood pressure. Mineralocorticoid receptor blockers inhibit the effects of aldosterone and can be effective in lowering proteinuria. A new concept that has emerged in this pathway is the role of the ACE 2 enzyme, which converts Ang II to a vasodilatory and potentially renoprotective mediator, Ang-(1–7). This enzyme may also prevent further production of Ang II by converting Ang I to Ang-(1–9).

oxide, which is synthesized in endothelial cells, binds to vascular smooth muscle cells to cause vasodilation. In vitro evidence from endothelial cells shows that increased glucose concentrations interfere with nitric oxide metabolism.[31] In animal models of diabetes, the significance of nitric oxide becomes evident from the exaggerated increase in blood pressure that inhibitors of nitric oxide synthase induce.[32] Beyond the potential role of hyperglycemia in inducing such dysfunction, CKD and diabetes are also both associated with an increased level of an endogenous inhibitor of nitric oxide synthase, asymmetric dimethylarginine (ADMA). Vascular resistance and blood pressure increase with infusion of ADMA into healthy individuals,[33] and ADMA levels in patients with diabetes or CKD are independently associated with increased risk for cardiovascular events.[34–37]

Alternatively, vascular tone could be influenced by increased activity of vasoconstrictive mediators related to endothelial cell dysfunction. Endothelin-1 (ET-1) is a vasoconstrictive peptide that exerts its actions through binding to tissue receptors throughout the body, including the glomerulus and vascular smooth muscle cells. Both animal and human studies show increased local renal tissue levels and plasma levels of ET-1,[38,39] and insulin resistance has been potentially implicated as playing a role.[40] Subsequently, increased ET-1 activity may have adverse effects on both systemic blood pressure and local renal hemodynamics and function. Pharmacologic inhibition of endothelin receptors can improve endothelial cell dysfunction in patients with diabetes,[41] and the application of such drugs in larger randomized trials is discussed in the management section.

Oxidative Stress

Increased oxidative stress is one mechanism that potentially unifies the role that the RAAS and endothelial cell function play in hypertension. Increased reactive oxidative species may be generated in the vasculature through the effects of Ang II on nicotinamide adenine dinucleotide hydrate/nicotinamide adenine dinucleotide phosphate oxidase.[42,43] Through interaction with free radicals, nitric oxide may (1) lose its capacity to properly induce vasodilation and (2) propagate further reactions to augment the overall level of oxidative stress in the vasculature. The inhibitor of nitric oxide synthase, ADMA, is also believed to be increased with levels of high oxidative stress secondary to decreased function of an inhibiting enzyme of ADMA, dimethylarginine dimethylaminohydrolase (DDAH). Consequently, oxidative stress has been implicated in part of the pathogenesis of hypertension. The high levels of oxidative stress seen in both diabetes and CKD are likely involved in the high prevalence of hypertension in these populations (**Fig. 2**).[44–46]

Sympathetic Nervous System Activity

Similar to the RAAS, the increased activity of the sympathetic nervous system (SNS) can affect blood pressure through multiple mechanisms. In addition to increasing renal sodium reabsorption, increased sympathetic nervous activity may influence blood pressure through centrally mediated processes in animal models of renal ablation.[47] In humans, increased SNS activity can be seen in CKD and ESRD caused by various etiologies.[48,49] As autonomic neuropathy is a potential microvascular complication of diabetes, it has been proposed that increased nocturnal blood pressure in patients with type 1 or type 2 diabetes may be explained by this phenomenon.[50–52] Thus, both diabetes and CKD may independently contribute to increased SNS activity. Given the previously described role of the RAAS in hypertension in diabetic kidney disease, it is of interest that the ACE inhibitor enalapril has been shown to reduce SNS activity compared with the effects of amlodipine in patients with CKD.[49]

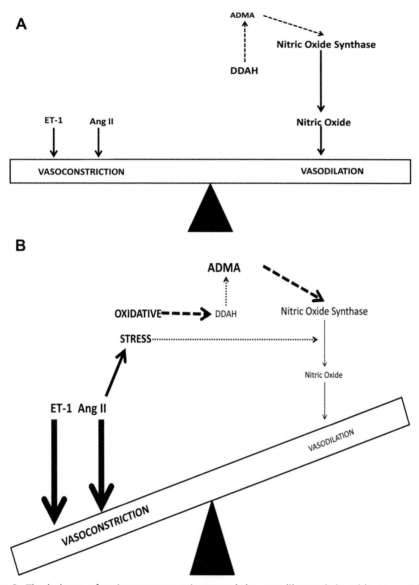

Fig. 2. The balance of various vasoconstrictors and the vasodilator nitric oxide on vascular smooth muscle tone is depicted in (*A*). Endothelial cell nitric oxide synthase should produce sufficient nitric oxide to balance out the effects of ET-1 and Ang II. Although ADMA can inhibit nitric oxide synthase activity, DDAH can sufficiently metabolize ADMA to restore balance. In the context of diabetic kidney disease (*B*), this entire balance can be disrupted owing in part to an increase level of oxidative stress. The RAAS system is inappropriately upregulated given the degree of extracellular volume overload, and Ang II can generate additional oxidative stress. This environment prevents adequate metabolism of ADMA by DDAH and promotes interaction of nitric oxide with free radicals. This ultimately results in inadequate nitric oxide production to counter the vasoconstriction caused by ET-1 and Ang II.

TREATMENT

Diabetic kidney disease develops and progresses over many years. In patients with type 2 diabetes, the presence of either albuminuria or microalbuminuria is the best predictor of rapid deterioration of GFR over the next several years.[53] The baseline GFR at the time of assessment is also an important predictor of ESRD.[54] Lowering blood pressure is one of the primary goals in the management of diabetic nephropathy. Blood pressure reduction slows decline in GFR in patients with type 1 diabetes and reduces the incidence of microalbuminuria in patients with type 2 diabetes.[55–58] The specific use of antihypertensive agents that offer additional renoprotective benefits, such as inhibitors of the RAAS, are considered to be the first-line antihypertensive agents in diabetic kidney disease.

RAAS Inhibition

The cardiovascular benefits of ACE inhibitors and angiotensin receptor blockers (ARBs) in diabetic patients have been extracted from clinical trials among more heterogeneous groups of high-risk patients.[59,60] One of these studies[59] further showed how ACE inhibitors may reduce the incidence of kidney disease. Appropriately, several large trials have been conducted to more specifically define the role RAAS inhibition in diabetic nephropathy.

Because of the potential for diabetic kidney disease to rapidly progress to ESRD once overt nephropathy is present, this stage of disease is expected to yield a large number of hard clinical end points that can be studied through clinical trials. The ACE inhibitor captopril, compared with placebo, reduced the risk for the primary end point doubling of serum creatinine among patients who are hypertensive with type 1 diabetes with more than 500 mg per day of proteinuria.[61] Therapy with captopril also resulted in a slower decline in creatinine clearance and a significant reduction in the composite end point of death and ESRD. Additionally, captopril therapy significantly attenuates the progression of albuminuria among patients with type 1 diabetes and overt nephropathy compared with standard antihypertensive therapy.[62] Inhibition of RAAS provides similar benefits for patients with type 2 diabetes and overt nephropathy. The Reduction in Endpoints in Non–insulin-dependent diabetes mellitus (RENAAL) trial and Irbesartan in Diabetic Nephropathy Trial (IDNT) both investigated the effects of ARBs versus placebo in this specific patient population.[63,64] The RENAAL trial showed the superior efficacy of losartan, and the IDNT showed superior efficacy of irbesartan.

Subsequent trials have investigated the effects of RAAS inhibition at earlier points in time including even before the onset of microalbuminuria. These studies have primarily used surrogate end points of disease progression, given the extended period that would be expected to generate hard clinical end points. Compared with placebo, irbesartan reduced the risk for incident diabetic nephropathy in a dose-dependent manner among patients who are hypertensive with type 2 diabetes and microalbuminuria.[65] Among patients with type 2 diabetes, trandolapril reduced the risk for developing microalbuminuria compared with both verapamil and placebo.[66] Most recently, olmesartan reduced the risk for microalbuminuria among a similar population compared with placebo.[67] These findings are in contrast to those from a study in patients who are normotensive with type 1 diabetes in which neither treatment with losartan nor enalapril resulted in any significant changes in mesangial fractional volume assessed on renal biopsy specimens compared with placebo.[68] Furthermore, in this study, more subjects receiving losartan developed microalbuminuria compared with those receiving placebo. Another analysis of studies including patients with type 1 and type 2 diabetes failed to show any benefit of candesartan in preventing microalbuminuria, although this was not the original primary end point that these studies were powered to investigate.[69]

In summary, several landmark trials have specifically investigated the effects of RAAS inhibition in diabetic kidney disease. The findings from these studies fortify the evidence from subgroup analyses in clinical trials among more heterogeneous groups of diabetic patients. The cumulative evidence thus suggests that these drugs are beneficial to most patients with diabetes along a wide spectrum of renal disease.

Combined RAAS inhibition

Despite the findings from these trials and the common practice to implement RAAS inhibition in diabetic patients with any evidence of kidney disease, diabetic nephropathy continues to result in ESRD in a substantial number of patients. Because of the improvements in outcomes that have been proven with either an ACE inhibitor or ARB, there remains speculation that further inhibition of RAAS through combination therapy may extend the benefits experienced with the use of a single agent. Such a strategy theoretically offers the ability to target (1) incomplete inhibition of the production or effects of Ang II, (2) increases in renin that can occur with ACE inhibitor use, or (3) "aldosterone escape" that can occur with ACE inhibitor or ARB use. The effects of these strategies on BP and albuminuria in patients with diabetic nephropathy are summarized in **Table 1**.

There is conflicting evidence of the effect of combining an ACE inhibitor and ARB in diabetic patients. In studies that individually studied type 1 and type 2 diabetic patients alone, combination therapy showed greater proteinuria reduction compared with single-agent RAAS blockade.[70,71] In a study that included both type 1 and type 2 diabetic patients, such an effect was not seen.[72] Given that this latter study followed patients for up to 1 year, the paucity of studies that are of sufficient duration to detect hard clinical end points must be emphasized in considering this option of therapy.

The Ongoing Telmisartan Alone and in Combination with Ramipril Global Endpoint Trial (ONTARGET) provides counterpoint evidence for combination RAAS inhibition in diabetes.[73] This trial used a composite of cardiovascular end points to compare ramipril, telmisartan, or combination therapy among a large population of subjects (with or without diabetes) considered at high risk for such events. Hyperkalemia and renal failure occurred more often in the combination therapy group despite both groups having similar results regarding the primary composite end point. A limitation in generalizing these findings to diabetic kidney disease is that (1) this study had relatively few subjects with diabetic kidney disease at baseline and (2) those with diabetic kidney disease were not found to be the subjects with the highest risk for renal outcomes in post hoc analysis.[74] Ultimately, the Combination Angiotensin Receptor Blocker and Angiotensin Converting Enzyme Inhibitor for Treatment of Diabetic Nephropathy VA NEPHRON-D Study: Nephropathy in Diabetes Study (VA NEPHRON) should answer the question of what role ACE inhibitor plus ARB therapy has in this population.[75] This active study includes patients with type 2 diabetes with overt nephropathy and is using a composite of renal outcomes and mortality as the primary end point in comparing lisinopril plus losartan therapy with losartan alone.

Addition of a mineralocorticoid receptor antagonist (MRA) to baseline therapy, including an ACE inhibitor or ARB, is another potential consideration that targets the specific renal and extrarenal effects of aldosterone. Two brief studies (one in patients with type 1 diabetes only) and a 1-year study in patients with type 1 and type 2 diabetes demonstrated that this strategy reduces proteinuria compared with single-agent therapy.[76–78] The long-term effects of combination therapy, including an MRA

Table 1
Clinical trials in diabetic nephropathy comparing dual RAAS inhibition to single-agent RAAS inhibition

Population/Baseline Medication Use	Intervention Groups	Renal End Point	BP Effect
ACE Inhibitor + ARB			
Type 2 DM Receiving maximum dose of ACE Inhibitor[71]	1. Candesartan 16 mg 2. Placebo	Albuminuria (mg/24 h) 1. Candesartan 706 2. Placebo 508 (28% reduction, P<.001)	24 h SBP (mm Hg): 1. Candesartan 135 vs 2. Placebo 138 (P = .21)
Type 1 DM[70]	1. Benazepril 20 mg 2. Valsartan 80 mg 3. Benazepril + Valsartan 4. Placebo	Albuminuria (mg/24 h) 1. Benazepril: 239 2. Valsartan: 225 3. Combination: 138 4. Placebo: 701 All P<.001 vs placebo; combination <.01 vs monotherapy	24 h SBP vs placebo: 1. Benazepril: –15 mm Hg 2. Valsartan: –15 mm Hg 3. Combination Therapy: –22 mm Hg
Type 1 or 2 DM[72]	1. Lisinopril 40 mg 2. Candesartan 16 mg + Lisinopril 20 mg	UACR change (mg/mmol) 1. Lisinopril: –0.16 2. Combination therapy: –0.42 (P = .38 vs lisinopril)	Mean difference between 24 h SBP: 3.9 mm Hg (P = .16)
Type 2 DM[75]	1. Losartan 2. Losartan + Lisinopril	ONGOING TRIAL (VA-NEPHRON)	

ACE Inhibitor or ARB + Mineralocorticoid Receptor Antagonist			
Type 1 DM ACE Inhibitor or ARB[76]	1. Spironolactone 25 mg 2. Placebo	Albuminuria (mg/d) 1. Spironolactone: 584 2. Placebo: 831 (P<.001)	24 h BP (mm Hg) 1. Spironolactone:136 2. Placebo: 144 (P = .08)
Type 1 and 2 DM Nephrotic Syndrome ACE Inhibitor or ARB[77]	1. Spironolactone 25 mg 2. Placebo	Albuminuria (g/d) 1. Spironolactone: 2.5 2. Placebo: 3.7 (P<.001)	24 h SBP (mm Hg) 1. Spironolactone:137 2. Placebo: 143 (P = .004)
Type 1 and 2 DM Lisinopril 80 mg[78]	1. Spironolactone 25 mg 2. Losartan 100 mg 3. Placebo	Albuminuria Reduction 1. Spironolactone: −51.6% (−38.2% vs placebo, P = .007) 2. Losartan −38.2% (−16.8% vs placebo, P = .2)	SBP (mm Hg) 1. Spironolactone: 132 2. Losartan: 134 3. Placebo: 136 (NS between groups)
ACE Inhibitor or ARB + Direct Renin Inhibitor			
Type 2 DM Losartan 100 mg[80]	1. Aliskiren 300 mg 2. Placebo	UACR 1. Aliskiren: −20% vs placebo (P<.001)	SBP (mm Hg) 1. Aliskiren: −2 vs placebo (P<.07)
Type 2 DM[81]	1. Aliskiren 300 mg 2. Irbesartan 300 mg 3. Aliskiren + Irbesartan 4. Placebo	Albuminuria reduction vs placebo: 1. Aliskiren: −48% (P<.001) 2. Irbesartan −58% (P<.001) 3. Combination therapy: −71% (P<.00 compared with placebo and this was significant compared with either monotherapy: P<.001 and P =.028)	24 h SBP reduction (mm Hg) 1. Aliskiren: −3 (NS) 2. Irbesartan −12 (P<.001) 3. Combination therapy: −10 (P = .001 vs placebo, NS vs Irbesartan)
Type 2 DM[82]	1. Aliskiren 300 mg 2. Placebo	TERMINATED secondary to adverse events in Aliskiren group	

Abbreviations: ACE, angiotensin converting enzyme; ARB, angiotensin receptor blocker; BP, blood pressure; DM, diabetes mellitus; RAAS, renin angiotensin aldosterone system; SBP, systolic blood pressure; UACR, urine albumin creatinine ratio.

on hard clinical end points remain unknown. Hyperkalemia is also a potential risk to be aware of with this strategy.

One final RAAS-inhibiting combination therapy that has been explored is the addition of a direct renin inhibitor (DRI) to either an ACE inhibitor or an ARB. Direct renin inhibitors are antihypertensive drugs that lower albuminuria in diabetic nephropathy compared with placebo, and they further reduce albuminuria when combined with an ARB[79–81]; however, there have been recent safety concerns for this strategy following the early termination of the Aliskiren Trial in Type 2 Diabetes Using Cardiovascular and Renal Disease Endpoints (ALTITUDE) trial. Inclusion criteria for this study were (1) type 2 diabetes, (2) current use of either an ACE inhibitor or ARB, and (3) either macroalbuminuria or reduced kidney function plus 1 additional cardiovascular risk factor.[82] The subjects were randomized to either aliskiren 300 mg daily or placebo. Early termination from the trial resulted from excessive incidents of hyperkalemia, renal failure, and hypotension in the aliskiren group.[83] There were not reported to be any beneficial effects of aliskiren on the primary outcome, and this combination strategy is currently contraindicated in patients with diabetes.

The role of dietary sodium in RAAS inhibition
Although the role of combination RAAS therapy continues to be explored, it is important to acknowledge RAAS inhibition can be optimized with judicious management of extracellular volume. Recently, a retrospective analysis of IDNT and RENAAL investigated the association of urinary sodium/creatinine ratio on renal and cardiovascular outcomes.[84] Among subjects who were randomized to an ARB, there were fewer renal events and fewer cardiovascular events among those with lower amounts of sodium excretion. This effect was not seen in the subjects who were not randomized to an ARB. Furthermore, the beneficial effects seen in subjects randomized to ARB compared with those not randomized to ARB were amplified in the subjects with the lowest sodium excretion. Dietary sodium ingestion has similarly been shown to influence outcomes in a retrospective analysis of nondiabetic patients with CKD. Among subjects from the Ramipril Efficacy in Nephropathy (REIN) studies receiving ramipril, the risk for ESRD increased with increases in urinary sodium excretion and appeared to be influenced by proteinuria.[85] Although these findings remain limited by the retrospective nature of the studies, dietary sodium restriction and judicious use of diuretics remain recommended strategies to enhance the effects of ACE inhibitors and ARB.

Vitamin D therapy
Vitamin D has also been identified as a potential mediator of RAAS activity in animal studies.[86,87] In animal models of diabetes, knockout of the vitamin D receptor resulted in more proteinuria and glomerulosclerosis.[88] Vitamin D is widely prescribed for patients with CKD and ESRD with secondary hyperparathyroidism. Recent evidence suggests that vitamin D may have additional therapeutic benefits among patients with diabetic nephropathy.[89] In a randomized clinical trial, paracalcitiol, 2 μg daily, significantly reduced both systolic blood pressure and urinary albumin excretion compared with placebo. Among subjects receiving either 1 or 2 μg daily, there remained a positive trend toward albuminuria reduction compared with placebo. The overall cardiovascular and renal effects of vitamin D remain to be further explored.

Mediators of Endothelial Cell Dysfunction

Inhibition of the RAAS does not completely eliminate proteinuria in all patients with diabetic kidney disease. Consequently, therapies that target other potential mechanisms for hypertension and renal disease progression offer alternative strategies to improve outcomes in these patients. Endothelial cell dysfunction plays a role in hypertension in this population, but likely also has an independent effect on kidney disease.[90] Several clinical trials have investigated the effects of various endothelin receptor antagonists on diabetic kidney disease.[41,91–93] Some of these medications differ in their specificity for inhibiting either the ET-A receptor or the ET-B receptor. On vascular smooth muscle cells, the ET-A receptor is responsible for vasoconstriction, whereas the ET-B receptor is more responsible for vasodilation and removal of circulating ET-1. Although these studies consistently show reduction in proteinuria regardless of the study medication, the different receptor specificities may be responsible for differences in adverse effects that have been noted among them.

Bosentan is an ET-1 receptor antagonist that binds to both ET-A and ET-B receptors. One small randomized trial in subjects with type 2 diabetes and microalbuminuria showed that 4 weeks of bosentan improved peripheral endothelial cell function compared with placebo. This short study failed to show improvement in macrovascular endothelial cell function assessed by brachial artery flow-mediated vasodilation or in microalbuminuria (not a specified end point) so that the clinical relevance of these results remains unclear.[41]

Larger studies with other endothelin receptor antagonists have overall shown positive results regarding proteinuria reduction in (**Table 2**), but have been limited by concurrent adverse events. Compared with placebo, avosentan achieved significant reductions in the primary end point of albuminuria reduction but resulted in peripheral edema in a dose-dependent manner.[91] A larger placebo-controlled trial with this drug in diabetic nephropathy was terminated early because of an increased incidence of congestive heart failure with avosentan, despite the proteinuria reduction.[92] A trial investigating the effects of a more ET-A–specific drug, atrasentan, showed a lower incidence of peripheral edema compared with those reported with avosentan while preserving the proteinuria-reducing effects of this drug class.[93] As this trial was of brief duration, further investigation is warranted to establish the efficacy and safety of this drug.

Other Novel Applications of Antihypertensives in Diabetic Kidney Disease

Lowering blood pressure with antihypertensive drugs has clearly been demonstrated to improve outcomes in diabetic kidney disease. As we have learned about the mechanisms responsible for not only hypertension, but also kidney disease progression itself, certain antihypertensive drugs, such as RAAS inhibitors, have stood out as offering renoprotection independent of their blood pressure–lowering effect. As the clinical research arena follows the basic science advancements in understanding diabetic kidney disease, there are likely to be more novel approaches to treating this disease.

Losartan established the role of ARBs in diabetic kidney disease in the RENAAL trial. Subsequent analysis of that study now demonstrates a significant reduction in serum uric acid in patients randomized to losartan compared with placebo and that the reduction in uric acid was independently associated with a reduction in the risk for renal end points.[94] At present, the adverse effects of endothelin receptor antagonists have hindered their acceptance as a safe option to treat diabetic nephropathy. However, therapeutic interventions that improve endothelial cell dysfunction are still sought after. One drug, nicorandil, is a nitrogen donor and is also believed to inhibit the production of free radicals within endothelial cells. When administered to rats with streptozocin-induced diabetes, there is a reduction in proteinuria that coincides with preservation of podocyte structure, although there was no evidence of systemic benefits on endothelial cell dysfunction.[95] There are currently available "third-generation"

Table 2
Clinical trials studying the effects of endothelin receptor antagonists in diabetic nephropathy

Population/Baseline Medication	Intervention Group	Renal End Point	BP End Point
Type 1 and 2 DM ACE inhibitor or ARB therapy[91]	1. Avosentan 5 mg 2. Avosentan 10 mg 3. Avosentan 25 mg 4. Avosentan 50 mg 5. Placebo	Mean relative percent change in UAER from baseline: 1. Avosentan 5 mg: −20.9% 2. Avosentan 10 mg: −16.3% 3. Avosentan 25 mg: −25% 4. Avosentan 50 mg: −29.9% 5. Placebo: +35.5 ($P<.01$ for all doses vs placebo)	SBP (mm Hg) (baseline, week 12 follow up): 1. Avosentan 5 mg: 146, 142 2. Avosentan 10 mg: 147, 144 3. Avosentan 25 mg: 140, 141 4. Avosentan 50 mg: 146, 144 5. Placebo: 144, 147 ($P<.01$ for all doses vs placebo)
Type 2 DM ACE Inhibitor or ARB[92]	1. Avosentan 25 mg 2. Avosentan 50 mg 3. Placebo	No effect seen on primary outcome of doubling serum creatinine, ESRD or death. terminated early albuminuria reduced with avosentan Median UACR −40%–50% in Avosentan Groups vs −8%–10% in placebo ($P<.0001$) Change in sitting SBP at 3 months and 6 months: Avosentan 25 mg: −4.1 and −4.3 mm Hg ($P = .09, .09$) Avosentan 50 mg: −4.4 and −6.1 mm Hg ($P = .02$ and $.02$); Placebo: 0.5, −0.5	
Type 2 DM ACE Inhibitor or ARB[93]	1. Atresentan 0.25 mg 2. Atresentan 0.75 mg 3. Atresentan 1.75 mg 4. Placebo	UACR Reduction 1. Atresentan 0.25 mg: 21% ($P = .03$ vs placebo) 2. Atresentan 0.75 mg: 42% ($P = .02$ vs placebo) 3. Atresentan 1.75 mg: 35% ($P = .07$ vs placebo) 4. Placebo: −11%	SBP Reduction (mm Hg) 1. Atresentan 0.25 mg: −0.3 ($P = .8$ vs placebo) 2. Atresentan 0.75 mg: −8.8 ($P = .05$ vs placebo) 3. Atresentan 1.75 mg: −7.6 ($P = .09$ vs placebo) 4. Placebo+ 0.7

Abbreviations: ACE, angiotensin converting enzyme; ARB, angiotensin receptor blocker; BP, blood pressure; DM, diabetes mellitus; ESRD, end stage renal disease; SBP, systolic blood pressure; UACR, urine albumin creatinine ratio; UAER, urinary albumin excretion ratio.

beta adrenergic receptor antagonists that possess properties that are believed to improve endothelial cell dysfunction.[96–98]

Blood Pressure Targets

Despite the Kidney Disease Outcomes Quality Initiative recommendations to target a blood pressure of 130/80[4], there is no randomized clinical trial that establishes this target for patients with diabetic kidney disease. In subgroup analysis of the Hypertension Optimal Treatment (HOT) trial, the 1500 subjects with diabetes had significant reductions in a composite of major cardiovascular events with randomization to lower diastolic blood pressure levels (80 vs 85 vs 90 mm Hg)[99]; however, the Action to Control Cardiovascular Risk in Diabetes (ACCORD) study did not show any benefit of lowering systolic blood pressure to lower than 120 mm Hg compared with lower than 140 mm Hg among patients with type 2 diabetes without significant proteinuria or renal impairment.[100] Among patients with diabetic nephropathy in retrospective analysis of IDNT, there was increased risk for all-cause and cardiovascular mortality with systolic blood pressure lower than 120 mm Hg and diastolic blood pressure lower than 85 mm Hg, respectively.[101] This is in contrast to analyses showing that lower blood pressure invariably improves renal outcomes in patients with diabetes, including those with diabetic nephropathy at baseline.[102,103] The potential cardiovascular risk of achieving too low of a blood pressure must be weighed against the apparent renal benefits of such a strategy, and thus some uncertainty remains as to what the absolute ideal blood pressure target should be for patients with diabetic kidney disease.

RECOMMENDATIONS

Regardless of the stage of kidney disease, an ACE inhibitor or ARB should be used as a first-line antihypertensive drug in all diabetic patients. This strategy offers cardioprotective effects in those with preserved kidney function and renoprotective effects in those with varying degrees of renal impairment. Blood pressure should be lowered to a target of 130/80, but further prospective research is required to further delineate more specific goals beyond that. Patients should be instructed to limit their dietary sodium ingestion and diuretics should be used in patients who remain hypertensive despite the use of a RAAS inhibitor or for patients susceptible to hyperkalemia. It is likely that many patients will require even further antihypertensive therapy, which should include beta blockers, calcium channel blockers, vasodilators, and centrally acting agents as guided by the underlying comorbidities of an individual patient. Regarding combination RAAS therapy, the use of an ACE inhibitor plus ARB requires completion of the VA NEPHRON study. Direct renin inhibitors should not be used with an ACE inhibitor or ARB in patients with diabetic nephropathy, but adding a mineralocorticoid receptor blocker remains a potentially viable strategy that requires further investigation.

SUMMARY

Hypertension commonly coexists with diabetes, and its prevalence is even higher in the presence of diabetic kidney disease. The pathogenesis of hypertension in this population stems from increased extracellular volume and increased vasoconstriction that results from mechanisms that may be attributed to both diabetes and the eventual impairment of renal function. Antihypertensive therapy aimed at reducing blood pressure remains a primary goal in preventing the incidence of diabetic kidney and slowing its progression. Initial therapy should consist of an ACE inhibitor or ARB titrated to the maximally tolerated dose. Using combination RAAS therapy further reduces proteinuria, but the benefits of this strategy compared with the potential risks of hyperkalemia and acute deterioration of renal function are still unknown. Endothelin receptor antagonists also lower proteinuria, but these can be associated with volume overload and edema with no clear long-term benefit on renal function yet identified. Further large clinical trials are needed to better understand how progression to ESRD can be slowed or halted in patients with diabetic kidney disease.

REFERENCES

1. Parving H, Gall M, Skott P, et al. Prevalence and causes of albuminuria in non insulin-dependent diabetic patients. Kidney Int 1992;4:758–62.
2. Chobanian A, Bakris G, Black H, et al. The Seventh Report of the Joint National Committee on Prevention, detection, evaluation, and treatment of high blood pressure. J Am Med Assoc 2003;289:2560–72.
3. American Diabetes Association. Treatment of hypertension in adults with diabetes. Diabetes Care 2003;26:S80–2.
4. National Kidney Foundation. KDOQI Clinical practice guidelines and clinical practice recommendations for diabetes and chronic kidney disease. Am J Kidney Dis 2007;49(Suppl 2):S1–180.
5. Norgaard K, Feldt-Rasmussen B, Johnsen K, et al. Prevalence of hypertension in type 1 (insulin dependent) diabetes mellitus. Diabetologia 1990;33:407–10.
6. Parving H, Hommel E, Mathiesen E, et al. Prevalence of microalbuminuria, arterial hypertension, retinopathy, and neuropathy in patients with insulin dependent diabetes. Br Med J (Clin Res Ed) 1988;296:156–60.
7. Lurbe E, Redon J, Kesani A. Increase in nocturnal blood pressure and progression to microalbuminuria in type 1 diabetes. N Engl J Med 2002;347:797–805.
8. Haffner S, Mykkanen L, Festa A, et al. Insulin-resistant prediabetic subjects have more atherogenic risk factors than insulin-sensitive prediabetic subjects: implications for preventing coronary heart disease during the prediabetic state. Circulation 2000;101:975–80.
9. Keller C, Bergis K, Filser D, et al. Renal findings in patients with short term type 2 diabetes. J Am Soc Nephrol 1996;7:2627–35.
10. Ismail N, Becker B, Strzelczyk P, et al. Renal disease and hypertension in non-insulin dependent diabetes mellitus. Kidney Int 1999;55:1–28.
11. Hypertension in Diabetes Study Investigators. Hypertension in Diabetes Study (HDS): II, increased risk of cardiovascular complications in hypertensive type 2 diabetic patients. J Hypertens 1993;11:319–25.
12. Mogensen C. Glomerular filtration rate and renal plasma flow in short-term and long-term juvenile diabetes mellitus. Scand J Clin Lab Invest 1971;28:91–100.
13. Vallon V, Richter K, Blantz R, et al. Glomerular hyperfiltration in experimental diabetes mellitus: potential role of tubular reabsorption. J Am Soc Nephrol 1999;10:2569–76.
14. Brands M, Bell T, Gibson B. Nitric oxide may prevent hypertension early in diabetes by counteracting renal actions of superoxide. Hypertension 2004;43:57–63.
15. Veelken R, Hilgers K, Hartner A, et al. Nitric oxide synthase isoforms and glomerular hyperfiltration in early diabetic nephropathy. J Am Soc Nephrol 2000;11:71–9.
16. Tuck M, Corry D, Trujillo A. Salt-sensitive blood pressure and exaggerated vascular reactivity in the hypertension of diabetes mellitus. Am J Hypertens 1990;88:210–6.

17. Anderson F, Jung F, Ingelfinger J. Renal rennin-angiotensin system in diabetes: functional, immunohistochemical, and molecular biologic correlations. Am J Physiol 1993;265(4 Pt 2):F477–86.
18. Konoshita T, Wakahara S, Mizuno EA. Tissue gene expression of rennin-angiotensin system in human type 2 diabetic nephropathy. Diabetes Care 2006;29:848–52.
19. Mizuiri S, Yoshikawa H, Tanegashima M, et al. Renal ACE immunohistochemical localization in NIDDM patients with nephropathy. Am J Kidney Dis 1998;31:301–7.
20. Mezzano S, Droguett A, Burgos M, et al. Renin-angiotensin system activation and interstitial inflammation in human diabetic nephropathy. Kidney Int Suppl 2003;86:S64–70.
21. Price D, Porter L, Gordon M. The paradox of the low renin state in diabetic nephropathy. J Am Soc Nephrol 1999;10:2382.
22. Price D, De'Oliveira J, Fisher N, et al. The state and responsiveness of the renin-angiotensin-aldosterone system in patients with type 2 diabetes mellitus. Am J Hypertens 1999;12:348.
23. Giani J, Burghi V, Veiras L, et al. Angiotensin-(1-7) attenuates diabetic nephropathy in Zucker diabetic fatty rats. Am J Physiol Renal Physiol 2012;302: F1606–15.
24. Ye M, Wysocki J, William J, et al. Glomerular localization and expression of angiotensin-converting enzyme 2 and angiotensin-converting enzyme: implications for albuminuria in diabetes. J Am Soc Nephrol 2006;17:3067–75.
25. Lely A, Hamming I, van Goor H, et al. Renal ACE2 expression in human kidney disease. J Pathol 2004;204:587–93.
26. Mizuiri S, Hemmi H, Arita M, et al. Expressio of ACE and ACE2 in individuals with diabetic kidney disease and healthy controls. Am J Kidney Dis 2008;51:613–23.
27. Soro-Paavonen A, Gordin D, Forsblom C, et al. Circulating ACE2 activity is increased in patients with type 1 diabetes and vascular complications. J Hypertens 2012;30:375–83.
28. Dogra G, Irish A, Chan D, et al. Insulin resistance, inflammation, and blood pressure determine vascular function in CKD. Am J Kidney Dis 2006;48:926–34.
29. Makino H, Doi K, Hiuge A, et al. Impaired flow-mediated vasodilation and insulin resistance in type 2 diabetic patients with albuminuria. Diabetes Res Clin Pract 2008;79:177–82.
30. Chan W, Chan N, Lai C, et al. Vascular defect beyond the endothelium in type II diabetic patients with overt nephropathy and moderate renal insufficiency. Kidney Int 2006;70:711–6.
31. Giugliano D, Marfella R, Coppola L, et al. Vascular effects of acute hyperglycemia in humans are reversed by L-arginine: evidence for reduced availability of nitric oxide during hyperglycemia. Circulation 1997;95:1783–90.
32. Fitzgerald S, Brands M. Nitric oxide may be required to prevent hypertension at the onset of diabetes. Am J Phys 2000;279:E762–8.
33. Achan V, Broadhead M, Malaki M, et al. Asymetric dimethylarginine causes hypertension and cardiac dysfunction in humans and is actively metabolized by dimethyl dimethylaminohydrolase. Arterioscler Thromb Vasc Biol 2003;23: 1455–9.
34. Kielstein J, Boger R, Bode-Boger S. Asymetric dimethylarginine concentrations differ in patients with end stage renal disease: relationship to treatment method and atherosclerotic disease. J Am Soc Nephrol 1999;10:594–600.
35. Zoccali C, Bode-Boger S, Mallamaci F, et al. Plasma concentrations of asymmetrical dimethylarginine and mortality in patients with end-stage renal disease: a prospective study. Lancet 2001;358:2113–7.

36. Tarnow L, Hovind P, Teerlink T, et al. Elevated plasma asymetric dimethylarginine as a marker of cardiovascular morbidity in early diabetic nephropathy in type 1 diabetes. Diabetes Care 2004;27:765–9.

37. Abbasi F, Asagmi T, Cooke J, et al. Plasma concentrations of asymetric dimethylarginine are increased in patients with type 2 diabetes mellitus. Am J Cardiol 2001;88:1201–3.

38. Kakizawa H, Itoh M, Itoh Y, et al. The relationship between glycemic control and plasma vascular endothelial growth factor and endothelin-1 concentration in diabetic patients. Metabolism 2004;53:550–6.

39. Minchenko A, Stevens M, White L, et al. Diabetes-induced overexpression of endothelin-1 and endothelin receptors in the rat renal cortex is mediated via poly (ADP-ribose) polymerase activation. FASEB 2003;17:1514–6.

40. Muniyappa R, Quon M. Insulin action and insulin resistance in vascular endothelium. Curr Opin Clin Nutr Metab Care 2007;10:523.

41. Rafnsson A, Bohm F, Settergren M, et al. The endothelin receptor antagonist bosentan improves peripheral endothelial cell function in patients with type 2 diabetes mellitus and microalbuminuria: a randomised trial. Diabetologia 2012;55:600–7.

42. Rajagopalan S, Kurz S, Munzel T, et al. Angiotensin II-mediated hypertension in the rate increases vascular superoxide production via membrane NADH/NADPH oxidase activation. J Clin Invest 1996;97:1916–23.

43. Griendling K, Ollernenshaw J, Minieri C, et al. Angiotensin II stimulates NADH and NADPH activity in cultured vascular smooth muscle cells. Circ Res 1994;74:1141–8.

44. Brownlee M. Biochemistry and molecular cell biology of diabetic complications. Nature 2001;414:813–20.

45. Spittle M, Hoenich N, Handelman G, et al. Oxidative stress and inflammation in hemodialysis patients. Am J Kidney Dis 2001;38:1408–13.

46. Ceballos-Picot I, Wtiko-Sarsat V, Merad-Boudia M, et al. Glutathione antioxidant system as a marker of oxidative stress in chronic renal failure. Free Radic Biol Med 1996;21:845–53.

47. Campese V, Kogosove E. Renal afferent denervation prevents hypertension in rats with chronic renal failure. Hypertension 1995;25:878–82.

48. Converse R, Jacobsen T, Toto R, et al. Sympathetic overactivity in patients with chronic renal failure. N Engl J Med 1992;327:1912–8.

49. Ligtenberg G, Blankestijn P, Oey P, et al. Reduction of sympathetic hyperactivity by enalapril in patients with chronic renal failure. N Engl J Med 1999;340:1321–8.

50. Spallone V, Gambardella S, Maiello M, et al. Relationship between autonomic neuropathy, 24-h blood pressure profile, and nephropathy in normotensive IDDM patients. Diabetes Care 1994;17:578–84.

51. Liniger C, Favre L, Assal J. Twenty-four hour blood pressure and heart rate profiles of diabetic patients with abnormal cardiovascular reflexes. Diabet Med 1991;8:420–7.

52. Nielsen F, Hansen H, Jacobsen P. Increased sympathetic activity during sleep and nocturnal hypertension in Type 2 diabetic patients with diabetic nephropathy. Diabet Med 1999;16:555–62.

53. Zoppini G, Targher G, Choncol M, et al. Predictors of estimated GFR decline in patients with type 2 diabetes and preserved kidney function. Clin J Am Soc Nephrol 2012;7:401–8.

54. Berhane A, Weil E, Knowler W, et al. Albuminuria and estimated glomerular filtration rate as predictors of diabetic end-stage renal disease and death. Clin J Am Soc Nephrol 2011;6:2444–51.

55. Mogensen C. Long-term antihypertensive treatment inhibiting progression of diabetic nephropathy. Br Med J 1982;285:685–8.
56. Parving H, Smidt U, Andersen A, et al. Early aggressive anithypertensive treatment reduces rate of decline of kidney function in diabetic nephropathy. Lancet 1983;321:1175–9.
57. Parving H, Andersen A, Smidt U, et al. Effect of antihypertensive treatment on kidney function in diabetic nephropathy. Br Med J 1987;294:1443–7.
58. UK Prospective Diabetes Study Group. Tight blood pressure control and risk of macrovascular and microvascular complications in type 2 diabetes: UKPDS 38. BMJ 1998;317:703–13.
59. Heart Outcomes Prevention Evaluation (HOPE) Study Investigators. Effects of ramipril on cardiovascular and microvascular outcomes in people with diabetes mellitus: results of the HOPE study and MICRO-HOPE substudy. Lancet 2000; 355:253–9.
60. Lindholm L, Ibsen H, Dahlof B, et al. Cardiovascular morbidity and mortality in patients with diabetes in the losartan intervention for endpoint reduction in hypertension study (LIFE): a randomised trial against atenolol. Lancet 2002; 359:1004–10.
61. Lewis EJ, Hunsicker LG, Bain RP, et al. The effect of angiotensin-converting-enzyme inhibition on diabetic nephropathy. The Collaborative Study Group. N Engl J Med 1993;329(20):1456–62.
62. Parving HH, Hommel E, Jensen BR, et al. Long-term beneficial effect of ACE inhibition on diabetic nephropathy in normotensive type 1 diabetic patients. Kidney Int 2001;60(1):228–34.
63. Lewis EJ, Hunsicker LG, Clarke WR, et al. Renoprotective effect of the angiotensin-receptor antagonist irbesartan in patients with nephropathy due to type 2 diabetes. N Engl J Med 2001;345(12):851–60.
64. Brenner BM, Cooper ME, de Zeeuw D, et al. Effects of losartan on renal and cardiovascular outcomes in patients with type 2 diabetes and nephropathy. N Engl J Med 2001;345(12):861–9.
65. Parving HH, Lehnert H, Brochner-Mortensen J, et al. The effect of irbesartan on the development of diabetic nephropathy in patients with type 2 diabetes. N Engl J Med 2001;345(12):870–8.
66. Ruggenenti P, Fassi A, Ilieva A, et al. Preventing microalbuminuria in type 2 diabetes. N Engl J Med 2004;351:1941–51.
67. Haller H, Ito S, Izzo J, et al. Olmesartan for the delay or prevention of microalbuminuria in type 2 diabetes. N Engl J Med 2011;364:907–17.
68. Mauer M, Zinman B, Gardiner R, et al. Renal and retinal effects of enalapril and losartan in type 1 diabetes. N Engl J Med 2009;361:40–51.
69. Bilous R, Chaturvedi N, Sjolie A, et al. Effect of candesartan on microalbuminuria and albumin excretion rate in diabetes. Ann Intern Med 2009;151: 11–20.
70. Jacobsen P, Andersen S, Jensen B, et al. Additive effect of ACE inhibition and angiotensin II receptor blockade in type 1 diabetic patients with diabetic nephropathy. J Am Soc Nephrol 2003;14:992–9.
71. Rossing K, Jacobsen P, Pietraszek L, et al. Renoprotective effects of adding angiotensin II receptor blocker to maximal recommended doses of ACE inhibitor in diabetic nephropathy. Diabetes Care 2003;26:2268–74.
72. Andersen N, Poulsen P, Knudson S, et al. Long-term dual blockade with candesartan and lisinopril in hypertensive patients with diabetes. Diabetes Care 2005; 28:273–7.

73. ONTARGET Investigators. Telmisartan, ramipril, or both in patients at high risk for vascular events. N Engl J Med 2008;358:1547–59.
74. Mann J, Schmieder R, McQueen EA. Renal outcomes with telmisartan, ramipril, or both in people at high vascular risk (the ONTARGET study): a multicentre, randomized, double-blind, controlled trial. Lancet 2008;372:547–53.
75. Department of Veteran Affairs; Combination Angiotensin Receptor Blocker and Angiotensin Converting Enzyme Inhibitor for Treatment of Diabetic Nephropathy; VA NEPHRON-D Study: Nephropathy iN Diabetes Study. In: Clinical Trials.gov [Internet]. Bethesda (MD): National Library of Medicine (US); 2000-[cited 2012 March 26]. Available at: http://www.clinicaltrials.gov/ct2/show/NCT00555217. Accessed on 26th March 2012.
76. Schjoedt K, Rossing K, Juhl T, et al. Beneficial impact of spironolactone in diabetic nephropathy. Kidney Int 2005;68:2829–36.
77. Schjoedt KJ, Rossing K, Juhl TR, et al. Beneficial impact of spironolactone on nephrotic range albuminuria in diabetic nephropathy. Kidney Int 2006;70(3): 536–42.
78. Mehdi U, Adams-Huet B, Raskin P, et al. Addition of angiotensin receptor blockade or a mineralocorticoid antagonism to maximal angiotensin-converting enzyme inhibition in diabetic nephropathy. J Am Soc Nephrol 2009;20:2641–50.
79. Persson F, Rossing P, Schjoedt K, et al. Time course of the antiproteinuric and anithypertensive effects of the direct rennin inhibition in type 2 diabetes. Kidney Int 2008;73:1419–25.
80. Parving H, Persson F, Lewis J, et al. Aliskiren combined with losartan in type 2 diabetes and nephropathy. N Engl J Med 2008;358:2433–46.
81. Persson F, Rossing P, Reinhard H. Renal effects of aliskiren compared with and in combination with irbesartan in patients with type 2 diabetes, hypertension, and albuminuria. Diabetes Care 2009;32:1873–9.
82. Parving H, Brenner B, McMurray J, et al. Aliskiren trial in type 2 diabetes using cardio-renal endpoints (ALTITUDE): rationale and study design. Nephrol Dial Transplant 2009;24:1663–71.
83. Aliskiren-containing medications: drug safety communication—new warning and contraindication. 2012. Available at: http://www.fda.gov/Safety/MedWatch/SafetyInformation/SafetyAlertsforHumanMedicalProducts/ucm301120.htm? source=govdelivery. Accessed May 4, 2012.
84. Heerspink H, Holtkamp F, Parving H, et al. Moderation of dietary sodium potentiates the renal and cardiovascular protective effects of angiotensin receptor blockers. Kidney Int 2012;82:330–7.
85. Vegter S, Perna A, Postma M, et al. Sodium intake, ACE inhibition, and progression to ESRD. J Am Soc Nephrol 2012;23:165–73.
86. Li Y, Kong J, Wei M, et al. 1,25-Dihydroxyvitamin D3 is a negative endocrine regulator of the renin-angiotensin system. J Clin Invest 2002;110:229–38.
87. Zhou C, Lu F, Cao K, et al. Calcium-independent and $1,25(OH)_2D_3$-dependent regulation of the renin-angiotensin system in 1 alpha-hydroxylase knockout mice. Kidney Int 2008;74:170–9.
88. Zhang Z, Sun L, Wang Y, et al. Renoprotective role of the vitamin D receptor in diabetic nephropathy. Kidney Int 2008;73:163–71.
89. de Zeeuw D, Agarwal R, Amdahl M, et al. Selective vitamin D receptor activation with paricalcitol for reduction of albuminuria in patients with type 2 diabetes (VITAL study): a randomised controlled trial. Lancet 2010;376:1543–51.
90. Jawa A, Nachimuthu M, Pendergrass M, et al. Impaired vascular reactivity in African American patients wtih type 2 diabetes mellitus and microalbuminuria

or proteinuria despite angiotensin converting enzyme inhibitor therapy. J Clin Endocrinol Metab 2006;91:31–5.

91. Wenzel R, Littke T, Kuranoff S, et al. Avosentan reduces albumin excretion in diabetics with macroalbuminuria. J Am Soc Nephrol 2009;20:655–64.

92. Mann J, Green D, Jamerson K, et al. Avosentan for overt diabetic nephropathy. J Am Soc Nephrol 2010;21:527–35.

93. Kohan D, Pritchett Y, Molitch M, et al. Addition of atrasentan to renin-angiotensin system blockade reduces albuminuria in diabetic nephropathy. J Am Soc Nephrol 2011;22:763–72.

94. Miao Y, Ottenbros S, Laverman G, et al. Effect of a reduction in uric acid on renal outcomes during losartan treatment. Hypertension 2011;58:2–7.

95. Tanabe K, Lanaspa M, Kitagawa W, et al. Nicorandil as a novel therapy for advanced diabetic nephropathy in the e-NOS deficient mouse. Am J Physiol Renal Physiol 2012;302:F1151–60.

96. Saijonmaa O, Metsarinne K, Fyhrquist F. Carvedilol and its metabolites suprress endothelin-1 production in endothelial cell culture. Blood Press 1997;6:24–8.

97. Inrig J, Van Buren P, Kim C, et al. Probing the mechanisms of intradialytic hypertension: a pilot study targeting endothelial cell dysfunction. Clin J Am Soc Nephrol 2012;7:1300–9.

98. Zepeda R, Castillo R, Rodrigo R, et al. Effect of Carvedilol and Nebivolol on Oxidative Stress-related Parameters and Endothelial Function in Patients with Essential Hypertension. Basic Clin Pharmacol Toxicol 2012;111:309–16.

99. Hansson L, Zanchetti A, Carruthers S, et al. Effects of intensive blood-pressure lowering and low-dose aspirin in patients with hypertension: principal results of the Hypertension Optimal Treatment (HOT) randomised trial. Lancet 1998;351:1755–62.

100. The ACCORD Study Group. Effects of intensive blood pressure control in type 2 diabetes mellitus. N Engl J Med 2010;362:1575–85.

101. Berl T, Hunsicker LG, Lewis J, et al. Impact of achieved blood pressure on cardiovascular outcomes in the irbesartan diabetic nephropathy trial. J Am Soc Nephrol 2005;16:2170–9.

102. Bakris GL, Weir MR, Shanifar S, et al. Effects of blood pressure level on progression of diabetic nephropathy: results from the RENAAL study. Arch Intern Med 2003;163(13):1555–65.

103. de Galan B, Perkovic V, Ninomiya T, et al. Lowering blood pressure reduces renal events in type 2 diabetes. J Am Soc Nephrol 2009;20:883–92.

Nonproteinuric Diabetic Nephropathy
When Diabetics Don't Read the Textbook

Jamie P. Dwyer, MD*, Julia B. Lewis, MD

KEYWORDS

- Diabetic nephropathy • Nonproteinuric • Normoalbuminuria

KEY POINTS

- The traditional clinical paradigm of diabetic nephropathy (DN) may not apply to all patients with diabetes and decreased renal function.
- A feature of the natural history of DN that is gaining renewed investigation is the progression from normoalbuminuria to proteinuria and then to renal failure.
- A subset of patients with presumed DN have minimal proteinuria.
- Mechanisms proposed to explain this finding include use of agents which block the renin-angiotensin system, bouts of acute kidney injury, genetic predisposition, and other non-diabetic kidney diseases.

INTRODUCTION

The term "diabetic nephropathy" (DN) refers to the structural and functional changes seen in the kidneys of patients because of either type 1 or type 2 diabetes mellitus (DM1 or DM2). The classically observed natural history of DN (summarized elsewhere in this article) follows a sequence of diabetes onset, hyperfiltration, microalbuminuria (MA), overt proteinuria, renal dysfunction, and renal or patient death,[1] which was first characterized for DM1[2] but has also been described in observational studies in patients with DM2.[3] However, the time of onset of DM2 is rarely known accurately, and cardiovascular events in a patient with DM2 can censor the natural history of DN.

Disclosures: Dr Dwyer reports grants and travel support from Keryx Biopharmaceuticals, Inc, Chemocentryx, Inc, Eli Lilly, Inc, and Nephrogenex, Inc; Dr Lewis reports grants and travel support from Keryx Biopharmaceuticals, Inc, Eli Lilly, Inc, and Nephrogenex, Inc.
Division of Nephrology and Hypertension, and Nephrology Clinical Trials Center, Vanderbilt University Medical Center, MCN S-3223, Nashville, TN 37232, USA
* Corresponding author. Division of Nephrology and Hypertension, Vanderbilt University Medical Center, MCN S-3223, Nashville, TN 37232.
E-mail address: Jamie.dwyer@vanderbilt.edu

Med Clin N Am 97 (2013) 53–58
http://dx.doi.org/10.1016/j.mcna.2012.10.006
0025-7125/13/$ – see front matter © 2013 Elsevier Inc. All rights reserved.

medical.theclinics.com

A feature of the natural history of DN that is gaining renewed investigation is the progression from normoalbuminuria to proteinuria and then to renal failure. In the classical paradigm, overt proteinuria precedes the decline in renal function. Recently, there have been several reports describing patients with primarily DM2 and presumed DN who have declining renal function with normoalbuminuria or MA and not the previously well-described proteinuria. Early observational studies that described the natural history of DN with proteinuria preceding declining renal function were largely conducted before availability of current therapeutic interventions to slow the progression of DN. Of course, the concept of natural history describes the course of a disease that has not been interrupted by treatment. In the case of DN, there are now interventions[4–8] that have been proved to delay the progression from one stage to the next. These treatments did not exist when the traditional paradigm was conceived. These therapeutic interventions may have changed the natural history, resulting in renal failure without preceding proteinuria. Alternatively, there are other possible explanations for the described subset of patients with DM2, DN, and declining renal function in the absence of proteinuria, including the following: patients with early DN (and hence only normoalbuminuria or MA) suffer loss of renal function because of unresolved episodes of acute kidney injury (AKI); because few patients without proteinuria and only presumed DN have been biopsied, they may in fact be misdiagnosed and another disease leads to progressive decline in renal function.

AN ANIMAL MODEL OF NONPROTEINURIC DN

The Cohen diabetic rat is a model of DM2; it consists of 2 strains, the diabetes-sensitive and the diabetes-resistant strain. When fed a diabetogenic diet, the sensitive strain develops a syndrome that looks clinically like DM2, but the resistant strain does not.[9] Sensitive rats fed a diabetogenic diet lost weight, failed to thrive, and exhibited a metabolic phenotype consistent with DM2 (increased blood glucose, insulin, and hemoglobin A1c levels).[10] The rats developed low glomerular filtration rate (GFR), but *without* proteinuria or hypertension despite classical DN histologic changes, including mesangial matrix expansion, thickened basement membranes, and increased deposition of type IV collagen. They also developed retinal changes consistent with nonproliferative diabetic retinopathy. The investigators postulated that there were genetic factors that determined the lack of proteinuria in these diabetic sensitive rats.

Although no animal model of DN satisfactorily mimics human disease, this model is similar to the subset of humans with presumed DN and the absence of proteinuria. However, unlike the Cohen rats, humans are hypertensive. This animal model nevertheless suggests it is possible to have DN without proteinuria.

HUMAN STUDIES

The existence of rare patients with diabetes and declining renal function in the absence of overt proteinuria has been recognized for many years. An early study[11] of glomerular structure in women with DM1 identified subjects with low GFR and normal urinary albumin excretion (UAE). The investigators compared them to subjects with normal GFR and MA, and low GFR and MA, and showed that renal morphometric measures were similar, and importantly, still showed the changes consistent with a diagnosis of DN. The investigators concluded that the concept of "incipient nephropathy" should be expanded beyond MA alone to include those with low GFR in the absence of MA, because the pathologic correlate of DN was present even when MA was not. In a small prospective observational study[12] of subjects with DM1 and DM2 and reduced GFR, the 15 of 89 subjects with normal UAE and reduced GFR had a slower further decline in renal function than those with proteinuria and reduced GFR. This parallels the finding in patients with proteinuric DN that the degree of proteinuria and the degree to which proteinuria is suppressible a few months after initiation of treatment with renin-angiotensin-aldosterone system (RAAS) blockade are the strongest predictors of progression of DN.[13–15] However, there were other differences between the normal UAE and proteinuric subjects that might have accounted for the slower rate of decline of renal function: the normal UAE group had more women, had a shorter duration of DM, and was older. Thus, although small in number of subjects examined, the data given earlier would suggest that patients with nonproteinuric DN indeed have histologic DN and may have a better clinical course.

The United Kingdom Prospective Diabetes Study was a prospective clinical trial designed to test the effect of improved glycemic or blood pressure (BP) control on the development of complications of DM2. As such, all subjects were newly diagnosed with DM2 and were followed prospectively for the development of complications. Of the subjects who developed renal insufficiency (defined as Cockcroft-Gault creatinine clearance <60 mL/min, or doubling of serum creatinine), 61% did not have documented preceding albuminuria.[16] Importantly, albumin excretion was measured only once per year on one sample, and the finding may represent detection bias. The investigators did not account for the effect of inhibitors of the RAAS, BP control, or other events in their analysis, but the sheer number of subjects in whom albuminuria was not present is noteworthy.

The first large cross-sectional analysis of the presence or absence of proteinuria in patients with DM and decreased GFR was generated from the Third National Health and Nutrition Examination Survey (NHANES III) conducted from 1988 to 1994 in the United States.[17] Spot urine albumin-to-creatinine ratio and serum creatinine were measured one time, and although this limits reproducibility, 20% of subjects with diabetes had advanced renal failure (defined as estimated GFR [eGFR] <30 mL/min/1.73 m^2) in the absence of albuminuria. Of 171 participants with DM2 and eGFR less than 60 mL/min/1.73 m^2, 30% had no retinopathy or albuminuria.[18] Based on those data, it is estimated that there are 300,000 US adults with DM2, chronic kidney disease, and no retinopathy or albuminuria. The NHANES authors suggested that these participants' decreased renal function may be caused by some pathologic lesion other than classic diabetic glomerulosclerosis.

The largest international cross-sectional study performed to date to screen patients with DM2 for the presence or absence of albuminuria and decreased renal function was the Developing Education on MA for Awareness of renal and cardiovascular risk iN Diabetes (DEMAND) study. DEMAND was a referred global cohort of 32,208 subjects with DM2 analyzed for MA.[19] Among 11,315 subjects with reported decreased kidney function, 20.5% were found to be normoalbuminuric and 30.7% microalbuminuric.[20] These data provide additional evidence that the clinical presentation of DM2 and normoalbuminuria or MA and decreased renal function is not rare.

POTENTIAL MECHANISMS

There are several postulated mechanisms to account for this clinical presentation.[12,16–18,20–24] One possibility is that the absence of proteinuria despite decreased renal function may be because of the use of inhibitors of RAAS or BP control that have been demonstrated to decrease proteinuria and preserve renal function.[4–7] The subjects in cross-sectional analyses found to have decreased renal function and normoalbuminuria or MA may have had proteinuria in their past, which decreased or resolved with BP control and the use of RAAS blockade. Also, although multiple trials have demonstrated that RAAS inhibitors delay the progression of renal disease and reduce proteinuria, there are still subjects whose proteinuria goes down but nonetheless have progression of their underlying renal disease.[5,6]

In an analysis of a clinical trial of sulodexide to slow the progression of DN,[24] among subjects screened for participation, 22% had eGFR less than 60 mL/min/1.73 m^2, but low levels of proteinuria (<500 mg/g creatinine). More than 10% of screened subjects with decreased GFR had extremely low levels of proteinuria (<300 mg/g). Ninety three percent of subjects were treated with RAAS inhibitors at the time of screening, which supports the hypothesis that the effects of RAAS inhibition contribute to the changing paradigm of DN, particularly on proteinuria.

Few patients with diabetes and decreased GFR in the absence of proteinuria have been biopsied and results reported.[11] Any number of other renal lesions could be present in these patients, including atheroembolism, renovascular disease, or tubulointerstitial disease from the many medications used to treat comorbidities. Lastly, patients with DM2 have a high risk for cardiovascular events and many comorbidities that confer great risk for AKI. It is possible that unresolved episodes of AKI account for the decreased GFR seen in many nonproteinuric patients with diabetes. Lastly, nonproteinuric diabetic kidney disease may represent a genetically different form of DN.

FUTURE DIRECTIONS

The traditional clinical paradigm of DN may not apply to all patients with diabetes and decreased renal function. If in fact there is a subset of diabetic patients who have a different renal diagnosis, we may need to consider biopsying more of them. However, it is not clear that in the absence of proteinuria, biopsy results would alter clinical care. A large prospective biopsy study of nonproteinuric subjects with renal failure and diabetes followed by longitudinal observation would be ideal, in which case the pathology could be well characterized. Genetic analysis of subjects in studies would be potentially rewarding, particularly if their natural history proves to be better that those with proteinuric DN. Finally, all the interventions that have been proved to benefit DN may not actually apply to some of these patients. Conversely, and perhaps perversely, these patients may be the ones who are benefitting the most from interventions like RAAS inhibition, because their proteinuria is "well-suppressed." A well-designed biopsy study and a series of intervention trials on large numbers of subjects will be needed to fully understand this phenomenon.

REFERENCES

1. Dwyer JP, Lewis JB. Clinical aspects of diabetic nephropathy. In: Schrier RW, Coffman TM, Falk RJ, et al, editors. Schrier's diseases of the kidney. 9th edition. Philadelphia: Wolters Kluwer Health/Lippincott Williams & Wilkins; 2013;1659–75.
2. Kussman MJ, Goldstein H, Gleason RE. The clinical course of diabetic nephropathy. JAMA 1976;236(16):1861–3.
3. Adler AI, Stevens RJ, Manley SE, et al. Development and progression of nephropathy in type 2 diabetes: the United Kingdom Prospective Diabetes Study (UKPDS 64). Kidney Int 2003;63(1):225–32.
4. Lewis EJ, Hunsicker LG, Bain RP, et al. The effect of angiotensin-converting-enzyme inhibition on diabetic nephropathy. The Collaborative Study Group. N Engl J Med 1993;329(20):1456–62.

5. Lewis EJ, Hunsicker LG, Clarke WR, et al. Renoprotective effect of the angiotensin-receptor antagonist irbesartan in patients with nephropathy due to type 2 diabetes. N Engl J Med 2001;345(12):851–60.
6. Brenner BM, Cooper ME, de Zeeuw D, et al. Effects of losartan on renal and cardiovascular outcomes in patients with type 2 diabetes and nephropathy. N Engl J Med 2001;345(12):861–9.
7. Parving HH, Lehnert H, Brochner-Mortensen J, et al. The effect of irbesartan on the development of diabetic nephropathy in patients with type 2 diabetes. N Engl J Med 2001;345(12):870–8.
8. Haller H, Ito S, Izzo JL, et al. Olmesartan for the delay or prevention of microalbuminuria in type 2 diabetes. N Engl J Med 2011;364(10):907–17.
9. Weksler-Zangen S, Yagil C, Zangen DH, et al. The newly inbred cohen diabetic rat: a nonobese normolipidemic genetic model of diet-induced type 2 diabetes expressing sex differences. Diabetes 2001;50(11):2521–9.
10. Yagil C, Barak A, Ben-Dor D, et al. Nonproteinuric diabetes-associated nephropathy in the Cohen rat model of type 2 diabetes. Diabetes 2005;54(5): 1487–96.
11. Lane PH, Steffes MW, Mauer SM. Glomerular structure in IDDM women with low glomerular filtration rate and normal urinary albumin excretion. Diabetes 1992; 41(5):581–6.
12. Rigalleau V, Lasseur C, Raffaitin C, et al. Normoalbuminuric renal-insufficient diabetic patients: a lower-risk group. Diabetes Care 2007;30(8):2034–9.
13. Atkins RC, Briganti EM, Lewis JB, et al. Proteinuria reduction and progression to renal failure in patients with type 2 diabetes mellitus and overt nephropathy. Am J Kidney Dis 2005;45(2):281–7.
14. de Zeeuw D, Remuzzi G, Parving HH, et al. Albuminuria, a therapeutic target for cardiovascular protection in type 2 diabetic patients with nephropathy. Circulation 2004;110(8):921–7.
15. de Zeeuw D, Remuzzi G, Parving HH, et al. Proteinuria, a target for renoprotection in patients with type 2 diabetic nephropathy: lessons from RENAAL. Kidney Int 2004;65(6):2309–20.
16. Retnakaran R, Cull CA, Thorne KI, et al. Risk factors for renal dysfunction in type 2 diabetes: U.K. Prospective Diabetes Study 74. Diabetes 2006;55(6):1832–9.
17. Garg AX, Kiberd BA, Clark WF, et al. Albuminuria and renal insufficiency prevalence guides population screening: results from the NHANES III. Kidney Int 2002;61(6):2165–75.
18. Kramer HJ, Nguyen QD, Curhan G, et al. Renal insufficiency in the absence of albuminuria and retinopathy among adults with type 2 diabetes mellitus. JAMA 2003;289(24):3273–7.
19. Parving HH, Lewis JB, Ravid M, et al. Prevalence and risk factors for microalbuminuria in a referred cohort of type II diabetic patients: a global perspective. Kidney Int 2006;69(11):2057–63.
20. Dwyer JP, Parving HH, Hunsicker LG, et al. Renal dysfunction in the presence of normoalbuminuria in type 2 diabetes: results from the DEMAND study. Cardiorenal Med 2012;2(1):1–10.
21. Caramori ML, Fioretto P, Mauer M. Low glomerular filtration rate in normoalbuminuric type 1 diabetic patients: an indicator of more advanced glomerular lesions. Diabetes 2003;52(4):1036–40.
22. Cirillo M, Laurenzi M, Mancini M, et al. Low glomerular filtration in the population: prevalence, associated disorders, and awareness. Kidney Int 2006;70(4): 800–6.

23. Leitao CB, Canani LH, Kramer CK, et al. Masked hypertension, urinary albumin excretion rate, and echocardiographic parameters in putatively normotensive type 2 diabetic patients. Diabetes Care 2007;30(5):1255–60.

24. Packham DK, Ivory SE, Reutens AT, et al. Proteinuria in type 2 diabetic patients with renal impairment: the changing face of diabetic nephropathy. Nephron Clin Pract 2011;118(4):c331–8.

Obesity and Diabetic Kidney Disease

Christine Maric-Bilkan, PhD

KEYWORDS

- Kidney • Obesity • Diabetes • Proteinuria • Hyperfiltration • Hypertension
- Glomerulopathy • Diabetic nephropathy

KEY POINTS

- The prevalence of obesity has risen to epidemic proportions and continues to be a major health problem worldwide.
- The high prevalence of obesity is closely linked to the increased incidence of several chronic diseases, including type 2 diabetes, hypertension, and cardiovascular disease.
- Obesity, type 2 diabetes, hypertension, and cardiovascular disease are all risk factors for chronic kidney disease (CKD) and end-stage renal disease (ESRD).
- The mechanisms by which obesity independently, or in concert with type 2 diabetes and hypertension, contributes to the development and/or progression of ESRD are not completely understood.

INTRODUCTION

The prevalence of obesity (body mass index [BMI] ≥ 30 kg/m^2) has risen to epidemic proportions and continues to be a major health problem worldwide.[1–3] The high prevalence of obesity is closely linked to the increased incidence of several chronic diseases, including type 2 diabetes, hypertension, and cardiovascular disease.[2,4–8] Obesity, type 2 diabetes, hypertension, and cardiovascular disease are all risk factors for chronic kidney disease (CKD) and end-stage renal disease (ESRD),[9–13] inasmuch as the presence of 1 or more of these risk factors multiplies the overall risk for disease development and progression (Fig. 1). In addition, evidence suggests that obesity may also increase the risk of ESRD independently of type 2 diabetes and hypertension.[14–16] However, the precise mechanisms by which obesity independently, or in concert with type 2 diabetes and hypertension, contributes to the development and/or progression of CKD and ESRD are not completely understood.

The authors acknowledge the financial support of NIH/NIDDK (RO1DK075832 to C. Maric-Bilkan.
Department of Physiology and Biophysics, University of Mississippi Medical Center, 2500 North State Street, Jackson, MS 39216-4505, USA
E-mail address: cmaric@umc.edu

Med Clin N Am 97 (2013) 59–74
http://dx.doi.org/10.1016/j.mcna.2012.10.010   **medical.theclinics.com**

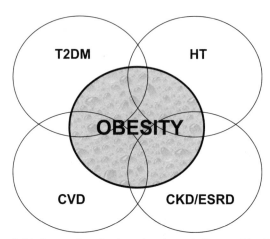

Fig. 1. Clustering of risk factors for obesity-related renal disease. Obesity, type 2 diabetes (T2DM), hypertension (HT), and cardiovascular disease (CVD) are all risk factors for chronic kidney disease (CKD) and end-stage renal disease (ESRD). The presence of 1 or more of these risk factors multiplies the overall risk for disease development and progression.

The two leading causes of ESRD are type 2 diabetes and hypertension, which together account for more than 70% of patients with ESRD.[17,18] Because the growing prevalence of obesity is a major driving force for the continued increase in the prevalence of type 2 diabetes,[7,19] it is often difficult to separate out the individual contribution of either obesity, type 2 diabetes, or hypertension to the development of ESRD. The pathophysiology of type 2 diabetes–related renal disease (ie, diabetic nephropathy) and obesity-related renal disease is almost identical. They both evolve in a sequence of stages beginning with initial increases in glomerular filtration rate (GFR) and intraglomerular capillary pressure (P_{Gc}), glomerular hypertrophy, and microalbuminuria.[20,21] Increased systolic blood pressure further exacerbates the disease progression to proteinuria, nodular glomerulosclerosis, and tubulointerstitial injury and a decrease in GFR leading to ESRD.[22,23] Diabetes-related and obesity-related renal disease also have common initiating events, which include interactions among multiple metabolic and hemodynamic factors that activate common intracellular signaling pathways that in turn trigger the production of cytokines and growth factors, leading to renal disease. The purpose of this review is to provide perspectives regarding the mechanisms by which obesity may lead to ESRD and to discuss prevention strategies and the treatment of obesity-related renal disease.

EPIDEMIOLOGY OF OBESITY AND DIABETES-RELATED KIDNEY DISEASE
Prevalence of Obesity and Type 2 Diabetes

Based on the most recent report from the National Health and Nutrition Examination Survey (NHANES) examining obesity prevalence among US adults, adolescents, and children, more than one-third of adults and almost 17% of children and adolescents were obese in 2009/2010.[24,25] Although there has been a significant increase in obesity prevalence among men and boys over the last decade, no changes were seen among women and girls. The prevalence of obesity is 35.5% among adult men, 35.8% among adult women, and 16.9% amongst children and adolescents of both sexes. Thus, the Healthy People 2010 goals of 15% obesity among adults and 5% obesity among children are far from being met.

Similar to obesity, the global prevalence of type 2 diabetes has more than doubled in the last 30 years and is predicted to continue to increase at an alarming rate. According to the World Health Organization, in 2008, almost 350 million people worldwide have diabetes, 90% of whom have type 2 diabetes.[26] Although the major driving force for the increase in the prevalence of type 2 diabetes is obesity, other factors, including genetic and environmental factors, are also important contributors to the development of type 2 diabetes. Accumulating evidence suggests that this markedly high prevalence of both obesity and type 2 diabetes contributes to the increased incidence of chronic diseases, including CKD and ESRD.[9–13]

Obesity, Diabetes, and CKD

Obesity is a well-recognized risk factor for both type 2 diabetes and hypertension, which are leading causes of CKD and ESRD.[27] Analysis of data from the Framingham Heart Study, which included more than 2600 patients with no CKD at baseline, showed an increased risk of developing stage 3 CKD in obese (BMI $\geq$30 kg/m^2) but not overweight (BMI 25–30 kg/m^2) patients after 18.5 years of follow-up.[9] However, this relationship was no longer significant after adjustment for known cardiovascular disease risk factors, including diabetes and hypertension. Numerous other studies have also demonstrated that the association between obesity and CKD is mediated through risk factors including diabetes, hypertension, and other elements of the metabolic syndrome.[10,16,28–30]

Although studies clearly indicate that the high risk of obesity-related CKD is driven by diabetes and hypertension, there are several other studies that suggest that obesity can lead to the development of CKD independently of either diabetes or hypertension. Specifically, the data from the Hypertension Detection and Follow-Up Program show that, in a cohort of 5897 patients with hypertension and no CKD at baseline, the incidence of CKD after a 5-year follow-up was 28% in patients with normal BMI, 31% in overweight patients, and 34% in obese patients.[16] This risk for CKD persisted in the overweight and obese patients even after adjustment for covariates, including type 2 diabetes, suggesting that obesity increases the risk of CKD independently of type 2 diabetes. Also supporting the notion that obesity increases the risk of CKD independently of diabetes and hypertension is the Physician's Health Study, a large cohort of initially healthy men, in which BMI was associated with increased risk for CKD over 14 years.[31] Furthermore, in 74,986 prehypertensive individuals participating in the first Health Study in Nord-Trøndelag in Norway, the risk of CKD over 21 years was shown to increase dramatically with obesity.[32] In addition to increasing the risk of CKD, obesity has also been suggested to have a higher rate of decline of GFR and progress faster to ESRD.[33]

Obesity, Diabetes, and ESRD

Several studies have shown that increased BMI is an independent risk factor for ESRD. In a cohort of 320,252 adult patients of Kaiser Permanente who were followed for 15 to 35 years, BMI was found to be a strong and common risk factor for ESRD.[10] This relationship between BMI and ESRD persisted even after controlling for baseline blood pressure and diabetes. Similarly, in a population-based, case-control study in Sweden, obesity was shown to be an important and potentially preventable risk factor for ESRD.[11] This study also showed that the coexistence of obesity and diabetes doubled the risk of new onset kidney disease. One study compared the temporal trends in mean BMI and obesity prevalence among incident ESRD by year of dialysis initiated between 1995 and 2002, and these trends were compared with those in the US population during this same period.[34] This study found that among incident patients with ESRD, mean BMI at the start of dialysis increased from 25.7 to 27.5 kg/m^2, and total obesity and stage 2 obesity increased by 33 and 63%, respectively. The slope of mean BMI at initiation of dialysis over the 8 years of follow-up was ~2-fold higher in the incident ESRD population compared with the US population for all age groups.[34]

In contrast to most of the studies suggesting that obesity is a risk factor for CKD and ESRD, some studies have reported that high BMI is associated with greater survival in patients on maintenance hemodialysis.[35,36] This phenomenon, commonly referred to as the obesity paradox, reasons that in patients receiving long-term hemodialysis, larger body size (ie, larger BMI) with more muscle mass (ie, higher serum creatinine concentration) is associated with greater survival. These observations indicate that it is the increase in muscle mass rather than increase in total body weight that confers protection, suggesting that BMI may not always be the most reliable index of CKD risk, at least in certain patient populations. Other studies indicate that visceral or central obesity, but not BMI, is associated with incident CKD[37] and increased cardiovascular disease in patients with CKD.[38] Thus, it is conceivable that overall weight loss with a concomitant increase in muscle mass may be an effective treatment strategy in preventing obesity-associated CKD and ESRD.

PATHOPHYSIOLOGY OF OBESITY AND DIABETES-RELATED KIDNEY DISEASE

Obesity-related renal disease, similar to diabetes-related renal disease, is associated with physiologic, anatomic, and pathologic changes in the kidney (**Fig. 2**). Both obesity and diabetes renal disease evolve in a sequence of stages beginning with initial increases in GFR and P_{Gc}, glomerular hypertrophy, and microalbuminuria.[20,21] Increased systolic blood pressure further exacerbates the disease progression to proteinuria, nodular glomerulosclerosis and tubulointerstitial injury, and a decline in GFR leading to ESRD.[22,23] Obesity-related and diabetes-related renal disease also share common initiating events, which include interactions among multiple metabolic

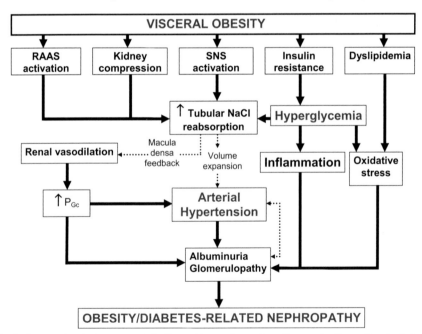

Fig. 2. Interaction between metabolic and hemodynamic pathways in the pathophysiology of obesity-related and diabetes-related renal disease. P_{Gc}, intraglomerular capillary pressure; RAAS, renin angiotensin aldosterone system; SNS, sympathetic nervous system.

and hemodynamic factors that activate common intracellular signaling pathways that in turn trigger the production of cytokines and growth factors, leading to renal disease (**Fig. 3**).

Obesity, Diabetes, and Glomerular Hemodynamics

Experimental studies in diet-induced obese dogs and genetically induced obese rats show that one of the earliest changes in renal hemodynamics in response to the obese state is glomerular hyperfiltration. Specifically, dogs fed a high-fat diet for only 5 to 6 weeks and obese Zucker rats show an increase in GFR.[39,40] These changes in GFR are reversible, at least in the obese Zucker rats, in which food restriction was associated with attenuation of glomerular hyperfiltration, possibly due to decreased protein intake or overall weight loss.[40] These observations in experimental models have also been confirmed in obese humans. Studies have shown that obese individuals have around 50% higher GFR compared with lean individuals.[41] Although there is still some debate about the mechanisms underlying obesity-related glomerular hyperfiltration, the most likely explanation is increased sodium reabsorption by the proximal tubule or loop of Henle, leading to tubuloglomerular feedback (TGF)–mediated reduction in afferent arteriolar resistance, increased P_{Gc}, and thus increased GFR.[42] This TGF-driven dilation of afferent arterioles and resultant impairment of renal autoregulation, in turn, allows increases in blood pressure to be transmitted to the glomerulus causing further increases in P_{Gc} and subsequent glomerular injury.[43] This may be especially important in individuals with a reduced number of nephrons in whom there is a greater risk of enhanced glomerular blood pressure transmission due to the substantially greater pre-glomerular vasodilation.[43] There is also evidence for increased activation of the renin-angiotensin-aldosterone system (RAAS) and increased renal sympathetic tone as important stimuli for increased sodium reabsorption exacerbating the renal hemodynamic changes associated with obesity.[44–46]

It is generally believed that the initial increase in GFR associated with obesity likely serves as an early compensatory response that allows for restoration of salt balance despite continued increases in tubular reabsorption. However, in the long term, glomerular hyperfiltration may contribute to the development of renal injury, especially

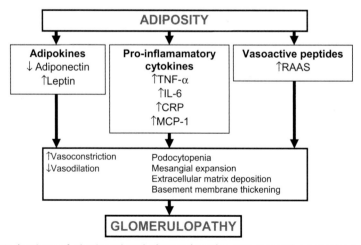

Fig. 3. Mechanisms of obesity-related glomerulopathy. CRP, C-reactive protein; IL-6, interleukin-6; MCP-1, monocyte chemoattractant protein-1; RAAS, renin angiotensin aldosterone system; TNF-α, tumor necrosis factor α.

if combined with hypertension. Studies supporting this notion show that weight loss reduces glomerular hyperfiltration and subsequent renal injury.[41,47]

Similar to obesity-associated glomerular hyperfiltration, renal vasodilation and increases in GFR and P_{Gc} also characterize the early stages of diabetes-associated renal disease.[48] Although the precise mechanisms underlying diabetes-associated glomerular hyperfiltration remain inconclusive, it is believed that mechanisms similar to those occurring in obesity drive the initial increase in GFR. Specifically, reduced delivery of salt to the macula densa, as a consequence of increased proximal reabsorption of glucose and sodium, reduces afferent arteriolar resistance leading to increased P_{Gc} and GFR via attenuated TGF.[49–51] In addition, afferent vasodilation and efferent vasoconstriction in response to circulating or locally formed vasoactive factors (eg, angiotensin II (Ang II) and endothelin) produced in response to hyperglycemia or shear stress are also believed to contribute to the development of diabetes-associated glomerular hyperfiltration.[52,53]

Although most studies suggest that the mechanisms underlying glomerular hyperfiltration due to obesity and diabetes are similar, there is some evidence to suggest that hyperglycemia and obesity may have at least partially additive effects on glomerular hemodynamics. Because obesity and diabetes coexist with elements of the metabolic syndrome, including hypertension, it is often difficult to separate the effects of each element on glomerular hemodynamics and progression of renal injury, at least in humans. However, experimental studies provide some mechanistic insights. Specifically, mice lacking the gene for the melanocortin-4 receptor are obese, hyperinsulinemic, and hyperleptinemic but normotensive at 55 weeks of age and exhibit moderately increased GFR compared with their wild-type counterparts.[54] However, when rendered hypertensive via treatment with N(G)-nitro-L-arginine methyl ester (L-NAME), they develop prominent glomerular hyperfiltration, suggesting that increases in blood pressure may exacerbate obesity-related increases in GFR. These data support the concept of a synergistic effect of various components of obesity, metabolic syndrome, diabetes, and hypertension on glomerular hemodynamics.

Although the early stages of obesity-related and diabetes-related renal disease are characterized by glomerular hyperfiltration, one of the hallmarks of the advanced stages of the disease is the decline in GFR. Unlike studies examining the mechanisms underlying glomerular hyperfiltration, much less is known about the mechanisms underlying the decline in GFR characteristic of advanced diabetic and obesity-related nephropathy. The main reason for this lack of knowledge is the lack of appropriate experimental models that mimic the advanced stages of the disease; most experimental models of obesity-related or diabetes-related renal injury never really develop overt nephropathy and are in a permanent state of glomerular hyperfiltration. However, the existing evidence suggests that obesity and diabetes are states of low-grade inflammation and oxidative stress, both of which may lead to kidney damage, progressive loss of nephrons, and decrease in GFR over time. In addition, hyperlipidemia has been linked to reduced GFR associated with advanced diabetic nephropathy. Several clinical studies have demonstrated the importance of lipid control in preserving GFR in patients with diabetes.[55] However, additional studies are warranted to examine whether the beneficial effects of lipid lowering in diabetes-related and obesity-related nephropathy are caused by improvement in the lipid profile or more direct renoprotection.

Hypertension as a Driving Force for Obesity-Related and Diabetes-Related Kidney Disease

The nearly linear relationship between BMI and blood pressure in diverse populations throughout the world[35,56–58] has led to the notion that obesity contributes to the development of hypertension. Numerous clinical, population, and basic research studies have shown that visceral obesity, the main driver of type 2 diabetes, increases blood pressure.[59,60] Data from the Framingham Heart Study and other population-based studies indicate that excess weight gain may account for as much as 78% of primary (essential) hypertension in men and 65% in women.[61,62] In addition, obese individuals have a 3.5-fold increase in the risk for developing hypertension.[56,63] Clinical studies also indicate that weight loss reduces blood pressure in most patients with hypertension and is effective in the primary prevention of hypertension.[60] Discussing the mechanisms underlying obesity-driven hypertension is beyond the scope of this review, but accumulating evidence suggests that physiologic, environmental, and genetic factors all contribute to obesity-related hypertension.[64] Given that the focus of this review is the contribution of obesity to the development of renal disease, the question to be asked is how does obesity-related hypertension lead to the development of renal disease?

Several studies have suggested that visceral (but not subcutaneous) obesity induces hypertension, initially by increasing renal tubular sodium reabsorption and causing a hypertensive shift of renal-pressure natriuresis via activation of multiple pathways including the sympathetic nervous system and the RAAS.[39,64,65] In addition, physical compression of the kidneys caused by visceral obesity has also been suggested to contribute to the increase in blood pressure, at least in some experimental models.[39] This increase in blood pressure, alongside increases in P_{Gc} and GFR (discussed later), and other metabolic abnormalities (eg, dyslipidemia, hyperglycemia) all likely interact to contribute to the initial renal insult. A similar sequence of events has been proposed to contribute to renal injury in the setting of type 2 diabetes, independent of obesity, suggesting that hypertension plays a major role in obesity as well as diabetes-associated renal disease. Hypertension, in addition to contributing to the initial development of renal injury is also an important factor in the disease progression. Progressive renal injury only occurs when hypertension is superimposed on obesity or diabetes.[54] The importance of tight blood pressure control for treating diabetic nephropathy is recognized in current guidelines, with a recommended target blood pressure of less than 130/80 mm Hg.[66] Several studies have shown clear renoprotection with respect to slowing progression of nephropathy in patients with type 2 diabetes by lowering blood pressure.[67–71]

Obesity, Diabetes, and Albuminuria

The earliest clinical manifestation of obesity-related and diabetes-related renal injury is microalbuminuria (30–300 mg/d) which, over time, can progresses to overt proteinuria (300–3000 mg/d).[72–74] Microalbuminuria, in turn, signifies increased risk of progression to ESRD and cardiovascular disease.[74] Studies in nondiabetic and diabetic overweight individuals have shown that increases in urine albumin excretion strongly correlate with increases in body weight and other markers of obesity, including BMI, waist circumference, and waist-to-hip ratio.[75–78] In the Prevention of Renal and Vascular End stage Disease (PREVEND) study, the prevalence of microalbuminuria in lean and obese individuals correlated with central obesity even after correction for confounding variables.[79] Retrospective analysis of the database of a population study showing that the prevalence of microalbuminuria increased from 9.5% in men with normal BMI to 18.3% in overweight men, and 29.3% in obese men further supports the notion of a direct correlation between BMI and microalbuminuria.[77] In a cross-sectional study of a cohort of African Americans, microalbuminuria was most prevalent in patients with newly diagnosed type 2 diabetes and was independently associated with BMI.[78] Others have shown that even moderate weight reduction in patients with type 2 diabetes with proteinuria reduces urine protein excretion by approximately 30%.[80] Furthermore, weight reduction achieved by either dietary caloric restriction or bariatric surgery has been shown to attenuate progression of proteinuria in obese nondiabetic individuals.[81,82]

The development of microalbuminuria in either nondiabetic or diabetic individuals was traditionally believed to result from damage to the glomerular filtration barrier as a consequence of an increase in blood pressure which is transmitted to the glomeruli, increasing P_{Gc} and GFR. In addition, in the setting of diabetes, hyperglycemia-associated inflammation and oxidative stress have been shown to contribute to the damage to the glomerular filtration barrier, contributing to increased leakage of protein across the membrane leading to the development of albuminuria.[72] In the setting of obesity, cytokines including adiponectin have been suggested to play a role in the development of albuminuria. Specifically, the adiponectin knockout mouse exhibits increased baseline albuminuria and podocyte foot process effacement, suggesting that adiponectin regulates podocyte function and thus contributes to the initial development of albuminuria.[83] Apart from the glomerulocentric view of the origin of albuminuria, a more recent theory on the mechanisms of albuminuria, especially in the setting of diabetes, is that the diabetic milieu also impairs proximal tubular reabsorption of albumin leading to increased urine albumin excretion.[84]

Obesity, Diabetes, and Glomerulopathy

Accompanying the hemodynamic changes, the early stage of obesity is associated with up to a 40% increase in kidney weight.[39,85] Histologically, the obese kidney is characterized by glomerulomegaly, mesangial expansion, and podocytopenia, leading to focal segmental glomerulosclerosis.[43,86,87] These features, which precede overt renal insufficiency, have been observed in biopsies from obese humans[88] and experimental models of obesity-related kidney disease, namely the obese Zucker rat[89,90] and dogs fed a high-fat diet.[39] However, the degree of glomerulosclerosis seems to be highly variable amongst different experimental models and obese individuals,[91] and some studies indicate that some obese individuals do not even develop glomerulosclerosis, despite the glomerulomegaly.[87] A review of native 6818 renal biopsies indicated that obesity-related glomerulopathy is characterized by lesser segmental sclerosis, less podocyte effacement, but more glomerulomegaly compared with idiopathic glomerulosclerosis.[91] However, despite the less pronounced glomerular lesions in obesity-related glomerulopathy, the long-term prognosis of the disease is just as poor. It has been reported that the probabilities of renal survival are 77% and 51% at 5 and 10 years, respectively,[92] and that nephron number may play a significant role in the renal prognosis.[93] Specifically, in patients with unilateral renal agenesis, the decline in renal function is most pronounced in obese patients, suggesting that obesity accelerates renal dysfunction in patients with severe reductions in renal mass.[93]

Similar to obesity-related glomerulopathy, early diabetic nephropathy is accompanied by hyperfiltration and microalbuminuria. Histologically, the diabetic kidney exhibits glomerular hypertrophy, widening of the glomerular basement membrane, mesangial expansion, podocytopenia leading to nodular (Kimmelstiel-Wilson) glomerulosclerosis, and tubulointerstitial fibrosis.[22] Thus, given the similarities in the histologic appearance of the renal lesions from diabetic and obese individuals, it is not surprising that the mechanisms underlying these changes have many similarities.

Mechanisms of Obesity-Related and Diabetes-Related Glomerulopathy

Obesity (ie, visceral adiposity) and diabetes (hyperglycemia) both promote a low-grade inflammatory state and are associated with infiltration of macrophages into the kidney.

The infiltrated macrophages, in turn, become a source of a whole host of proinflammatory mediators such as tumor necrosis factor-α (TNF-α), interleukin-6 (IL-6), C-reactive protein, monocyte chemoattractant protein-1, and macrophage migration inhibitory factor.[94,95] In addition, visceral fat releases adipokines such as adiponectin and leptin into the circulation which also play a role in the pathophysiology of renal injury.[95] Apart from adipokines and inflammatory mediators, vasoactive peptides such as Ang II also contribute to obesity-associated and diabetes-associated glomerulopathy.

Adiponectin

Obese humans are characterized by consistently low levels of circulating adiponectin. However, in patients with CKD and ESRD due to obesity or diabetes, adiponectin levels are increased, possibly because of impaired renal function.[96,97] Experimental studies have shown that genetic deletion of adiponectin is associated with albuminuria and podocyte effacement, which are further exacerbated by diabetes.[98] Treatment of these mice with exogenous adiponectin results in normalization of albuminuria, improvement of podocyte foot process effacement, increased activation of glomerular AMP-activated kinase, and reduced urinary and glomerular markers of oxidative stress.[83] These observations suggest that adiponectin may have a renoprotective effect.

Leptin

Although the primary action of leptin is to act on the satiety center to limit food intake, leptin has also been linked to renal disease. Circulating leptin levels are increased in CKD and in patients on hemodialysis.[99,100] Leptin levels are also typically increased in obese individuals. Mice overexpressing leptin have more renal disease than leptin-deficient mice.[101] Long-term infusion of recombinant leptin in rats is associated with proteinuria, increased expression of extracellular matrix proteins (collagen type IV), transforming growth factor-beta (TGF-β) and other proinflammatory cytokines, macrophage infiltration, and glomerulosclerosis.[102] These observations suggest that, unlike adiponectin, leptin promotes the development of renal injury in both obese and lean individuals.

Inflammatory markers

Both obesity and diabetes are characterized by increased levels of circulating cytokines, including TNF-α and IL-6,[103,104] and markers of inflammation are inversely associated with measures of kidney function and positively with albuminuria. It is believed that the major source of proinflammatory cytokines in obese and diabetic individuals that directly contribute to renal injury are infiltrated macrophages.[101] In addition, renal parenchyma has also been shown to release proinflammatory cytokines in response to hyperglycemia or locally active vasoactive peptides, such as Ang II.[105] Once released, these proinflammatory mediators contribute to a low-grade chronic inflammatory state that contributes to obesity-associated and diabetes-associated glomerulopathy. In particular, TNF-α has been shown to reduce the expression of key components of the slit diaphragm, nephrin and podocin, thus contributing to podocytopathy.[106] Similarly, IL-6 promotes the expression of adhesion molecules and subsequent oxidative stress,[107] whereas blocking the IL-6 receptor prevents progression of proteinuria, renal lipid deposition, and mesangial cell proliferation associated with severe hyperlipoproteinemia.[108] Thus, there is strong evidence for the contribution of inflammation in obesity-associated and diabetes-associated renal disease.

Other factors

Although several vasoactive peptides have been implicated in the pathogenesis of obesity-associated and diabetes-associated glomerulopathy, the most prominent, and certainly the best described vasoactive hormonal pathway is the RAAS; Ang II is the most biologically active component. Both obesity and persistent hyperglycemia are associated with upregulation of the intrarenal RAAS.[109,110] Activation of the RAAS leads to both hemodynamic and cellular effects. Ang II leads to increases in efferent arteriolar vasoconstriction and glomerular pressure, sodium retention, and cell proliferation.[111–113] On a cellular level, Ang II activates protein kinase C and mitogen-activated protein kinase, and transcription factors such as nuclear factor-κB that lead to alteration in the gene expression of several growth factors and cytokines including TGF-β. TGF-β, in turn, promotes podocyte apoptosis, mesangial cell proliferation, and extracellular matrix synthesis, cellular events that are important in the development of obesity-associated and diabetes-associated glomerulopathy.[114]

Although there are many similarities between the obese and diabetic kidney, there are some features unique to obesity in the absence of diabetes. Glomerular/mesangial lipid deposits (foam cells) are frequently seen in the kidneys of obese individuals, supporting the concept of lipotoxicity (ie, lipid-induced renal injury). This lipid accumulation in the glomerulus then leads to upregulation of the sterol-regulatory element-binding proteins (SREBP-1 and -2), which, in turn, promote podocyte apoptosis and mesangial cell proliferation and cytokine synthesis.[115]

SUMMARY

Obesity and diabetes are major causes of CKD and ESRD, and are thus enormous health concerns worldwide. Both obesity and diabetes, along with other elements of the metabolic syndrome including hypertension, are highly interrelated and contribute to the development and progression of renal disease. Studies show that multiple factors act in concert to initially cause renal vasodilation, glomerular hyperfiltration, and albuminuria, leading to the development of glomerulopathy. The coexistence of hypertension contributes to the disease progression, which, if not treated, may lead to ESRD. Although early intervention and management of body weight, hyperglycemia, and hypertension are imperative, novel therapeutic approaches are also necessary to reduce the high morbidity and mortality associated with both obesity-related and diabetes-related renal disease.

REFERENCES

1. Yanovski SZ, Yanovski JA. Obesity prevalence in the United States–up, down, or sideways? N Engl J Med 2011;364(11):987–9.
2. Flegal KM, Carroll MD, Ogden CL, et al. Prevalence and trends in obesity among US adults, 1999-2008. JAMA 2010;303(3):235–41.
3. World Health Organization. Obesity and overweight fact sheet. 2012. Available at: http://www.who.int/mediacentre/factsheets/fs311/en/index.html. Accessed on October 2nd, 2012.
4. Kopelman P. Health risks associated with overweight and obesity. Obes Rev 2007;8(Suppl 1):13–7.
5. Eknoyan G. Obesity, diabetes, and chronic kidney disease. Curr Diab Rep 2007;7(6):449–53.
6. Hall JE, Crook ED, Jones DW, et al. Mechanisms of obesity-associated cardiovascular and renal disease. Am J Med Sci 2002;324(3):127–37.
7. Ogden CL, Carroll MD, Curtin LR, et al. Prevalence of overweight and obesity in the United States, 1999-2004. JAMA 2006;295(13):1549–55.
8. Neeland IJ, Turer AT, Ayers CR, et al. Dysfunctional adiposity and the risk of prediabetes and type 2 diabetes in obese adults. JAMA 2012;308(11):1150–9.

9. Foster MC, Hwang SJ, Larson MG, et al. Overweight, obesity, and the development of stage 3 CKD: the Framingham Heart Study. Am J Kidney Dis 2008; 52(1):39–48.

10. Hsu CY, McCulloch CE, Iribarren C, et al. Body mass index and risk for end-stage renal disease. Ann Intern Med 2006;144(1):21–8.

11. Ejerblad E, Fored CM, Lindblad P, et al. Obesity and risk for chronic renal failure. J Am Soc Nephrol 2006;17(6):1695–702.

12. Praga M, Morales E. Obesity, proteinuria and progression of renal failure. Curr Opin Nephrol Hypertens 2006;15(5):481–6.

13. Wang Y, Chen X, Song Y, et al. Association between obesity and kidney disease: a systematic review and meta-analysis. Kidney Int 2008;73(1):19–33.

14. Ogden CL, Yanovski SZ, Carroll MD, et al. The epidemiology of obesity. Gastroenterology 2007;132(6):2087–102.

15. Coresh J, Selvin E, Stevens LA, et al. Prevalence of chronic kidney disease in the United States. JAMA 2007;298(17):2038–47.

16. Kramer H, Luke A, Bidani A, et al. Obesity and prevalent and incident CKD: the hypertension detection and follow-up program. Am J Kidney Dis 2005;46(4):587–94.

17. de Zeeuw D, Ramjit D, Zhang Z, et al. Renal risk and renoprotection among ethnic groups with type 2 diabetic nephropathy: a post hoc analysis of RENAAL. Kidney Int 2006;69(9):1675–82.

18. Remuzzi G, Macia M, Ruggenenti P. Prevention and treatment of diabetic renal disease in type 2 diabetes: the BENEDICT study. J Am Soc Nephrol 2006; 17(4 Suppl 2):S90–7.

19. US Renal Data System. USRDS 2009 annual data report: atlas of chronic kidney disease and end-stage renal disease in the United States. Bethesda (MD): National Institutes of Health, National Institute of Diabetes and Digestive and Kidney Diseases; 2009.

20. Thomson SC, Vallon V, Blantz RC. Kidney function in early diabetes: the tubular hypothesis of glomerular filtration. Am J Physiol Renal Physiol 2004;286(1):F8–15.

21. Hostetter TH. Hyperfiltration and glomerulosclerosis. Semin Nephrol 2003;23(2):194–9.

22. Caramori ML, Mauer M. Diabetes and nephropathy. Curr Opin Nephrol Hypertens 2003;12(3):273–82.

23. Leon CA, Raij L. Interaction of haemodynamic and metabolic pathways in the genesis of diabetic nephropathy. J Hypertens 2005;23(11):1931–7.

24. Ogden CL, Carroll MD, Kit BK, et al. Prevalence of obesity and trends in body mass index among US children and adolescents, 1999-2010. JAMA 2012; 307(5):483–90.

25. Flegal KM, Carroll MD, Kit BK, et al. Prevalence of obesity and trends in the distribution of body mass index among US adults, 1999-2010. JAMA 2012; 307(5):491–7.

26. Danaei G, Finucane MM, Lin JK, et al. National, regional, and global trends in systolic blood pressure since 1980: systematic analysis of health examination surveys and epidemiological studies with 786 country-years and 5.4 million participants. Lancet 2011;377(9765):568–77.

27. US Renal Data System. USRDS 2006 annual data report: atlas of end-stage renal disease in the United States. Bethesda (MD): National Institutes of Health, National Institute of Diabetes and Digestive and Kidney Diseases; 2006.

28. Kurella M, Lo JC, Chertow GM. Metabolic syndrome and the risk for chronic kidney disease among nondiabetic adults. J Am Soc Nephrol 2005;16(7):2134–40.

29. Chen J, Muntner P, Hamm LL, et al. The metabolic syndrome and chronic kidney disease in U.S. adults. Ann Intern Med 2004;140(3):167–74.

30. Stengel B, Tarver-Carr ME, Powe NR, et al. Lifestyle factors, obesity and the risk of chronic kidney disease. Epidemiology 2003;14(4):479–87.

31. Gelber RP, Kurth T, Kausz AT, et al. Association between body mass index and CKD in apparently healthy men. Am J Kidney Dis 2005;46(5):871–80.

32. Munkhaugen J, Lydersen S, Wideroe TE, et al. Prehypertension, obesity, and risk of kidney disease: 20-year follow-up of the HUNT I study in Norway. Am J Kidney Dis 2009;54(4):638–46.

33. Iseki K, Ikemiya Y, Kinjo K, et al. Body mass index and the risk of development of end-stage renal disease in a screened cohort. Kidney Int 2004;65(5):1870–6.

34. Kramer HJ, Saranathan A, Luke A, et al. Increasing body mass index and obesity in the incident ESRD population. J Am Soc Nephrol 2006;17(5):1453–9.

35. Kalantar-Zadeh K, Kopple JD. Obesity paradox in patients on maintenance dialysis. Contrib Nephrol 2006;151:57–69.

36. Kalantar-Zadeh K, Streja E, Kovesdy CP, et al. The obesity paradox and mortality associated with surrogates of body size and muscle mass in patients receiving hemodialysis. Mayo Clin Proc 2010;85(11):991–1001.

37. Elsayed EF, Sarnak MJ, Tighiouart H, et al. Waist-to-hip ratio, body mass index, and subsequent kidney disease and death. Am J Kidney Dis 2008;52(1):29–38.

38. Elsayed EF, Tighiouart H, Weiner DE, et al. Waist-to-hip ratio and body mass index as risk factors for cardiovascular events in CKD. Am J Kidney Dis 2008; 52(1):49–57.

39. Henegar JR, Bigler SA, Henegar LK, et al. Functional and structural changes in the kidney in the early stages of obesity. J Am Soc Nephrol 2001;12(6):1211–7.

40. Maddox DA, Alavi FK, Santella RN, et al. Prevention of obesity-linked renal disease: age-dependent effects of dietary food restriction. Kidney Int 2002; 62(1):208–19.

41. Chagnac A, Weinstein T, Herman M, et al. The effects of weight loss on renal function in patients with severe obesity. J Am Soc Nephrol 2003;14(6):1480–6.

42. Hall JE. The kidney, hypertension, and obesity. Hypertension 2003;41(3 Pt 2): 625–33.

43. Griffin KA, Kramer H, Bidani AK. Adverse renal consequences of obesity. Am J Physiol Renal Physiol 2008;294(4):F685–96.

44. Hall JE, Kuo JJ, da Silva AA, et al. Obesity-associated hypertension and kidney disease. Curr Opin Nephrol Hypertens 2003;12(2):195–200.

45. Esler M, Rumantir M, Wiesner G, et al. Sympathetic nervous system and insulin resistance: from obesity to diabetes. Am J Hypertens 2001;14(11 Pt 2):304S–9S.

46. Blanco S, Bonet J, Lopez D, et al. ACE inhibitors improve nephrin expression in Zucker rats with glomerulosclerosis. Kidney Int Suppl 2005;(93):S10–4.

47. Chagnac A, Herman M, Zingerman B, et al. Obesity-induced glomerular hyperfiltration: its involvement in the pathogenesis of tubular sodium reabsorption. Nephrol Dial Transplant 2008;23(12):3946–52.

48. Yip JW, Jones SL, Wiseman MJ, et al. Glomerular hyperfiltration in the prediction of nephropathy in IDDM: a 10-year follow-up study. Diabetes 1996;45(12): 1729–33.

49. Vallon V, Schroth J, Satriano J, et al. Adenosine A(1) receptors determine glomerular hyperfiltration and the salt paradox in early streptozotocin diabetes mellitus. Nephron Physiol 2009;111(3):p30–8.

50. Woods LL, Mizelle HL, Hall JE. Control of renal hemodynamics in hyperglycemia: possible role of tubuloglomerular feedback. Am J Physiol 1987;252(1 Pt 2):F65–73.

51. Persson P, Hansell P, Palm F. Tubular reabsorption and diabetes-induced glomerular hyperfiltration. Acta Physiol (Oxf) 2010;200(1):3–10.
52. Cherney DZ, Scholey JW, Miller JA. Insights into the regulation of renal hemodynamic function in diabetic mellitus. Curr Diabetes Rev 2008;4(4):280–90.
53. Carmines PK. The renal vascular response to diabetes. Curr Opin Nephrol Hypertens 2010;19(1):85–90.
54. do Carmo JM, Tallam LS, Roberts JV, et al. Impact of obesity on renal structure and function in the presence and absence of hypertension: evidence from melanocortin-4 receptor-deficient mice. Am J Physiol Regul Integr Comp Physiol 2009;297(3):R803–12.
55. Fried LF, Orchard TJ, Kasiske BL. Effect of lipid reduction on the progression of renal disease: a meta-analysis. Kidney Int 2001;59(1):260–9.
56. Must A, Spadano J, Coakley EH, et al. The disease burden associated with overweight and obesity. JAMA 1999;282(16):1523–9.
57. Wilson PW, D'Agostino RB, Sullivan L, et al. Overweight and obesity as determinants of cardiovascular risk: the Framingham experience. Arch Intern Med 2002;162(16):1867–72.
58. Doll S, Paccaud F, Bovet P, et al. Body mass index, abdominal adiposity and blood pressure: consistency of their association across developing and developed countries. Int J Obes Relat Metab Disord 2002;26(1):48–57.
59. Hall JE, Jones DW, Kuo JJ, et al. Impact of the obesity epidemic on hypertension and renal disease. Curr Hypertens Rep 2003;5(5):386–92.
60. Neter JE, Stam BE, Kok FJ, et al. Influence of weight reduction on blood pressure: a meta-analysis of randomized controlled trials. Hypertension 2003;42(5):878–84.
61. Garrison RJ, Kannel WB, Stokes J 3rd, et al. Incidence and precursors of hypertension in young adults: the Framingham Offspring Study. Prev Med 1987;16(2):235–51.
62. Kannel WB, Zhang T, Garrison RJ. Is obesity-related hypertension less of a cardiovascular risk? The Framingham Study. Am Heart J 1990;120(5):1195–201.
63. Mokdad AH, Ford ES, Bowman BA, et al. Prevalence of obesity, diabetes, and obesity-related health risk factors, 2001. JAMA 2003;289(1):76–9.
64. Kotchen TA. Obesity-related hypertension: epidemiology, pathophysiology, and clinical management. Am J Hypertens 2010;23(11):1170–8.
65. Hall JE, Henegar JR, Dwyer TM, et al. Is obesity a major cause of chronic kidney disease? Adv Ren Replace Ther 2004;11(1):41–54.
66. Van Buren PN, Toto R. Hypertension in diabetic nephropathy: epidemiology, mechanisms, and management. Adv Chronic Kidney Dis 2011;18(1):28–41.
67. Mancia G. Effects of intensive blood pressure control in the management of patients with type 2 diabetes mellitus in the Action to Control Cardiovascular Risk in Diabetes (ACCORD) trial. Circulation 2010;122(8):847–9.
68. Heerspink HJ, de Zeeuw D. The kidney in type 2 diabetes therapy. Rev Diabet Stud 2011;8(3):392–402.
69. Rayner HC, Hollingworth L, Higgins R, et al. Systematic kidney disease management in a population with diabetes mellitus: turning the tide of kidney failure. BMJ Qual Saf 2011;20(10):903–10.
70. Williams ME. The goal of blood pressure control for prevention of early diabetic microvascular complications. Curr Diab Rep 2011;11(4):323–9.
71. Grossman E, Messerli FH. Management of blood pressure in patients with diabetes. Am J Hypertens 2011;24(8):863–75.

72. Jauregui A, Mintz DH, Mundel P, et al. Role of altered insulin signaling pathways in the pathogenesis of podocyte malfunction and microalbuminuria. Curr Opin Nephrol Hypertens 2009;18(6):539–45.

73. de Boer IH, Sibley SD, Kestenbaum B, et al. Central obesity, incident microalbuminuria, and change in creatinine clearance in the epidemiology of diabetes interventions and complications study. J Am Soc Nephrol 2007;18(1):235–43.

74. Eijkelkamp WB, Zhang Z, Remuzzi G, et al. Albuminuria is a target for renoprotective therapy independent from blood pressure in patients with type 2 diabetic nephropathy: post hoc analysis from the Reduction of Endpoints in NIDDM with the Angiotensin II Antagonist Losartan (RENAAL) trial. J Am Soc Nephrol 2007; 18(5):1540–6.

75. Klausen KP, Parving HH, Scharling H, et al. Microalbuminuria and obesity: impact on cardiovascular disease and mortality. Clin Endocrinol (Oxf) 2009; 71(1):40–5.

76. Savage S, Nagel NJ, Estacio RO, et al. Clinical factors associated with urinary albumin excretion in type II diabetes. Am J Kidney Dis 1995;25(6):836–44.

77. de Jong PE, Verhave JC, Pinto-Sietsma SJ, et al. Obesity and target organ damage: the kidney. Int J Obes Relat Metab Disord 2002;26(Suppl 4):S21–4.

78. Kohler KA, McClellan WM, Ziemer DC, et al. Risk factors for microalbuminuria in black Americans with newly diagnosed type 2 diabetes. Am J Kidney Dis 2000; 36(5):903–13.

79. Pinto-Sietsma SJ, Navis G, Janssen WM, et al. A central body fat distribution is related to renal function impairment, even in lean subjects. Am J Kidney Dis 2003;41(4):733–41.

80. Morales E, Valero MA, Leon M, et al. Beneficial effects of weight loss in overweight patients with chronic proteinuric nephropathies. Am J Kidney Dis 2003;41(2):319–27.

81. Praga M, Morales E. Obesity-related renal damage: changing diet to avoid progression. Kidney Int 2010;78(7):633–5.

82. Mohan S, Tan J, Gorantla S, et al. Early improvement in albuminuria in non-diabetic patients after Roux-en-Y bariatric surgery. Obes Surg 2012;22(3): 375–80.

83. Sharma K, Ramachandrarao S, Qiu G, et al. Adiponectin regulates albuminuria and podocyte function in mice. J Clin Invest 2008;118(5):1645–56.

84. Comper WD, Russo LM. The glomerular filter: an imperfect barrier is required for perfect renal function. Curr Opin Nephrol Hypertens 2009;18(4):336–42.

85. Kasiske BL, Cleary MP, O'Donnell MP, et al. Effects of genetic obesity on renal structure and function in the Zucker rat. J Lab Clin Med 1985;106(5):598–604.

86. Tran HA. Obesity-related glomerulopathy. J Clin Endocrinol Metab 2004;89(12): 6358.

87. Ritz E, Koleganova N, Piecha G. Is there an obesity-metabolic syndrome related glomerulopathy? Curr Opin Nephrol Hypertens 2011;20(1):44–9.

88. Kasiske BL, Napier J. Glomerular sclerosis in patients with massive obesity. Am J Nephrol 1985;5(1):45–50.

89. Coimbra TM, Janssen U, Grone HJ, et al. Early events leading to renal injury in obese Zucker (fatty) rats with type II diabetes. Kidney Int 2000;57(1):167–82.

90. O'Donnell MP, Kasiske BL, Cleary MP, et al. Effects of genetic obesity on renal structure and function in the Zucker rat. II. Micropuncture studies. J Lab Clin Med 1985;106(5):605–10.

91. Kambham N, Markowitz GS, Valeri AM, et al. Obesity-related glomerulopathy: an emerging epidemic. Kidney Int 2001;59(4):1498–509.

92. Praga M, Hernandez E, Morales E, et al. Clinical features and long-term outcome of obesity-associated focal segmental glomerulosclerosis. Nephrol Dial Transplant 2001;16(9):1790–8.

93. Praga M. Synergy of low nephron number and obesity: a new focus on hyperfiltration nephropathy. Nephrol Dial Transplant 2005;20(12):2594–7.

94. King GL. The role of inflammatory cytokines in diabetes and its complications. J Periodontol 2008;79(Suppl 8):1527–34.

95. Tang J, Yan H, Zhuang S. Inflammation and oxidative stress in obesity-related glomerulopathy. Int J Nephrol 2012;2012:608397.

96. Guebre-Egziabher F, Bernhard J, Funahashi T, et al. Adiponectin in chronic kidney disease is related more to metabolic disturbances than to decline in renal function. Nephrol Dial Transplant 2005;20(1):129–34.

97. Saraheimo M, Forsblom C, Thorn L, et al. Serum adiponectin and progression of diabetic nephropathy in patients with type 1 diabetes. Diabetes Care 2008; 31(6):1165–9.

98. Ma K, Cabrero A, Saha PK, et al. Increased beta-oxidation but no insulin resistance or glucose intolerance in mice lacking adiponectin. J Biol Chem 2002; 277(38):34658–61.

99. Kastarinen H, Kesaniemi YA, Ukkola O. Leptin and lipid metabolism in chronic kidney failure. Scand J Clin Lab Invest 2009;69(3):401–8.

100. Sharma K, Considine RV, Michael B, et al. Plasma leptin is partly cleared by the kidney and is elevated in hemodialysis patients. Kidney Int 1997;51(6):1980–5.

101. Mathew AV, Okada S, Sharma K. Obesity related kidney disease. Curr Diabetes Rev 2011;7(1):41–9.

102. Wolf G, Ziyadeh FN. Leptin and renal fibrosis. Contrib Nephrol 2006;151: 175–83.

103. Park HS, Park JY, Yu R. Relationship of obesity and visceral adiposity with serum concentrations of CRP, TNF-alpha and IL-6. Diabetes Res Clin Pract 2005;69(1): 29–35.

104. Gupta J, Mitra N, Kanetsky PA, et al. Association between albuminuria, kidney function, and inflammatory biomarker profile. Clin J Am Soc Nephrol 2012. http://dx.doi.org/10.2215/CJN.03500412.

105. Ruiz-Ortega M, Ruperez M, Lorenzo O, et al. Angiotensin II regulates the synthesis of proinflammatory cytokines and chemokines in the kidney. Kidney Int Suppl 2002;(82):S12–22.

106. Ikezumi Y, Suzuki T, Karasawa T, et al. Activated macrophages down-regulate podocyte nephrin and podocin expression via stress-activated protein kinases. Biochem Biophys Res Commun 2008;376(4):706–11.

107. Patel NS, Chatterjee PK, Di Paola R, et al. Endogenous interleukin-6 enhances the renal injury, dysfunction, and inflammation caused by ischemia/reperfusion. J Pharmacol Exp Ther 2005;312(3):1170–8.

108. Tomiyama-Hanayama M, Rakugi H, Kohara M, et al. Effect of interleukin-6 receptor blockage on renal injury in apolipoprotein E-deficient mice. Am J Physiol Renal Physiol 2009;297(3):F679–84.

109. Ahmed SB, Fisher ND, Stevanovic R, et al. Body mass index and angiotensin-dependent control of the renal circulation in healthy humans. Hypertension 2005;46(6):1316–20.

110. Kennefick TM, Anderson S. Role of angiotensin II in diabetic nephropathy. Semin Nephrol 1997;17(5):441–7.

111. Zhuo JL, Li XC. Novel roles of intracrine angiotensin II and signalling mechanisms in kidney cells. J Renin Angiotensin Aldosterone Syst 2007;8(1):23–33.

112. Griffin KA, Bidani AK. Progression of renal disease: renoprotective specificity of renin-angiotensin system blockade. Clin J Am Soc Nephrol 2006;1(5):1054–65.
113. Crowley SD, Gurley SB, Coffman TM. AT(1) receptors and control of blood pressure: the kidney and more. Trends Cardiovasc Med 2007;17(1):30–4.
114. Ziyadeh FN. Mediators of diabetic renal disease: the case for tgf-Beta as the major mediator. J Am Soc Nephrol 2004;15(Suppl 1):S55–7.
115. Jiang G, Li Z, Liu F, et al. Prevention of obesity in mice by antisense oligonucleotide inhibitors of stearoyl-CoA desaturase-1. J Clin Invest 2005;115(4):1030–8.

Diabetic Kidney Disease in Elderly Individuals

Mark E. Williams, MD

KEYWORDS

- Diabetes • Kidney disease • Elderly individuals

KEY POINTS

- Elderly individuals represent the fastest growing subgroup of the US general population, and diabetes mellitus is now a major health issue affecting them.
- Chronic kidney disease complicates diabetes and also has an increased prevalence in elderly individuals.
- The kidneys are among the most prominent body organs affected by both the aging process and by diabetes.

INTRODUCTION

Elderly individuals represent the fastest growing subgroup of the US general population, and diabetes mellitus is now a major health issue affecting them. The reported incidence of diagnosed diabetes in this elderly cohort is 10% to 18%, compared with roughly 8% of the general population. In the decade between 1994 and 2004, the prevalence of diabetes in persons more than 65 in the United States increased by 62%.[1] A recent report documented that the prevalence of both diabetes and prediabetes have reached new levels,[2] with total crude prevalence (diagnosed and undiagnosed cases) reported as 30% for those older than 60 years. This growing epidemic has been linked to obesity, tobacco use, urbanization, physical inactivity, poor nutrition, and improved survival of diabetic patients, and aging.[3] The number of individuals globally with diabetes and older than 65 years, which doubled between 1900 and 2000, is projected to double again by 2030 (**Fig. 1**).[4]

Chronic kidney disease (CKD) complicates diabetes and also has an increased prevalence in elderly individuals. Particularly in those older than 60 years, the most common cause of CKD and end-stage renal disease (ESRD) in the United States is diabetic kidney disease.[5] A third of new ESRD cases in people older than 75 years are caused by diabetic nephropathy. According to prevalence estimates from the Third National Health and Nutrition Examination Survey (NHANES III), approximately a third of older diabetic individuals have microalbuminuria, the earliest clinical stage

Renal Unit, Joslin Diabetes Center, 1 Joslin Place, Boston, MA 02215, USA
E-mail address: mark.williams@joslin.harvard.edu

Med Clin N Am 97 (2013) 75–89
http://dx.doi.org/10.1016/j.mcna.2012.10.011   medical.theclinics.com
0025-7125/13/$ – see front matter © 2013 Elsevier Inc. All rights reserved.

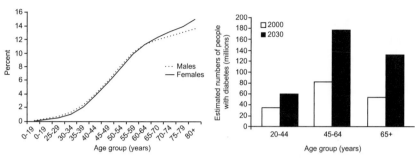

Fig. 1. Global diabetes prevalence by age and sex in 2000 (*left*), and estimated number of adults with diabetes by age group worldwide in 2000 and 2030 (*right*). (*Data from* Wild S, Roglic G, Gren A, et al. Global prevalence of diabetes: estimates for the year 2000 and projections for 2030. Diabetes Care 2004;27:1047–53.)

of diabetic kidney disease (although a nonspecific finding). Among 2570 older patients with diabetes in the US Veterans' Integrated Service Network, nearly half (48%) were afflicted with CKD, most of the time mild to moderate in severity.[6] A recent report on the prevalence of CKD and comorbid illness in elderly persons determined from 3 sources: laboratory tests in the Kidney Early Evaluation Program (KEEP) (a free community-based health screening program that targets adults at high risk of kidney disease based on personal or family history), NHANES (the cross-sectional probability samples of the civilian noninstitutionalized US population), and the prevalence of diagnosed CKD determined from billing codes of a random 5% sample of the US Medicare population. In all 3 data sets, the prevalence of CKD was higher in individuals suffering with diabetes (KEEP 48% vs 40%, NHANES 58% vs 41%, Medicare 14% vs 4%).[7]

Over the past quarter century, the fraction of patients with diabetic renal disease in the total population initiating dialysis in the United States has increased from about one-sixth to almost half, related to the epidemic of diabetics and the increased acceptance of diabetic patients into dialysis programs. Patients with diabetes as the primary causes of kidney failure now account for 45% of the incident (ie, new) ESRD population annually, up to a third of patients with type 2 diabetes develop ESRD and require renal replacement therapy for survival.[8] Internationally, Malaysia, Mexico, and the United States have the highest percentage of incident patients with ESRD with diabetes. Diabetes is responsible for half of all ESRD cases in New Zealand and Singapore, and is the fastest growing cause of ESRD in Europe.[9] Diabetes was present in 37% of elderly patients with ESRD in Canada.[10] This growing population represents unique challenges in multidisciplinary medical management. Many carry multiple comorbid conditions, such as ischemic heart disease, congestive heart failure, and peripheral vascular disease. Patients have hearing and visual disabilities, coexisting cognitive[11] and psychiatric disorders, frequently require nursing home care or assisted living, and may be unwilling or unable to comply with their proposed treatment. Diabetic ESRD is also associated with increased risk of dementia, especially as a result of vascular disease, leading to adverse outcomes. Both elderly and diabetic patients are less likely to have an arteriovenous fistula, the dialysis access recommended to cause fewer complications.[12]

PATHOPHYSIOLOGY

The kidneys are among the most prominent body organs affected by both the aging process and by diabetes. Kidney function and morphology are known to change with age. The kidney biopsy of a healthy elderly individual may include pathologic findings that have been considered a nonspecific part of the normal aging process.[13] Common findings in kidney biopsies of elderly individuals, variable in severity, include advanced vascular changes, fibrosis related to collagen accumulation and global sclerosis.[14] increases in mesangial and endothelial cell numbers, and relative podocyte depletion. Age-related increase in kidney fibrosis has been related to increased collagen accumulation.[15]

Pathologically, the aging kidney may be associated with mesangial matrix expansion and basement membrane thickening, nonspecific findings that are also recognized as key features of diabetic glomerulopathy. The contribution made by the aging process itself to age-associated CKD carries the potential that it could be accelerated by super-imposed conditions such as diabetes.[16] In older diabetic patients, classic findings of diabetic glomerulopathy (mesangial expansion, glomerular basement membrane thickening, Kimmelstiel-Wilson nodules) are compounded by advanced vascular changes,[17] which may be accompanied by adaptations that produce glomerular hyperperfusion injury. As an age-associated disease, it has been proposed that diabetes may accelerate cell and organ senescence in humans. It has recently been proposed that age-associated glomerulopathy may be understood as a senescence process affecting kidney cells such as the podocyte and accelerated by superimposed conditions such as diabetes, so that age-related changes are aggravated by diabetes. In the diabetic kidney, these changes would hinder the already limited ability of aged kidney tissue to repair itself. Verzola reported that diabetic nephropathy is associated with an acceleration of a senescent phenotype in kidney cells, using assays for senescence markers in kidney biopsies of patients with type 2 diabetic nephropathy.[18] The investigators propose that hyperglycemia may trigger the loss of repair capabilities, promote the early occurrence of senescence, and contribute to nephron loss in diabetic kidney disease. Hyperglycemia may also trigger oxidant stress and make it more difficult for kidney cells to undergo repair, leading to a state of accelerated senescence. A recent study by Tsaih and colleagues[19] suggested a common pathway for diabetic-related and age-related renal disease by finding genetic overlap of loci associated with albuminuria in aging mice and with proteinuria in human diabetic patients. Using a haplotype-association mapping approach was used to identify quantitative trait locus linkage. One significant and 8 suggestive loci were found. These loci were then compared with genome-wide association scans for diabetic nephropathy from a previously reported genome-wide association study.[20] Two of the 9 mouse loci for age-associated albuminuria were significantly associated with diabetic nephropathy.

Pathologic changes of aging may also reflect accumulation of advanced glycation end products (AGEs) in kidney tissues in aging and diabetes. Increasing evidence indicates that AGEs do accumulate during normal aging and contribute to the aging phenotype.[21,22] Glycation is a slow, nonenzymatic reaction between free amino groups in proteins and reducing sugars such as glucose that leads to the formation of heterogeneous end products. The expression for receptor for AGE (RAGE), an important transducer of AGE effects, is increased in both aging and diabetes. AGEs accumulate at an accelerated rate during the course of diabetes[22] and have been implicated in diabetic complications. AGEs are believed to be important contributors to inflammation in aging.[23] AGEs promote oxidation and inflammation through cell surface RAGE receptors. It has been recently proposed by Vlassara and colleagues[24] that the decline in kidney function with aging may be linked to oxidative stress and inflammation. In aging mice, greater oxidant intake is associated with increased age-related CKD.[25] Diabetic patients also have high serum AGE levels and increased oxidative stress and inflammation in the diabetic kidney. The role of AGE deposition in elderly humans with diabetic kidney disease remains to be determined.

Natural History

The classic presentation of CKD caused by diabetes mellitus is albuminuria initially, followed later by a decline in glomerular filtration rate (GFR). The typical course of diabetic nephropathy from microalbuminuria to CKD to ESRD is shown in **Fig. 2**.[26] However, compared with the classic presentation for diabetic nephropathy in younger individuals (heightened function then albuminuria followed by loss of function), it is known that there may be a higher prevalence of atypical presentations of diabetic kidney disease in this population (for example, decreased GFR without albuminuria). In 1 study, two-thirds of elderly diabetic patients with age-adjusted kidney impairment were lacking albuminuria.[27] Conversely, the presence of albuminuria in the elderly diabetic patient is often caused by conditions other than diabetic kidney disease.

Accurate assessment of kidney function is required for determining the prevalence and natural progression of kidney impairment, for morbidity and mortality risk stratification associated with CKD, and for evaluating the impact of new therapies in elderly populations. Moderate reductions in kidney function with aging have been shown both in cross-sectional and longitudinal surveys such as NHANES, and also in a series of healthy potential kidney donors.[28] The decline is associated with a proportionate decrease in renal blood flow. According to cross-sectional and longitudinal studies, GFR decreases by about 1 mL/min/1.73 m^2 after about age 30 years as a result of physiologic aging[29] (without diabetes). The age-related decline in kidney function seems to continue after age 60 years, so that normal GFR when measured as inulin clearance is about 80 mL/min/1.73 m^2 for those aged 75 to 79 years, and 65 mL/min/1.73 m^2 for those 80 to 89 years of age. Nonetheless, as a result of the typical age-related loss of function, elderly patients may be mislabeled as having moderate CKD despite the fact

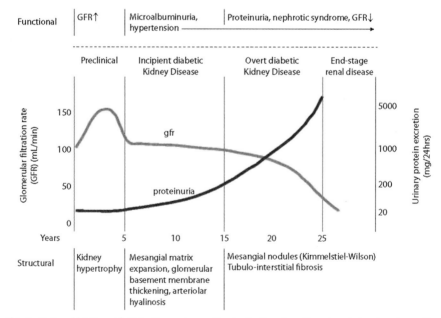

Fig. 2. Natural history of diabetic nephropathy, including functional and structural manifestations (course typical of type 1 diabetes). (*From* Vora JP, Chattington PD, Ibrahin H. Clinical manifestations and natural history of diabetic nephropathy. In: Comprehensive clinical nephrology. Elsevier; 2000; with permission.)

that their GFR corrected for age is not reduced.[30] Although most individuals have a decline in kidney function after age 30 years, up to a third did not in a recent longitudinal study. The natural history of the disease must be interpreted with this reality in mind, and the additional effect of disease progress on kidney function should be age-adjusted.[31]

Glomerular hyperfiltration is a well-characterized feature of type 1 diabetes that may be regarded as a potential risk factor for nephropathy complications in those patients. Age-unadjusted definitions of hyperfiltration range from 125 to 140 mL/min/1.73 m². In a survey of 662 patients with type 2 diabetes, GFR was measured by 99-tech-DTPA, and hyperfiltration determined using an age-unadjusted threshold of more than 130 mL/min/1.73 m² and incorporating a decline of 1 mL/min/1.73 m²/y after age 40 years (**Fig. 3**).[32] The prevalence of hyperfiltration was 7.4% with age-unadjusted and 16.6% with age-adjusted definitions. In those older than 65 years, adjusting for age increased the prevalence of hyperfiltration from 0.3% to 9.0%. Its pathogenic significance continues to be explored.

The natural history of elderly diabetic patients with CKD is also dominated by the cardiovascular complications of diabetes and diabetic kidney disease. Substantial observational evidence indicates that albuminuria is associated with increased risk of cardiovascular disease.[33] In a recent report of patients older than 65 years with and without hypertension and diabetes, a close correlation was found between micro-albuminuria and cardiovascular disease, inflammatory markers such as C-reactive protein, and systolic blood pressure.[34] Other factors may be a long history of hypertension, preexisting kidney disease, exposure to nephrotoxic medications, and renal ischemia caused by atherosclerotic occlusive disease.

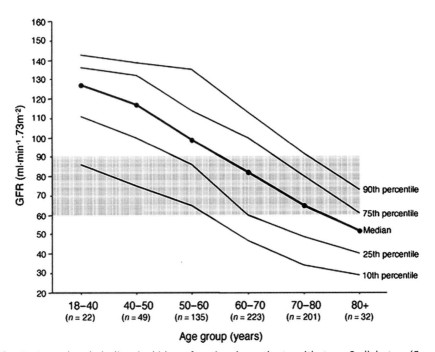

Fig. 3. Age-related decline in kidney function in patients with type 2 diabetes. (*From* Premaratne E, MacIsaac RJ, Tsalamandris C, et al. Renal hyperfiltration in type 2 diabetes: effect of age-related decline in glomerular filtration rate. Diabetologia 2005;48:2486–93; with permission.)

Diagnosis

There are few studies on which to base a diagnostic approach to diabetic kidney disease in elderly individuals. For example, how often diabetic retinopathy is absent, what the proper duration of diabetes is, and how commonly microscopic hematuria is present, are not clear. Screening for diabetic complications such as nephropathy should therefore be individualized in older adults. Evaluation of the elderly diabetic patient with kidney disease must take into account the different and frequently over-lapping histologic changes of diabetic glomerulopathy and aging, the increase in nondiabetic glomerular diseases, progression occurring independent of albuminuria, and an increased incidence of renovascular disease; a second factor is the likelihood that loss of function may be instead caused by aging itself. There could be a higher prevalence of unusual presentations of diabetic kidney disease in the elderly patients (for example, decreased GFR without albuminuria), although there are no studies that have addressed this issue. Another factor that needs to be considered in elderly indi-viduals is the existence of renal artery stenosis related primarily to atherosclerotic disease (renin-angiotensin-aldosterone system [RAS]). Indications for a kidney biopsy should include an active urinary sediment (many red blood cells or white blood cells or casts), high quantity of proteinuria (especially greater than 3 g/24 h), or a rapidly declining estimated GFR (eGFR).

TREATMENT

The standards of therapy for diabetic nephropathy in the general population are the triad of blood glucose control, blood pressure control, and administration of angiotensin-converting enzyme inhibitors (ACEI) or angiotensin receptor blockers (ARBs). The goals that have been established through clinical studies are a hemoglobin A1c (HbA1c) of less than 7%, a blood pressure of less than 130/80, and reduction of total urine protein to less than 500 mg/g of creatinine, or of urine albumin to less than 300 mg/g of creat-inine. These goals have been validated in a young to middle-aged population, but not in the elderly population. As a result, although CKD care of the elderly diabetic patient is central to their management, guidelines in the United States as well as Europe only marginally address this difficult population.[35]

To what extent should issues of CKD treatment and outcomes be addressed differ-ently in the geriatric diabetic population? Significant drawbacks in their application to the elderly diabetic population do exist: (1) the goals have been validated in young to middle-aged diabetic kidney patients and they do not distinguish between different age groups. Neither the efficacy nor safety of these goals may take into account the special needs of elderly patients with diabetes. For example, the risks of tight glycemic control have emerged in several recent studies of the general diabetic population.[36–39] (2) The guideline-based approach emphasizes primary and secondary prevention of diabetic kidney disease as a microvascular complication, although the elderly diabetic population may have more advanced microvascular disease, mixed renal pathophys-iology, and advanced macrovascular disease; and (3) data are not available to prior-itize the recommended interventions, a problem of greater relevance to the elderly population. Elderly diabetic patients with CKD may have different needs emanating from their greater frailty, higher comorbidity index, and shorter life expectancy, and may warrant a lower renoprotection treatment intensity than a younger population.[40] As noted in a recent review by Abatteruso and colleagues,[41] neither the EDAC (Euro-pean Diabetes and Aging Guidelines), the ADAG (American Diabetes and Aging Guidelines), the National Kidney Foundation Disease Outcomes Quality Initiative (KDOQI) Clinical Practice Guidelines and Clinical Practice Recommendations for

Diabetes and CKD, nor the Quality Indicators for the Care of Vulnerable Elders 3 (ACOVE-3) adequately address diabetic CKD in elderly individuals. For example, a time horizon (time to expected benefit) of glycemic management could exceed that of RAS blockade or hypertension control and must be measured against life expectancy in elderly individuals. Glycemic control may take as long as 8 years to positively affect microvascular complications.[40]

Nonetheless, evidence that benefit of treatment is occurring has emerged from a recent analysis from the Centers for Disease Control and Prevention, which determined that the decline in diabetes-related ESRD incidence included all age groups, including those older than 75 years (**Fig. 4**).[42] Using US Renal Data System data, Burrows and colleagues analyzed patients with incident ESRD who had diabetes listed as their primary diagnosis between 1990 and 2006. Incidence was calculated using the estimated US population with diabetes from the National Health Survey, followed by age adjustment. Whereas the number of those with diabetes-related ESRD treatment almost tripled between 1990 and 2006, the age-adjusted diabetes-related ESRD incidence decreased from 1996 to 2006, by 3.9% per year. Among individuals aged 65 to 74 years, rates decreased by 3.4% (beginning in 1998), and for those 75 years or older, by 2.1% (beginning in 1999). (Previously reported data had shown declining incidence only for those younger than 65 years.)

Glycemic Control

A recent report on the management of diabetes in elderly patients complicated by CKD[40] reviewed recent guidelines and data limitations on the matter. Regarding glycemic control, the KDOQI 2005 guidelines on diabetes and CKD emphasized the benefit of strict metabolic control early in progression, (ie, prevention of microalbuminuria), with evidence weak in later stages.[43] Although improved glycemic control may significantly reduce the risk of microvascular complications, the benefit on cardiovascular outcomes remains uncertain. No studies have prospectively evaluated the impact of intense glycemic control in patients older than 65 years. The UKPDS (United Kingdom Prospective Diabetes Study) is usually cited as the major large randomized

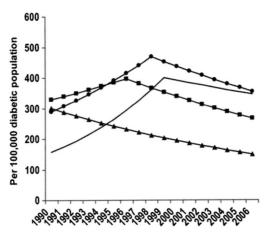

Fig. 4. Age-specific incidence of diabetes-related ESRD in the US population with diabetes mellitus, from 1990 to 2006. Symbols: triangles, <45 years; squares, 45–64 years; circles, 65–74 years; line, ≥75 years. (*From* Burrows NR, Li Y, Geiss LS. Incidence of treatment for end-stage renal disease among individuals with diabetes in the U.S. continue to decline. Diabetes Care 2010;33:73–7; with permission.)

controlled study in type 2 diabetes (patients 53.4 ± 8 years) to confirm the benefit of glycemic control in reducing microvascular complications.[44]

On the other hand, the risks of tight glycemic control in the general diabetes population have emerged in several recent studies. Collectively, 3 large trials (ACCORD [Action to Control Cardiovascular Risk in Diabetes], mean age 62 years[45]; ADVANCE, mean age 66 years[46]; and VADT, mean age 60 years[47]) have evaluated nearly 23,000 individuals with type 2 diabetes. Renal benefit varied among the studies, whereas cardiovascular benefit was lacking in all 3 trials. In ADVANCE, for example, the renal benefit involved a 21% reduction in the incidence of kidney disease (albuminuria) in the intensive treatment group. Importantly, hypoglycemia affected a significant proportion of patients in the intensive treatment groups of all 3 studies. The ACCORD study compared a strategy of intensive control (HbA1c target <6.0%) or standard control (hemoglobin target 7%–7.9%). The targeting of normal glycemic levels for 3.5 years led to increased mortality and did not significantly reduce major cardiovascular events or renal outcomes. In the ADVANCE study, severe hypoglycemia occurred occasionally but more commonly in the intensive control group. Intensification of therapy in older patients should be approached cautiously.

Definitive studies on the effects of glycemic control on progression of kidney disease in elderly individuals are lacking. Hyperglycemia leading to symptoms or risk of acute hyperglycemia complications should be avoided in all patients, including elderly patients. Recent guidelines regarding older patients with diabetes now recommend individualized care based on comorbid conditions, projected life expectancy, health care goals, and treatment preferences.[48] Only adults who are functional and have significant life expectancy should have the same diabetes treatment goals as younger adults.[49] The presence of advanced CKD further complicates management and requires prudence because of increasing comorbidities, limited life expectancy, and effects of kidney impairment on drug metabolism. Oral hypoglycemic agents to be avoided include chlorpropamide and glyburide (severe hypoglycemia) and metformin (fatal lactic acidosis).[50]

Blood Pressure Control

Hypertension is a hallmark of diabetic CKD in general, and in elderly patients may be present before kidney disease becomes evident. Central mechanisms are believed to involve the additive consequences of increased extracellular volume and enhanced vascular tone. Hypertension management of the elderly diabetic kidney patient suffers many of the same uncertainties as does glycemic control, although benefits to be derived from blood pressure control could occur significantly earlier. Hypertension is associated with worsening kidney function in diabetes, as well as cardiovascular complications such as stroke, major cardiovascular events, and heart failure. The importance of blood pressure control in slowing progression of diabetic kidney disease in younger individuals has been established in many studies.

The threshold for high blood pressure treatment is generally defined as 140/80 for elderly type 2 diabetic patients, whereas the Seventh Report of the Joint National Committee on Prevention, Detection, Evaluation, and Treatment of High Blood Pressure[51] defines hypertension as greater than 130/80 in the setting of diabetes or CKD. High blood pressure is presents in 40% to more than 90% of diabetic patients suffering from kidney complications. Its prevalence increases as kidney disease progresses, from microalbuminuria to kidney impairment. In addition, systolic pressure tends to increase, whereas diastolic blood pressure decreases after 66 to 69 years. Isolated systolic hypertension is the most common hypertension pattern in the elderly population. Furthermore, data from the Systolic Hypertension in the Elderly Population study, which included a small percentage of diabetic patients, showed a stronger correlation of systolic pressure with declining kidney function.[52] Over the full range of systolic pressures, the risk of kidney disease progression increased 2-fold.

Although several hypertension guidelines published in recent years have included management of hypertensive diabetic patients, specific recommendations for the elderly subgroup are lacking. Many studies that provide evidence for the guidelines have had limited sample sizes of diabetic patients, particularly those older than 70 years. Evidence for basing medical conclusions for the benefit/risk of tight blood pressure control on CKD progression in elderly diabetic patients is inadequate. Controlling blood pressure may be more important for prevention of cardiovascular risks, with potential benefits to reduce the risk of cardiac and neurologic events. Because of this situation, cardiovascular risk assessment should be completed at the time of diagnosis of hypertension. There are no randomized clinical trials to establish target blood pressures for elderly diabetic patients with CKD, so that uncertainty persists. For frail elderly patients, a goal of 150/80 may be acceptable. Likewise, there is no specific mix of blood pressure medications that is better in elderly patients compared with other groups. However, the selection of antihypertensive agents that provide renoprotection, such as RAS blockers, are recommended as first-line agents. Guidelines in general support the use of renin-angiotensin blockade and diuretics as initial therapy.[53] For cardiovascular risk, ACEI are viewed as the most beneficial agents. For hypertension control, more than 1 agent is typically necessary.

There remains debate as to how low the blood pressure should be decreased. The debate centers in part around uncertainty as to whether there is a J-shaped curve in mortality (ie, whether there could be an increase in mortality and worsening of kidney disease when blood pressure decreases less than a certain level). Diabetic elderly patients are clearly at higher risk for significant decreases in blood pressure for several reasons. Elderly patients tend to have decreased intake of salt and water, and may have higher losses of salt and water through perspiration and urine/stool losses. In addition, elderly individuals, and especially diabetic elderly patients, tend to have some degree of autonomic dysfunction. This situation prevents an increase in both heart rate and vasoconstriction with upright posture, leading to postural hypotension. Further risks of excessive decrease of blood pressure may occur with antihypertensive agents, so that physicians managing patients with diabetic kidney disease need to be aware of such risks, in order to prescribe drugs appropriately and to determine the age-appropriate blood pressure goal. In general, it seems that less than 140/90 mm Hg is a reasonable target.

RAS Blockade

Another important therapeutic intervention is the use of ACEI and ARBs in diabetic elderly patients. The value of these drugs in slowing progression of diabetic kidney disease has been established for both type 1[54] and type 2[55,56] diabetic patients. The acknowledged current standard of care is to start an ACEI or ARB in any patient with microalbuminuria or overt proteinuria even if blood pressure is at goal. Based on pathophysiologic evidence that overactivity of RAS is a dominant factor in the disease, clinical trials have led to the use of ACEI and ARBs as standard agents for diabetic kidney disease since the late 1990s. RAS activation is now known to lead to hemodynamic, biochemical, and histologic effects in diabetic glomerulopathy. RAS blockade improves systemic and intrarenal hemodynamics and the glomerular filtration barrier, and reduces intraglomerular pressures.

Current practice guidelines promulgated by the American Diabetes Association, the Joint National Commission, and the National Kidney Foundation support the use of both ACEI and ARBs as initial therapies for diabetic kidney disease. Both ACEI and ARBs are more effective than other antihypertensives in reducing proteinuria[57] and slowing the progression to kidney failure in patients with diabetic CKD. Both agents have superior antiproteinuric effects compared with other agents. In this largely hypertensive population, RAS blockers are more advantageous than other agents when blood pressure remains more than goal and achieve less superiority when blood pressure has been normalized. One important caveat is that kidney function may initially decline, because angiotensin blockade effectively lowers systemic pressures. However, mild initial loss of glomerular filtration (25%) may reflect effective RAS blockade and need not require cessation of ACEI or ARB therapy. In addition to stabilization of kidney function, a principal outcome target of RAS blockers and an earlier sign of efficacy is reduction in proteinuria. Clinical trial data do indicate that worse proteinuria is associated with a greater likelihood of progressive loss of function in diabetic kidney disease.[58]

Nonetheless, direct evidence of the benefit of RAS blockers in elderly patients remains unproved, and their use is an extrapolation from adult clinical trials of mostly middle-aged patients. There have been no large-scale clinical trials using ACEI to prevent kidney failure in type 2 patients. In the primary trials using ARBs, the mean age of participants was about 60 years. Regulatory trials indicated that in patients who already have progressed to overt nephropathy and have impaired GFR, ARBs can slow the progression to ESRD, albeit not stopping or reversing the decline. RENAAL was a large-scale randomized placebo-controlled trial evaluating losartan 50 to 100 mg daily against placebo in 1513 type 2 patients who were followed for 3.4 years.[55] The benefit was significant, with assignment to the ARB arm reducing the risk of doubling of serum creatinine by 25% and of ESRD by 28%. Furthermore, proteinuria was reduced by 35%, and reduction in ESRD risk was proportional to the decrease in proteinuria achieved. In those who did have a doubling of serum creatinine, the later development of ESRD was still less likely with the study drug. Confirmation of the RAS blockade benefit for CKD occurred in the IDNT trial,[56] a second landmark RAS blockade trial, and for slowing of microalbuminuria in the IRMA trial.[59]

Of importance to geriatric kidney disease, a recent follow-up report evaluated the safety and efficacy of losartan in the roughly one-quarter of patients in the RENAAL study who were 65 years of age. The investigators tested for effect modification by age of the impact of losartan on the incidence of the predefined end points (doubling of serum creatinine, ESRD, or death). The incidence of adverse events was also analyzed. The older group had the same benefit as the younger participants, even with no more risk for worsening of creatinine or potassium levels. Losartan reduced the risk of a composite outcome of creatinine doubling, ESRD, and death in this group.[60] Furthermore, in the oldest tertile, the rate of doubling of baseline serum creatinine was reduced by 38% with losartan, and the event rate of ESRD by 50%. Although not specifically conducted in an elderly population, the study provides the best clinical trial evidence available in support of ARB blockade of the RAS in older patients. However, CKD in the elderly diabetic population may frequently lack proteinuria and therefore be less responsive to RAS blockade. In NHANES III, a third of those surveyed with type 2 diabetes aged 60 to 70 years and with normal urinary albumin excretion nonetheless had a GFR of less than 30 mL/min, and almost half were between 30 and 60 mL/min.[61] Many studies have shown that increases in protein in the urine increase the risk of progressing to renal failure.[58]

Many elderly diabetic patients are apparently not prescribed ACEI or ARBs. In a study of Medicare patients in 2002 in Pennsylvania,[57] most of whom were 75 to 84 years of age, only about half of the hypertensive kidney patients were on either an ACEI or ARB. The investigators reviewed Medicare data for 2002 on patients residing in Pennsylvania who had diabetes. Of 30,750 patients identified, 21,053 had hypertension and 1243 were identified as having proteinuria or proteinuria and kidney disease. Most patients were 75 to 84 years old. Of the hypertensive only patients, 50.5% were on an ACEI or ARB; of the proteinuria patients, 40%; and for those with both hypertension and proteinuria, 54.7%. In each diagnostic category, roughly 25% fewer were under ACEI/ARB therapy than in a separate report regarding a younger cohort.[55] The investigators speculate that safety concerns about hyperkalemia and reduction in kidney function either acutely or during progression to ESRD, and lack of efficacy data in elderly individuals, underlie the prescription pattern. A recent study of a large community-based cohort in Canada also provided data on ACEI/ARB use.[62] The study evaluated the impact of estimated GFR reporting with nephrology visits and health care resource use. After the implementation of eGFR reporting, the rate of first outpatient nephrology visits for CKD increased by 68.4%, and referral rates were even higher for elderly patients with diabetes. Reporting of eGFR was not associated with an increase in ACEI/ARB use, perhaps because most (77.5%) of the elderly patients with diabetes were already under treatment.

Preventing cardiovascular morbidity and mortality may be a more important factor than delaying progression to ESRD, and may affect the selection of ACEI/ARBs in elderly patients. Existing guidelines suggest that when reducing cardiovascular risk is the priority, ACEI should be considered first-line therapy, and ARBs the first alternative. In addition, many studies have showed that microalbuminuria and proteinuria are strong risk factors for cardiovascular disease.[63–65] A recent study by Barzilay[34] explored the association of microalbuminuria in patients with and without hypertension and diabetes in a group that was 65 years and older. This investigator evaluated a wide range of variables, including endothelial dysfunction and inflammatory markers, in an effort to determine why there is a close association between microalbuminuria and cardiovascular disease. The results showed that there was a close correlation of microalbuminuria and cardiovascular disease with increasing age, inflammatory markers (such as C-reactive protein), and systolic blood pressure. These results underscore the importance of implementing blood pressure control and other approaches (blood glucose control and the use of ACE inhibitors and ARBs) in patients with microalbuminuria in order to reduce the risk of cardiovascular disease.

COMPREHENSIVE THERAPY

It should not be surprising, based on this information, that little is known about the risks/benefits of multiple combined therapies for diabetic CKD in elderly individuals. One study from Scotland by Joss and colleagues[66] of 90 patients whose mean age was 63 years (57% men and 43% women) showed the potential importance of aggressive intervention. The study was a prospective randomized controlled study. Patients with type 2 diabetes and nephropathy were randomly allocated to an intensive group ($n = 47$) or control group ($n = 43$) and followed for 2 years. Treatment targets were the same for both groups, but the intensive group were seen as often as required to meet the targets; controls were seen at their normal clinics. Specifically the treatment goals were: systolic blood pressure less than 140 mm Hg, diastolic blood pressure less than 80 mm Hg, HbA1c less than 8%, sodium intake less than 120 mmol/d, protein intake 0.7 to 1 g/kg of ideal body weight per day, and cholesterol less than 4 mmol/L or cholesterol/high-density lipoprotein cholesterol ratio less than 4. The primary end point was the rate of progression of renal disease in the second year. The results showed that the median rate of loss of kidney function (creatinine clearance) in the intensive group decreased from 0.44 mL/min/mo in the first year to 0.14 mL/min/mo in the second year, compared with 0.49 mL/min/mo and 0.53 mL/min/mo in the control group (P = .04 for second year). In this study, the intensively treated group achieved a rate of decline similar to the nondiabetic, healthy population, which is 1 mL/min/y or 0.083 mL/min/mo. Considering that the mean creatinine clearance at the start of the trial was 55 mL/min, these results if sustainable could delay the onset of dialysis by several years in the intensive group compared with the control group.

For other treatment considerations of diabetic CKD, it is reasonable to assume that treatment approaches considered for younger patients may not apply to elderly individuals. These approaches include drugs already approved for hypertension (aldosterone blockers, renin inhibitors) or for other indications (vitamin D analogues, thiazoledinediones, statins). The risk/benefit ratios of existing therapies for diabetic CKD as applied to the elderly population remain largely undetermined. For emerging therapies, inclusion of elderly patients in regulatory trials, taking into account the GFR decline caused by aging, the prevalence of nondiabetic kidney disease, and the potential for excessive risk, is a desirable goal.

SUMMARY

The treatment of diabetic nephropathy in elderly individuals is based primarily on data from younger age groups. However, the assumption that the same treatment approaches for the younger age groups can be uniformly applied to elderly individuals is likely to be incorrect. The cornerstones of aggressive therapy for diabetic kidney disease in general may have drawbacks in elderly patients. For example, significant risks of tight glycemic control have emerged in recent studies. Excessive decrease of blood pressure to existing targets may be unsafe in elderly individuals. Limited data do indicate that renin-angiotensin blockade may be as effective and no riskier than in middle-aged diabetic kidney patients. Until further studies are carried out, it is prudent to treat the elderly patient with similar approaches as in younger patients, but tempered by the issues reviewed in this article. There is a growing need for the development of clinical guidelines to retool CKD management in the elderly diabetic population using both current and emerging therapies.

REFERENCES

1. Sloan FA, Bethel A, Ruiz D Jr, et al. The growing burden of diabetes mellitus in the U.S. elderly population. Arch Intern Med 2008;168:192–9.
2. Covie CC, Rust KF, Ford ES, et al. Full accounting of diabetes and pre-diabetes in the U.S. population in 1988-1994 and 2005-2006. Diabetes Care 2009;32: 287–94.
3. Zimmet P, Alberti KG, Shaw J. Global and societal implications of the diabetes epidemic. Nature 2001;414:782–7.
4. Wild S, Roglic G, Gren A, et al. Global prevalence of diabetes: estimates for the year 2000 and projections for 2030. Diabetes Care 2004;27:1047–53.
5. Rosner M, Abdel-Rahman E, Williams ME. Geriatric nephrology: a new ASN priority. Clin J Am Soc Nephrol 2010;5:936–42.
6. Coresh J. Prevalence of chronic kidney and decreased kidney function in the adult US population: third National Health and Nutrition Examination Survey. Am J Kidney Dis 2003;41:1–12.
7. Stevens LA, Li S, Wang C, et al. Prevalence of CKD and comorbid illness in elderly patients in the United States: results from the Kidney Early Evaluation Program (KEEP). Am J Kidney Dis 2010;55(Suppl 2):S23–33.

8. Kurella M, Covinsky KE, Collins AJ, et al. Octogenarians and nonagenarians starting dialysis in the United States. Ann Intern Med 2007;146:177–83.

9. Van Dijk PC, Jager KJ, Stengel B, et al. Renal replacement therapy for diabetic end-stage renal disease: data from 10 registries in Europe (1991-2000). Kidney Int 2005;67:1489.

10. Letourneau I, Ouimet D, Dumont M, et al. Renal replacement in end-stage renal disease patients over 75 years old. Am J Nephrol 2003;23(2):71–7.

11. Kurella M, Chertow GM, Fried LF, et al. Chronic kidney disease and cognitive impairment in the elderly: the health, aging, and body composition study. J Am Soc Nephrol 2005;16(7):2127–33.

12. Loc CE, Oliver MJ, Su J, et al. Arteriovenous fistula outcomes in the era of the elderly dialysis population. Kidney Int 2005;67:2462–9.

13. Jefferson JA, Alpers CE. Should renal biopsies be performed in the very elderly? Nat Rev Nephrol 2009;5:561–2.

14. Martin JE, Sheaff MT. Renal ageing. J Pathol 2007;21:198–205.

15. Zhou XJ, Rakheja D, Yu X, et al. The ageing kidney. Kidney Int 2008;74:710–20.

16. Wiggins RC. The spectrum of podocytopathies: a unifying view of glomerular diseases. Kidney Int 2007;71:1205–14.

17. Nair R, Bell JM, Walker PD. Renal biopsy in patients 80 years and older. Am J Kidney Dis 2004;44:618–26.

18. Verzola D, Gandolfo MT, Gaetani G, et al. Accelerated senescence in the kidneys of patients with type 2 diabetic nephropathy. Am J Physiol Renal Physiol 2008; 295:F1563–73.

19. Tsaih SW, Pezzolesi MG, Yuan R, et al. Genetic analysis of albuminuria in ageing mice and concordance with loci for human diabetic nephropathy found in a genome-wide association scan. Kidney Int 2010;77:201–10.

20. Pezzolesi ZM, Poznik GD, Mychaleckyj JC. Genome-wide association scan for diabetic nephropathy susceptibility genes in type 1 diabetes. Diabetes 2009; 58:1403–10.

21. Semba RD, Nicklett EJ, Ferrucci L. Does accumulation of advanced glycation end products contribute to the ageing phenotype? J Gerontol A Biol Sci Med Sci 2010;65(9):963–75.

22. Kasper M, Funk RH. Age-related changes in cells and tissues due to advanced glycation end products (AGEs). Arch Gerontol Geriatr 2001;32:233–43.

23. Mei C, Zheng F. Chronic inflammation potentiates kidney ageing. Semin Nephrol 2009;29:555–68.

24. Vlassara H, Uribarri J, Ferrucci L, et al. Identifying advanced glycation end products as a major source of oxidants in ageing: implications for the management and/or prevention of reduced renal function in elderly persons. Semin Nephrol 2009;29:594–603.

25. Vlassara H, Torreggiani M, Post JB, et al. Role of oxidants/inflammation in declining renal function in chronic kidney disease and normal ageing. Kidney Int 2009;76(Suppl 114):S3–11.

26. Vora JP, Chattington PD, Ibrahin H. Clinical manifestations and natural history of diabetic nephropathy. In: Comprehensive clinical nephrology. Elsevier; 2000.

27. Wasen E, Isoaho R, Mattila K, et al. Renal impairment associated with diabetes in the elderly. Diabetes Care 2004;27:2648–53.

28. Ibrahim HN, Foley R, Tan L, et al. Long-term consequences of kidney donation. N Engl J Med 2009;360:459–69.

29. Rodriguez-Puyol D. The aging kidney. Kidney Int 1998;56:2247–55.

30. Raymond NT, Zehnder D, Smith SC, et al. Elevated relative mortality risk with mild-to-moderate chronic kidney disease decreases with age. Nephrol Dial Transplant 2007;22:3214–20.

31. Kausz AT. Chronic kidney disease in the older patient. Clin Geriatr 2004;12:39–47.

32. Premaratne E, MacIsaac RJ, Tsalamandris C, et al. Renal hyperfiltration in type 2 diabetes: effect of age-related decline in glomerular filtration rate. Diabetologia 2005;48:2486–93.

33. de Zeeuw D. Albuminuria, a therapeutic target for cardiovascular protection in type 2 diabetic patients with nephropathy. Circulation 2004;110:921–7.

34. Barzilay J. The relationship of cardiovascular risk factors to microalbuminuria in older adults with or without diabetes mellitus or hypertension: the cardiovascular health study. Am J Kidney Dis 2004;44:25–34.

35. Williams ME. Diabetic kidney disease in the older adult: an update. Aging Health 2009;5:625–33.

36. United Kingdom Prospective Diabetes Study (UKPDS) Group. Intensive blood-glucose control with sulphonylureas or insulin compared with conventional treatment and risk of complications in patients with type 2 diabetes (UKPDS 33). Lancet 1998;352:837–53.

37. Shorr RI, Franse LV, Resnick HE, et al. Glycemic control of older adults with type 2 diabetes: findings from the Third National Health and Nutrition Examination Survey, 1988-1994. J Am Geriatr Soc 2000;48:264–7.

38. Whitmer RA, Karter AJ, Yaffe K, et al. Hypoglycemic episodes and risk of dementia in older patients with type 2 diabetes mellitus. JAMA 2009;301:1565–72.

39. Kahn SE. Glucose control in type 2 diabetes: still worthwhile and worth controlling. JAMA 2009;301:1590–2.

40. Brown AF, Mangione CM, Saliba D, et al. Guidelines for improving the care of the older person with diabetes mellitus. J Am Geriatr Soc 2003;51:S265–80.

41. Abaterusso C, Lupo A, Ortalda V, et al. Treating elderly people with diabetes and Stages 3 and 4 chronic kidney disease. Clin J Am Soc Nephrol 2008;3:1185–94.

42. Burrows NR, Li Y, Geiss LS. Incidence of treatment for end-stage renal disease among individuals with diabetes in the U.S. continue to decline. Diabetes Care 2010;33:73–7.

43. KDOQI. KDOQI Clinical Practice Guidelines and Clinical Practice Recommendations for Diabetes and Chronic Kidney Disease. Am J Kidney Dis 2007;49(2 Suppl 2): S12–154.

44. Tkac I. Effect of intensive glycemic control on cardiovascular outcomes and all-cause mortality in type 2 diabetes: overview and metaanalysis of five trials. Diabetes Res Clin Pract 2009;86(Suppl 1):S57–62.

45. The Action to Control Cardiovascular Risk in Diabetes Study Group. Effects of intensive glucose lowering in type 2 diabetes. N Engl J Med 2008;358:2545–59.

46. The ADVANCE Collaborative Group. Intensive blood glucose and vascular outcomes in patients with type 2 diabetes. N Engl J Med 2008;358:2560–72.

47. Duckworth W, Abraira C, Moritz T, et al, for the VADT Investigators. Glucose control and vascular complications in veterans with type 2 diabetes. N Engl J Med 2009;360:129–39.

48. Abrahamson M. A 74-year-old woman with diabetes. Clinical Crossroads. JAMA 2007;297:196–204.

49. O'Hare AM, Bertenthal D, Covinsky KE, et al. Mortality risk stratification in chronic kidney disease: one size for all ages? J Am Soc Nephrol 2006;17:846–53.

50. Abbatecola AM, Paolisso G, Corsonello A, et al. Antidiabetic oral treatment in older people: does frailty matter? Drugs Aging 2009;26(Suppl 1):53–62.

51. Chobanian AV, Bakris GL, Black HR, et al. The seventh report of the Joint National Committee on Prevention, Detection, Evaluation, and Treatment of High Blood Pressure. JAMA 2003;289:19–29.
52. Young J. Blood pressure and decline in kidney function: findings from the Systolic Hypertension in the Elderly Program (SHEP). J Am Soc Nephrol 2002;13:276–82.
53. Kidney Disease Outcomes Quality Initiative (K/DOQI). KDOQI Clinical Practice Guidelines on hypertension and antihypertensive agents. Am J Kidney Dis 2004;43(Suppl 1):4–194.
54. Lewis E, Hunsicker LG, Bain RP, et al. The effect of angiotensin-converting-enzyme inhibition on diabetic nephropathy. N Engl J Med 1993;329:1456–62.
55. Brenner B, Cooper ME, de Zeeuw D, et al. Effects of losartan on renal and cardio-vascular outcomes in patients with type 2 diabetes and nephropathy. N Engl J Med 2001;345:861–9.
56. Lewis E, Hunsicker LG, Clarke WR, et al. Renoprotective effect of the angiotensin-receptor antagonist irbesartan in patients with nephropathy due to type 2 diabetes. N Engl J Med 2001;345:851–60.
57. Rosen AB, Karter AJ, Liu JY, et al. Use of angiotensin-converting enzyme inhibitors and angiotensin receptor blockers in high-risk clinical and ethnic groups with diabetes. J Gen Intern Med 2004;19:669–75.
58. Shahinfar S, Dickson T, Zhang Z, et al. Baseline predictors of end-stage renal disease risk in patients with type 2 diabetes and nephropathy: new lessons from the RENAAL study. Kidney Int 2005;67(Suppl 93):S48–51.
59. Parving HH, Lehnert H, Brochner-Mortensen J, et al. The effect of irbesartan on the development of diabetic nephropathy in patients with type 2 diabetes. N Engl J Med 2001;345:870–8.
60. Winkelmayer WC, Zhang Z, Shahinfar S, et al. Efficacy and safety of angiotensin II receptor blockade in elderly patients with diabetes. Diabetes Care 2006;29:2210–7.
61. Kramer HJ, Nguyen QD, Curhan G, et al. Renal insufficiency in the absence of albuminuria and retinopathy among adults with type 2 diabetes mellitus. JAMA 2003;289(24):3273–7.
62. Hemmelgarn BR, Zhang J, Manns B. Nephrology visits and health care resource use before and after reporting estimated glomerular filtration rate. JAMA 2010;303(12):1151–8.
63. Basi S, Lewis J. Microalbuminuria as a target to improve cardiovascular and renal outcomes. Am J Kidney Dis 2006;47(6):927–46.
64. Borch-Johnsen K, Feldt-Rasmussen B, Strandgaard S, et al. Urinary albumin excretion: an independent predictor of ischemic heart disease. Arterioscler Thromb Vasc Biol 1996;19:1992–7.
65. Miettinen H, Haffner SM, Lehto S, et al. Proteinuria predicts stroke and other atherosclerotic vascular disease events in nondiabetic and non–insulin-dependent diabetic subjects. Stroke 1996;27:2033–9.
66. Joss N, Ferguson C, Brown C, et al. Intensified treatment of patients with type 2 diabetes mellitus and overt nephropathy. QJM 2004;97(4):219–27.

The Genetic Risk of Kidney Disease in Type 2 Diabetes

Marcus G. Pezzolesi, PhD, MPH[a,b,]*,
Andrzej S. Krolewski, MD, PhD[a,b]

KEYWORDS

- Type 2 diabetes • Diabetic nephropathy • Kidney disease • Genetic risk

KEY POINTS

- Evidence in favor a genetic basis for the susceptibility of diabetic nephropathy (DN) in type 2 diabetes (T2D) has provided a foundation for studies aimed at identifying the causal genes responsible for its development.
- During this period, strategies used to map genes for DN have been driven by our understanding of variation across our genome and the technologies available to interrogate it; as both have evolved, so to have our approaches.
- The advent of next-generation sequencing technology and increased interest in the search for rare variants has begun to swing the pendulum of these efforts toward studies of pedigrees.
- Family based approaches should greatly facilitate efforts to identify variants in genes that have a major effect on the risk of DN in T2D. To be successful, the ascertainment and comprehensive study of families with multiple affected members is critical.

INTRODUCTION

Diabetic nephropathy (DN) is a major late complication of diabetes that affects approximately 40% of all patients with diabetes and remains the leading cause of end-stage renal disease (ESRD) in the United States.[1–3] As the incidence of type 2 diabetes (T2D) continues to increase in the United States and across the globe, so to are the personal and societal burdens associated with this complication.

Investigations on the familial clustering of DN in T2D and the heritability of DN and its related traits provide compelling evidence that genetic factors contribute to its susceptibility and have motivated studies aimed at identifying the causal genes

We acknowledge grant support from the National Institutes of Health (DK090125 to MGP and DK58549, DK77532 and DK53534 to ASK).

a Section on Genetics and Epidemiology, Research Division, Joslin Diabetes Center, One Joslin Place, Boston, MA 02215, USA; b Department of Medicine, Harvard Medical School, 25 Shattuck Street, Boston, MA 02115, USA

* Corresponding author. Section on Genetics and Epidemiology, Joslin Diabetes Center, Room 445C, One Joslin Place, Boston, MA 02215.
E-mail address: marcus.pezzolesi@joslin.harvard.edu

responsible for its development. For more than 20 years, investigators have been working to identify the genes that underlie its susceptibility. During this period, advances in genomics have expanded our understanding of genetic variation across our genome and its contribution to disease and facilitated cutting-edge technologies that have revolutionized our ability to identify the genes that underlie these conditions.

In this review, we discuss the approaches used to identify DN susceptibility genes in T2D, including their key findings, and present our perspective on future studies in this field.

FAMILIAL CLUSTERING OF NEPHROPATHY AND ESTIMATES OF ITS HERITABILITY IN T2D

Evidence of familial aggregation supports the notion that genetic factors play a major role in the susceptibility of DN in T2D.[4–7] In the earliest investigation of familial clustering of DN among families with T2D, Pettitt and colleagues[4] examined the risk of proteinuria among 316 Pima Indian families with diabetes in 2 generations. In this study, the risk of proteinuria among offspring with diabetes with a parent with proteinuria was 1.8 times higher than that of offspring of parents with diabetes without proteinuria. The adjusted prevalence of proteinuria among individuals with one parent with diabetes with proteinuria was 23%, compared with only 14% among offspring with 2 parents with diabetes with normoalbuminuria. The prevalence of proteinuria among offspring with 2 parents with diabetes with proteinuria was even greater, with 46% of these individuals having this complication.

In 52 multigenerational African American families, Freedman and colleagues[5] found that 37% of the patients with T2D-induced ESRD had either a first-, second-, or third-degree relative with ESRD, compared with only 7% of T2D controls. Individuals with diabetes from these families with a relative with ESRD were at an eightfold increased risk of developing ESRD. Studies by Faronato and colleagues[6] and Canani and colleagues[7] similarly demonstrated that siblings with T2D of probands with DN from Caucasian families had 3 to 4 times the risk of developing microalbuminuria and macroalbuminuria compared with a sibling of normoalbuminuic probands. Faronato and colleagues[6] also confirmed a previous report by Gruden and colleagues[8] that demonstrated that the albumin excretion rate (AER) was increased in nondiabetic family members of patients with T2D.

To more precisely determine the relative contribution of genetic factors to DN in T2D, we and others have estimated the heritability (h^2; ie, the proportion of total variation of a trait caused by genetic effects) of its correlated traits (ie, urinary AER and estimated glomerular filtration rate [eGFR]) in families with T2D.[9–13] In 96 large multigenerational families that included 630 individuals with T2D and 639 individuals with normoglycemia enrolled in the Joslin Study on the Genetics of Type 2 Diabetes, Fogarty and colleagues[9] estimated that 27% of the variance in the albumin-to-creatinine ratio (ACR) was genetically determined among all family members regardless of their diabetes status. In analyses restricted to individuals with diabetes, this estimate increased slightly to 31% and, supporting previous reports of familial clustering of AER among nondiabetic family members, h^2 was estimated to be 0.20 in nondiabetic individuals from this collection.

A subsequent analysis of the Joslin Study on the Genetics of Type 2 Diabetes collection restricted to families with a middle age at the onset of T2D (46 ± 16 years) reported similar estimates of heritability with ACR, ranging from 0.20 in all family members to 0.39 in relatives without diabetes.[11] An important strength of the Joslin T2D family collection is that its members were ascertained for studies on the genetics of T2D, not kidney complications. As such, these estimates of heritability are unlikely to be biased because of an enrichment of DN cases. Reinforcing the estimates obtained from this collection, Forsbolm and colleagues[10] and Langefeld and colleagues[12] reported similar heritability for AER in 267 nuclear families with T2D from Finland ($h^2 = 0.30$) and for ACR in 310 sibling pairs with T2D from the United States ($h^2 = 0.46$ in members with T2D and $h^2 = 0.35$ in all family members).

To evaluate the possible mode of inheritance of ACR in families with T2D, we performed a formal quantitative segregation analysis of this trait in members of the Joslin Study on the Genetics of Type 2 Diabetes collection.[14] In this analysis, evidence for the genetic effects on ACR was derived from its transmission between relatives across large pedigrees, which is an approach that provides substantial power in assessing this effect over studies limited to nuclear families. In models whereby the genetic effect was assessed separately in all members and in members with T2D members, the model that most completely described the control of ACR levels in these pedigrees combined the effects of at least one major locus (with a relatively common allele frequency between 0.25–0.40) with significant residual genetic variation that could be caused by multiple other genetic factors. These results are consistent with a previous segregation analysis of overt nephropathy by Imperatore and colleagues[15] that also supported the existence of a major DN gene with a common allele frequency in a collection of 715 nuclear Pima Indian families.

eGFR has also been shown to be a significantly heritable trait in families with T2D.[12,13] The first study to investigate this estimated the heritability of eGFR to be 0.75 among Caucasian sibling pairs with T2D and 0.69 in analyses that included all available family members.[12] Similarly, we found eGFR to be highly heritable in patients with T2D (h^2 ranging from 0.29–0.47) and all family members (h^2 ranging from 0.28–0.31) from the Joslin Study on the Genetics of Type 2 Diabetes collection.[13] To date, no formal segregation analysis of eGFR in T2D has been published.

Strong evidence of familial aggregation and the heritability of DN in T2D provides compelling evidence that DN and its related traits are influenced by genetic factors and suggest a complex, multifactorial mode of inheritance with one or more major susceptibility genes. Although a shared environment might contribute to some of the familial clustering of renal disease in T2D, these studies support the hypothesis that the increased risk of DN in T2D is partly caused by a shared gene or set of genes among affected family members. Together, these data have motivated investigations aimed at identifying the specific chromosomal regions that harbor genes contributing to its susceptibility. In the next 2 sections, we discuss the major approaches that are currently being used to identify DN susceptibility genes and highlight the salient findings from studies where they have been implemented.

GENOME-WIDE LINKAGE ANALYSES IDENTIFY SEVERAL SUSCEPTIBILITY LOCI FOR DN IN T2D

The major efforts to identify genes that cause DN in T2D have come from family based genome-wide linkage studies. These studies entail genotyping polymorphic genetic markers in families, typically either small nuclear families or multigenerational extended families, and evaluating the correlation between the phenotype of interest and the pattern of inheritance of these markers. Earlier studies used a set of approximately 300 to 400 highly polymorphic microsatellite markers dispersed across the genome. Conventional studies now use dense linkage panels comprised of 5000 or more single nucleotide polymorphisms (SNPs). An advantage of linkage-based approaches is that they offer a model-free screen of markers across the genome; however, linkage studies are limited with respect to the magnitude of the underlying genetic effect and the resolution with which they are able to pinpoint susceptibility loci. Linkage studies are generally powered to identify major disease loci (ie, those with effect sizes greater than 2.0) and typically localize linkage signals to regions several megabase pairs in length.

To date, a total of 11 complete genome-wide linkage scans have been published for DN in T2D.[11,13,15–23] The major findings from these studies are summarized in **Tables 1** and **2**. Although several distinct regions across the genome provide some evidence of linkage, consistent linkage with DN and its related phenotypes has been localized to several potential candidate loci.

The strongest evidence of linkage with DN was identified on chromosome 18q (maximum logarithm of odds score [MLS] = 6.1) in 18 extended Turkish families with 115 members with T2D.[16] Evidence of linkage to this same region was shown in both African American patients with T2D with ESRD[17] and with eGFR in 378 multiethnic families from the Family Investigation of Nephropathy and Diabetes (FIND) collection.[23] In the FIND study, the findings at this locus were primarily driven by Mexican American families who composed 52% of the families enrolled in this collection. Resequencing efforts in 135 patients with T2D DN and 107 T2D non-DN controls later identified a significant association at a trinucleotide repeat in exon 2 of the carnosinase 1 gene (CNDP1) that encodes a variable stretch of leucine residues (5, 6, or 7 leucines).[24] In this study, the 5-leucine allele was present in only 59% of chromosomes in patients with DN compared with 88% in those without DN. Functional studies confirmed the protective effects of this allele by demonstrating its ability to inhibit the production of extracellular matrix components in cultured human podocytes exposed to high glucose. Similarly, transforming growth factor (TGF)-β production was reduced in cultured mesangial cells exposed to high glucose. Additional support of this polymorphism's role in DN was provided by its association in 858 European American patients (294 patients with ESRD with T2D, 258 controls with T2D, and 306 healthy controls).[25]

A second locus with consistent support of linkage to DN in T2D localizes to chromosome 3q. Bowden and colleagues[17] provided significant evidence of linkage to this region with early onset ESRD in an optimum subset analysis of 48 African American families. we reported suggestive evidence of linkage with eGFR near this same region in a genome-wide linkage scan performed in 63 multigenerational European American families from the Joslin Study on the Genetics of Type 2 Diabetes collection.[13] Linkage has also been reported on chromosome 3q in separate studies of sibling pairs concordant for type 1 diabetes (T1D) but discordant for DN from the Joslin Study of Genetics in Type 1 Diabetes collection and Finland.[26,27] As part of a targeted linkage study of candidate loci performed in 66 sibling pairs, we identified a strong linkage signal approximately 15-kg basepair downstream from the angiotensin II type 1 receptor gene (AGTR1).[27] A genome-wide linkage scan of 83 Finnish sibling pairs reported evidence of linkage at this same region.[26] Although the candidate gene underlying these signals has yet to be defined, these studies, as well as a recent effort to fine map this region in unrelated patients with T1D and controls,[28] reinforce the likelihood that this region harbors a gene (or genes) that contribute to the risk of DN and suggests that this susceptibility locus may be common to both T1D and T2D.

Evidence of linkage with DN phenotypes is also mounting at loci on chromosomes 7p and 22q.[11,13,17,22] On chromosome 7p, significant linkage (MLS = 3.6) was first reported in an ordered subset analysis (OSA) of African American families with patients with ESRD and a long duration of T2D.[17] In a study by Placha and colleagues,[13] a linkage scan for genes controlling variation in eGFR in 406 members with T2D and 428 nondiabetic members from 63 extended families in the Joslin Study on the

Table 1
Summary of loci with significant evidence of linkage with DN in T2D

Chromosome	Position (Mb)[a]	MLS/P Value	Phenotype	Population	Study Design	References
1	11.60–36.00	3.81	eGFR	European and African American	Families	Freedman et al[21]
1	233.96–242.13	3.78	eGFR	Mexican American	Sibling Pairs	Schelling et al[23]
2	44.70–66.60	4.31	eGFR	European and African American	Families	Freedman et al[21]
2	195.00–213.00	4.1	eGFR, T2D relatives	Primarily European (94%)	Sibling Pairs	Placha et al[13]
3	103.66–118.89	4.55	early onset ESRD	African American	Sibling Pairs	Bowden et al[17,b]
5	41.07–67.27	3.4	ACR	European American	Families	Krolewski et al[11]
7	6.00–26.00	4.0	eGFR, all relative-pairs	Primarily European American (94%)	Sibling Pairs	Placha et al[13]
7	151.20–154.20	4.23	eGFR	Mexican American	Sibling Pairs	Schelling et al[23]
8	66.23–87.24	8.7×10^{-6}	eGFR	Mexican American	Sibling Pairs	Schelling et al[23]
10	85.00–101.00	3.6	eGFR	European American	Sibling Pairs	Placha et al[13]
14	53.44–69.29	2.0×10^{-5}	Proteinuria/ESRD	American Indian	Primarily Sibling Pairs	Iyengar et al[20]
16	74.60–86.50	3.56	Creatinine Clearance	West African	Sibling Pairs	Chen et al[19]
18	56.97–71.24	3.72	ESRD, early onset T2D	African American	Sibling Pairs	Bowden et al[17,b]
18	68.95–73.23	6.1	Proteinuria	Turkish	Families	Vardarli et al[16]
18	71.24–75.95	6.4×10^{-6}	eGFR	Mexican American	Sibling Pairs	Schelling et al[23]
22	27.19–35.08	3.7	ACR	Primarily European American (94%)	Families	Krolewski et al[11]

MLS $\geq$ 3.3, $P < 4.9 \times 10^{-5}$.

Abbreviations: Mb, megabase pairs; MLS, maximum logarithm of odds pairs; MLS, maximum logarithm of odds score.

[a] Approximate positions for reported logarithm of odds (LOD)-1 intervals are provided in megabase pairs relative to the National Center for Biotechnology Information Build 36.1. For studies not reporting LOD-1 intervals, the approximated position of the peak/flanking markers is provided if available.

[b] Bowden and colleagues[17] also identified 1 significant (logarithm of odds [LOD] = 3.59, chromosome 7p) and 2 suggestive loci (LOD = 2.94, chromosome 12 and LOD = 2.85, chromosome 16) in OSA among patients with ESRD with a long duration of DM; however, these findings could potentially be spurious.

Data from Rogus JJ, Warram JH, Krolewski AS. Genetic studies of late diabetic complications: the overlooked importance of diabetes duration before complication onset. Diabetes 2002;51:1655–62.

Table 2
Summary of loci with suggestive evidence of linkage

Chromosome	Position (Mb)[a]	MLS/P Value	Phenotype	Population	Study Design	References
1	237.00	2.00	DN	American Indian	Primarily Sibling Pairs	Igo et al[22]
2	50.69–68.09	3.02	eGFR	Mexican American	Sibling Pairs	Schelling et al[23]
2	146.24	2.04	ACR	African American	Primarily Sibling Pairs	Igo et al[22]
2	213.38–236.13	2.7	eGFR	Mexican American	Families	Puppala et al[18]
3	71.61	2.76	ACR	African American	Primarily Sibling Pairs	Igo et al[22]
3	118.89	2.52	ESRD, early onset T2D	African American	Sibling Pairs	Bowden et al[17]
3	138.00–152.00	2.2	eGFR, non-T2D relatives	Primarily European American (94%)	Sibling Pairs	Placha et al[13]
3	188.62–198.53	2.21	Serum creatinine	West African	Sibling Pairs	Chen et al[19]
6	10.63	2.84	DN	European American	Primarily Sibling Pairs	Igo et al[22]
6	102.68–150.80	2.08	eGFR	West African	Sibling Pairs	Chen et al[19]
7	8.00	2.00	DN	American Indian	Primarily Sibling Pairs	Igo et al[22]
7	29.66–96.38	2.42	eGFR	European and African American	Families	Freedman et al[21]
7	68.19–82.63	6.0×10^{-4}	ACR	European American	Primarily Sibling Pairs	Iyengar et al[20]
7	82.63–95.90	6.0×10^{-5}	Proteinuria/ESRD	African American	Primarily Sibling Pairs	Iyengar et al[20]
7	91.34	2.96	ACR	European American	Primarily Sibling Pairs	Igo et al[22]
7	131.93–134.76	2.73	DN	Pima Indian	Sibling Pairs	Imperatore et al[15]
7	151.20–155.68	3.1	ACR	Primarily European American (94%)	Families	Krolewski et al[11]
9	78.97–90.00	2.9	eGFR	Mexican American	Families	Puppala et al[18]

10	4.87	2.10	DN	American Indian	Primarily Sibling Pairs	Igo et al[22]
10	43.37–92.40	2.53	Serum creatinine	West African	Sibling Pairs	Chen et al[19]
10	129.43	2.65	DN, late-onset T2D	African American	Sibling Pairs	Bowden et al[17]
11	11.00	2.28	DN	Mexican American	Primarily Sibling Pairs	Igo et al[22]
11	17.04–24.08	2.3	eGFR	African American	Sibling Pairs	Schelling et al[23]
11	36.00–53.00	2.1	eGFR, non-T2D relatives	Primarily European American (94%)	Sibling Pairs	Placha et al[13]
11	122.14–133.61	2.4	eGFR	Mexican American	Families	Puppala et al[18]
12	16.91	2.86	ESRD, late-onset T2D	African American	Sibling Pairs	Bowden et al[17]
12	113.58–127.91	2.69	eGFR	Europe American	Families	Freedman et al[21]
13	26.22–39.84	2.28	eGFR	European and African American	Families	Freedman et al[21]
15	45.46	2.04	DN	American Indian	Primarily Sibling Pairs	Igo et al[22]
15	63.13–68.97	2.98	eGFR	American Indian	Sibling Pairs	Schelling et al[23]
16	55.67	2.31	ACR	African American	Primarily Sibling Pairs	Igo et al[22]
17	0.00–14.60	2.08	Creatinine clearance	West African	Sibling Pairs	Chen et al[19]
18	6.00–10.00	2.2	eGFR, T2D relatives	Primarily European American (94%)	Sibling Pairs	Placha et al[13]
19	6.06	3.13	ESRD, late-onset T2D	African American	Sibling Pairs	Bowden et al[17]
20	17.32	2.5	ESRD, late-onset T2D	African American	Sibling Pairs	Bowden et al[17]
21	20.57	2.3	ACR	European American	Families	Krolewski et al[11]
21	46.86	2.59	ESRD, late-onset T2D	African American	Sibling Pairs	Bowden et al[17]
22	35.20	2.29	ACR	Mexican American	Primarily Sibling Pairs	Igo et al[22]

$3.3 > \text{MLS} \geq 2.0$, $4.9 \times 10^{-5} < P < 7.4 \times 10^{-4}$.

Abbreviations: Mb, megabase pairs; MLS, maximum logarithm of odds score.

a Approximate positions for reported logarithm of odds (LOD)-1 intervals are provided in megabase pairs relative to National Center for Biotechnology Information Build 36.1. For studies not reporting LOD-1 intervals, the approximated position of the peak/flanking markers is provided if available.

Genetics of Type 2 Diabetes collection identified strong evidence for linkage at this same region (MLS = 4.0). Most recently, suggestive evidence for linkage on chromosome 7p (MLS = 2.81) has also been reported in an expanded linkage scan of the FIND collection that now includes 1235 multiethnic T2D families.[22] In the Joslin collection, a second scan for regions linked with variation in urinary albumin excretion found a significant linkage on chromosome 22q (MLS = 3.7).[11] Support for this region has also recently been confirmed in Mexican American families from the FIND collection.[22]

On chromosome 22q, the nonmuscle myosin heavy chain 9 gene (*MYH9*), expressed in both glomerular podocytes and mesangial cells, represents a particularly interesting candidate gene.[29,30] Genetic variation at the *MYH9* locus is strongly associated with nondiabetic nephropathy, including focal segmental glomerulosclerosis, hypertensive nephropathy, and nondiabetes-associated ESRD.[31–33] As first demonstrated by Freedman and colleagues,[33] *MYH9* SNPs also seem to contribute to the risk of nephropathy in African American patients with T2D. In this study, a comparison of 751 patients with ESRD with clinically diagnosed T2D and 227 controls with T2D identified significant associations at 3 *MYH9* SNPs (rs4821480, rs2032487, and rs4821481). In a subsequent study, these same variants trended toward an association with ESRD in 536 patients with T2D and 467 controls with T2D of European American ancestry.[34] These observations, however, were not confirmed in a recent study of patients with T2D from the United Kingdom.[35] An important distinction between the study by McKnight and colleagues[35] and the 2 previous reports is that the former examined these associations in patients with T2D nephropathy with chronic kidney disease less than 100 of whom had ESRD. In consideration of this fact, and the support garnered from multiple linkage studies of DN in T2D, continued investigation of the role of variants in the *MYH9* region in T2D-associated DN is warranted.

GENOME-WIDE ASSOCIATION SCANS FOR DN GENES IN T2D

Overall, linkage-based approaches have been quite successful in mapping loci that contribute to the risk of DN in T2D. Because of the limited resolution of this approach, however, efforts to definitively identify the genes underlying these signals continue to be challenging. Driven both by the limitations of linkage-based approaches and advances in genotyping technology, genome-wide association scans (GWASs) have generated a great deal of optimism among researchers working to identify susceptibility genes for DN. This approach to mapping genes uses commercially available genotyping arrays to readily interrogate millions of common SNPs, with minor allele frequencies (MAFs) generally ranging from 5.0% to 45%, across the genome, which is a feature that offers significantly improved resolution compared with linkage studies. The underlying hypothesis of GWASs is that common variants increase susceptibility to common disease.

GWASs have proven to be extremely powerful in detecting disease loci that are associated with many complex human traits and diseases, including coronary heart disease, T1D, T2D, bipolar disorder, Crohn disease, and rheumatoid arthritis.[36] Over the past several years, such studies have become an increasingly attractive approach to identify DN susceptibility genes. To date, 3 formal GWASs have been conducted in patients with T2D with DN (**Table 3**).[37–39]

The first such report was the gene-based analysis of 81 315 SNPs in 188 Japanese patients with T2D (94 patients with either proteinuria or ESRD and 94 normoalbuminuric controls).[39] From this discovery panel, 1615 SNPs were selected for replication in a larger collection that included 466 patients with T2D DN and 266 controls with T2D. Using this 2-stage approach, rs741301, located in intron 18 of the engulfment and cell

Table 3
Summary of loci identified through genome-wide association analyses

Chromosome	Position (Mb)[a]	SNP	Gene	Phenotype	Population	P Value	References
6	133.19	rs7769051[b]	RPS12	ESRD	African Americans (1674 patients with ESRD and 1246 normoalbuminuric controls)	3.60×10^{-3}	McDonough et al[37]
6	148.75	rs6930576[b]	SASH1	ESRD	African Americans (1674 patients with ESRD and 1246 normoalbuminuric controls)	5.30×10^{-3}	McDonough et al[37]
7	36.89	rs741301	ELMO1	Proteinuria/ESRD	Japanese (94 patients with proteinuria/ESRD and 94 normoalbuminuric controls)	8.0×10^{-6}	Shimazaki et al[39]
8	129.14	rs2648875	PVT1	ESRD	Pima Indians (105 patients with ESRD and 102 normoalbuminuric/microalbuminuric controls)	2.0×10^{-6}	Hanson et al[38]
9	93.02	rs773506[b]	AUH	ESRD	African Americans (1674 patients with ESRD and 1246 normoalbuminuric controls)	2.57×10^{-4}	McDonough et al[37]
12	64.40	rs2358944[b]	MSRB3/HMGA2	ESRD	African Americans (1674 patients with ESRD and 1246 normoalbuminuric controls)	4.70×10^{-3}	McDonough et al[37]
22	29.98-30.23	rs2106294, rs4820043, rs5749286[b]	LIMK2/SFI1	ESRD	African Americans (1674 patients with ESRD and 1246 normoalbuminuric controls)	1.62×10^{-2}–2.74×10^{-2}	McDonough et al[37]

Abbreviation: Mb, megabase pairs.
[a] Approximate positions for leading SNPs in megabase pairs relative to National Center for Biotechnology Information Build 36.1.
[b] In combined analyses of 1674 patients with T2D ESRD and 1719 non-T2D controls, these SNPs achieved P values less than 1.0×10^{-5}.

motility 1 (*ELMO1*) gene on chromosome 7p, emerged as the most strongly DN-associated SNP in these collections ($P = 8.0 \times 10^{-6}$). Subsequent functional studies by Shimazaki and colleagues[39,40] demonstrated an increased expression of *ELMO1* in the presence of high glucose. Supporting its potential role in the pathogenesis of DN, *ELMO1* has also been shown to contribute to the progression of chronic glomerular injury by promoting excess TGF-β, collagen type 1, fibronectin, and integrin-linked kinase expression and dysregulation of renal extracellular matrix metabolism.

Since the initial report by Shimazaki and colleagues, variants at *ELMO1* have been shown to be associated with DN in multiple independent collections.[41–43] Confirmation of *ELMO1*'s potential role in the susceptibility of DN was first demonstrated in a study by Leak and colleagues[43] that identified strong associations between multiple variants located in intron 13 of *ELMO1* and ESRD in 2 large African American cohorts with T2D. Variants located in intron 13 were also associated with overt proteinuria in a family based study of Pima Indians with T2D.[41] Of note, the associations observed in Pima Indians were in the opposite direction of those observed in African Americans. Additionally, in a comprehensive investigation of variants across this locus using GWAS data from the Genetics of Kidneys in Diabetes (GoKinD) collections, we further established *ELMO1*'s role in conferring increased susceptibility to DN by demonstrating that *ELMO1* variants are also associated with its risk in Caucasian patients with T1D.[42] The strongest associations in this study mapped to intron 16 of *ELMO1*.

Evidence from each of these studies is consistent with *ELMO1*'s role in DN and suggests that extensive allelic heterogeneity, contributed by the diverse ancestral genetic backgrounds of the different ethnic groups examined in each of these studies, exists across this locus. we hypothesize that rare polymorphisms in *ELMO1*, either the same variants or variants in strong or complete linkage disequilibrium, may be common to each ethnic group and merely tagged by the common variants identified in each study. Further investigation of rare SNPs at the *ELMO1* locus is likely necessary to fully understand the commonality of these associations and to elucidate the mechanisms underlying their role in DN.

In a second GWAS aimed at identifying DN genes in T2D, Hanson and colleagues[38] used a pooled genomic DNA approach to genotype 115 352 SNPs in 105 Pima Indians with T2D and ESRD and 102 Pima Indians with T2D and either normoalbuminuria or microalbuminuria. This analysis identified strong associations at variants in the plasmacytoma variant translocation (*PVT1*) gene on chromosome 8. Subsequent fine mapping of this locus revealed the strongest evidence for association at rs2648875 ($P = 2.0 \times 10^{-6}$) located in intron 8 of *PVT1*. Confirmation of this association was later shown by Millis and colleagues[44] in a subset of patients with ESRD from the GoKinD collections.

In the largest GWAS to date, a multistage approach that included African American individuals with and without T2D identified several novel regions with evidence of association with T2D-associated ESRD.[37] As part of their approach, McDonough and colleagues[37] used comparisons of T2D-ESRD cases and nondiabetic, non-nephropathy controls to identify 67 candidate SNPs that were then genotyped in controls with T2D to discriminate between T2D-ESRD loci and T2D loci. In combined analyses of 1674 patients with T2D ESRD and 1719 non-T2D controls, a total of 5 loci achieved P values less than 1.0×10^{-5}. Among these, rs9493454 at AU RNA binding protein/enoyl–coenzyme A hydratase (*AUH*) on chromosome 9 and rs7735506 at ribosomal protein S12 (*RPS12*) on chromosome 6 were highly significant in comparisons between patients with T2D-ESRD and T2D non-DN controls (n = 1216; $P = 3.60 \times 10^{-3}$ and 8.79×10^{-4}, respectively).

Lastly, in conjunction with their linkage analysis, Igo and colleagues[22] also performed a sparse GWAS of DN and ACR in the FIND collection using approximately 5500 SNPs from their linkage panel. In this study, the strongest association with DN was observed on chromosome 18 in the American Indian subgroup (rs1241893; $P = 3.0 \times 10^{-5}$). On chromosome 11, associations with ACR were found at rs722317 in both European American and Mexican American samples ($P = 4.6 \times 10^{-4}$ and 2.6×10^{-3}, respectively; combined $P = 7.3 \times 10^{-5}$). A complete GWAS was recently completed in this same collection that includes approximately 935 000 SNPs (B. Freedman, personal communication, 2012). we anticipate that this study will offer a great deal of insight to these and several other loci that contribute to DN in T2D.

The ascent of GWASs in investigations on the genetic basis of DN in T2D has shifted gene-mapping strategies from family based linkage approaches to population-based studies, primarily centered on unrelated DN case and control subjects. In identifying multiple common variants with modest effect (ie, effect size generally less than 1.4) on its risk, these studies have improved our overall understanding of the allelic architecture that underlies DN and provided an alternative approach to identifying genetic variants associated with DN that are potentially distinct from those identified using linkage-based approaches. In comparison with other diseases, relatively few GWASs in DN have been published. Those that have been published have been largely underpowered; to date, no strong DN susceptibility loci have emerged from these studies. Nonetheless, given the polygenic nature of this complex disease, we expect that as more data are generated, associations will be identified at multiple loci. As has been demonstrated in other diseases, these loci, however, will likely explain only a modest proportion of the overall heritability of DN, leaving much of its genetic basis yet to be defined.[45]

NEXT-GENERATION SEQUENCING AND THE SEARCH FOR DN GENES IN T2D

Genes that contain variants with a major effect (ie, those with effect sizes greater than 2.0) on the risk of DN in T2D have not been identified by GWAS-based approaches. This circumstance is caused by the small effect sizes (less than 1.4) attributable to common variants and the existence of other genetic factors in DN's risk and disease cause. An important source of genetic variation that has not thoroughly been assessed through GWASs is variants located in the genome's coding regions. Coding variants may have important protein-altering consequences that significantly affect a protein's function. In studies of rare forms of kidney disease, including nephrotic syndrome and familial focal segmental glomerulosclerosis, several missense and nonsense mutations have been identified as genes that play a critical role in the structure and/or proper functioning of the glomerular filtration barrier, including nephrin (*NPHS1*), podocin (*NPHS2*), actinin alpha 4 (*ACTN4*), transient receptor potential cation channel subfamily C (*TRPC6*), and phospholipase C, epsilon 1 (*PLCE1*), in families with multiple affected members.[46–50] Similarly, studies of maturity-onset diabetes of the young present additional examples whereby the ascertainment of large affected pedigrees has facilitated the identification of rare, highly penetrant variants that cosegregate with the disease and cause this form of noninsulin-dependent diabetes.[51]

Although such progress has not yet been seen in DN, the recent emergence of next-generation sequencing technology (that allows large genomic regions or entire genomes to be sequenced rapidly and accurately) and advances in target enrichment technologies (that allow specific subregions of the genome to be selected for resequencing) are beginning to facilitate these efforts.

Because low-frequency disease predisposing variants are more common among affected relatives compared with unrelated individuals, we think that family based studies offer the best opportunity to detect the rare functional variants that contribute to DN susceptibility. In support of this, we recently initiated a family based targeted resequencing project to comprehensively survey rare variants that underlie the linkage signals at several previously identified chromosomal loci shown to contribute to variation in urinary albumin excretion and renal function in the Joslin Study on the Genetics of Type 2 Diabetes collection.[52] One hundred twenty-six patients with DN from 42 families with an excess of renal disease (approximately 3.0 cases per family) were selected for resequencing of the coding region of 361 protein-coding genes located at 4 genomic regions with evidence for linkage of urinary albumin excretion levels (chromosomes 5q, 7q, 21p, and 22q) and 2 genomic regions linked to variation in renal function (chromosomes 2q and 7p). To date, we have completed sequencing and analysis of 63 patients with DN from 21 of the selected families.

In **Table 4**, we have provided a summary of variants identified in 74 genes across the 20–megabase pair (Mb) region on chromosome 7p where we previously reported significant evidence of linkage with eGFR.[13] In this preliminary dataset, we identified a total of 385 nonreference variants, including 42 novel variants (ie, those not annotated in the current release of the National Center for Biotechnology Information's [NCBI] SNP database [dbSNP, build 135; www.ncbi.nlm.nih.gov/projects/SNP/] or present in data from the 1000 Genomes Project [www.1000genomes.org/]) and 170 (44.2%) nonsynonymous SNPs (ie, missense and nonsense).

Although the analysis of this data is still ongoing, to illustrate the utility of combining evidence from family based linkage analysis with targeted sequencing to uncover rare functional genetic variants that may contribute to DN, additional data are presented for the collagen type XXVIII alpha 1 (*COL28A1*) (**Fig. 1**), which is a gene located at position 7.36 to 7.54 Mb on chromosome 7 and a member of the extracellular matrix molecule family of collagens that is known to be expressed in kidney.[53] Our resequencing efforts identified 10 variants in *COL28A1*'s coding sequence, including 8 nonsynonymous SNPs and 2 synonymous SNPs. Two of these have not previously been reported in

Table 4	
Summary of variants identified in the chromosome 7p linkage region	
Total number of variants	385
Number of known variants	343
Number of novel variants	42
Variant class	*N*
Missense	162
Synonymous	80
Intronic	79
Downstream	36
Nonsense	8
Frameshift	7
Codon deletion	4
Stop lost	3
Codon insertion	2
Splice acceptor/donor	2
5′ untranslated region	1
Start lost	1

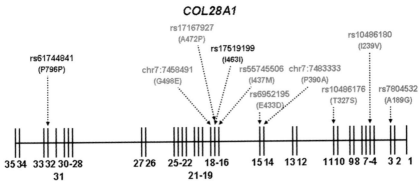

Fig. 1. Coding variants in *COL28A1* in patients with DN from the Joslin Study on the Genetics of Type 2 Diabetes collection. Ten variants identified in *COL28A1*'s coding sequence are shown, including 8 nonsynonymous SNPs and 2 synonymous SNPs. The reference SNP (rs) identification numbers for variants reported in dbSNP build 135 are provided. Variants not in dbSNP build 135 are identified by their chromosome and position relative to NCBI build 36.1.

dbSNP or in data from the 1000 Genomes Project. All 8 nonsynonymous SNPs are present in data from 4300 European Americans included in the National Heart, Lung, and Blood Institute's recent Exome Sequencing Project's (ESP, evs.gs.washington.edu/EVS). Two nonsynonymous SNPs shown in **Fig. 1** (chr7:7458491 and chr7:7483333) are extremely rare in the ESP dataset (MAFs = 0.02% and 0.2%, respectively). Of particular interest, chr7:7483333 was observed in 2 siblings with T2D with ESRD from a single family. Analysis of chr7:7483333 in all available members of this family is currently underway.

As we continue our analysis of all 361 genes across the 6 linkage regions in the Joslin Study on the Genetics of Type 2 Diabetes collection, we anticipate that this approach will allow the identification of variants in genes that contribute to variation in urinary albumin excretion and renal function decline in T2D at regions linked with each of these traits.

This preliminary analysis highlights some important concepts. First, next-generation resequencing coupled with target enrichment is an efficient and cost-effective approach to comprehensively interrogate tens to hundreds of genes within an area of known linkage. As their associated costs continue to come down, these technologies will become increasingly vital in identifying rare functional variants associated with complex disease. Second, although a far-reaching benefit from the ESP is the recent development of commercial genotyping arrays that contain more than 250 000 to 319 000 rare putative functional exonic variants that were generated as part of this project, resequencing in specific populations provides a more extensive catalog of the variation that may be relevant to a particular disease. For example, among the 170 nonsynonymous SNPs we identified in the chromosome 7p linkage region, only approximately 61% are represented on the Infinium HumanExome Beadchip that was derived from the ESP. Although commercial exome genotyping arrays offer previously unavailable coverage of rare variants at a very reasonable cost, resequencing, although more costly, is the most comprehensive approach to assess genomic variation both across a region of interest and in the population of interest. Finally, as illustrated by our analysis of *COL28A1*, family based approaches are well designed to identify functional variants that are extremely rare in the general population but that are common among related affected individuals. Renewed interest in such studies will help define the spectrum of genetic variation that accounts for the heritability of DN in T2D and its related traits.

SUMMARY

For more than 20 years, evidence in favor of a genetic basis for the susceptibility of DN in T2D has provided a foundation for studies aimed at identifying the causal genes responsible for its development. During this period, strategies used to map genes for DN have been driven by our understanding of variation across our genome and the technologies available to interrogate it; as both have evolved, so to have our approaches. The advent of next-generation sequencing technology and increased interest in the search for rare variants has begun to swing the pendulum of these efforts away from population-based studies and back to studies of pedigrees. As the field moves forward, family based approaches should greatly facilitate efforts to identify variants in genes that have a major affect on the risk of DN in T2D. To be successful, the ascertainment and comprehensive study of families with multiple affected members is critical.

REFERENCES

1. Parving HH, Mauer M, Ritz E. Diabetic nephropathy. In: Brenner BM, editor. Brenner and rector's the kidney. Philadelphia: Elsevier; 2004. p. 1777–818.
2. Krolewski AS, Warram JH. Clinical features and epidemiology of diabetic nephropathy. In: Pickup JC, Williams G, editors. Textbook of diabetes, vol. 2. Oxford (United Kingdom): Blackwell Scientific Publications; 1997. p. 53.1–53.13.
3. Jones CA, Krolewski AS, Rogus J, et al. Epidemic of end-stage renal disease in people with diabetes in the United States population: do we know the cause? Kidney Int 2005;67:1684–91.
4. Pettitt DJ, Saad MF, Bennett PH, et al. Familial predisposition to renal disease in two generations of Pima Indians with type 2 (non-insulin-dependent) diabetes mellitus. Diabetologia 1990;33:438–43.
5. Freedman BI, Tuttle AB, Spray BJ. Familial predisposition to nephropathy in African-Americans with non-insulin-dependent diabetes mellitus. Am J Kidney Dis 1995;25:710–3.
6. Faronato PP, Maioli M, Tonolo G, et al. Clustering of albumin excretion rate abnormalities in Caucasian patients with NIDDM. The Italian NIDDM Nephropathy Study Group. Diabetologia 1997;40:816–23.
7. Canani LH, Gerchman F, Gross JL. Familial clustering of diabetic nephropathy in Brazilian type 2 diabetic patients. Diabetes 1999;48:909–13.
8. Gruden G, Cavallo-Perin P, Olivetti C, et al. Albumin excretion rate levels in non-diabetic offspring of NIDDM patients with and without nephropathy. Diabetologia 1995;38:1218–22.
9. Fogarty DG, Rich SS, Hanna L, et al. Urinary albumin excretion in families with type 2 diabetes is heritable and genetically correlated to blood pressure. Kidney Int 2000;57:250–7.
10. Forsblom CM, Kanninen T, Lehtovirta M, et al. Heritability of albumin excretion rate in families of patients with Type II diabetes. Diabetologia 1999;42:1359–66.
11. Krolewski AS, Poznik GD, Placha G, et al. A genome-wide linkage scan for genes controlling variation in urinary albumin excretion in type II diabetes. Kidney Int 2006;69:129–36.

12. Langefeld CD, Beck SR, Bowden DW, et al. Heritability of GFR and albuminuria in Caucasians with type 2 diabetes mellitus. Am J Kidney Dis 2004;43:796–800.
13. Placha G, Canani LH, Warram JH, et al. Evidence for different susceptibility genes for proteinuria and ESRD in type 2 diabetes. Adv Chronic Kidney Dis 2005;12:155–69.
14. Fogarty DG, Hanna LS, Wantman M, et al. Segregation analysis of urinary albumin excretion in families with type 2 diabetes. Diabetes 2000;49:1057–63.
15. Imperatore G, Hanson RL, Pettitt DJ, et al. Sib-pair linkage analysis for susceptibility genes for microvascular complications among Pima Indians with type 2 diabetes. Pima Diabetes Genes Group. Diabetes 1998;47:821–30.
16. Vardarli I, Baier LJ, Hanson RL, et al. Gene for susceptibility to diabetic nephropathy in type 2 diabetes maps to 18q22.3-23. Kidney Int 2002;62:2176–83.
17. Bowden DW, Colicigno CJ, Langefeld CD, et al. A genome scan for diabetic nephropathy in African Americans. Kidney Int 2004;66:1517–26.
18. Puppala S, Arya R, Thameem F, et al. Genotype by diabetes interaction effects on the detection of linkage of glomerular filtration rate to a region on chromosome 2q in Mexican Americans. Diabetes 2007;56:2818–28.
19. Chen G, Adeyemo AA, Zhou J, et al. A genome-wide search for linkage to renal function phenotypes in West Africans with type 2 diabetes. Am J Kidney Dis 2007;49:394–400.
20. Iyengar SK, Abboud HE, Goddard KA, et al. Genome-wide scans for diabetic nephropathy and albuminuria in multiethnic populations: the family investigation of nephropathy and diabetes (FIND). Diabetes 2007;56:1577–85.
21. Freedman BI, Bowden DW, Rich SS, et al. Genome-wide linkage scans for renal function and albuminuria in Type 2 diabetes mellitus: the Diabetes Heart Study. Diabet Med 2008;25:268–76.
22. Igo RP Jr, Iyengar SK, Nicholas SB, et al. Genomewide linkage scan for diabetic renal failure and albuminuria: the FIND study. Am J Nephrol 2011;33:381–9.
23. Schelling JR, Abboud HE, Nicholas SB, et al. Genome-wide scan for estimated glomerular filtration rate in multi-ethnic diabetic populations: the Family Investigation of Nephropathy and Diabetes (FIND). Diabetes 2008;57:235–43.
24. Janssen B, Hohenadel D, Brinkkoetter P, et al. Carnosine as a protective factor in diabetic nephropathy: association with a leucine repeat of the carnosinase gene CNDP1. Diabetes 2005;54:2320–7.
25. Freedman BI, Hicks PJ, Sale MM, et al. A leucine repeat in the carnosinase gene CNDP1 is associated with diabetic end-stage renal disease in European Americans. Nephrol Dial Transplant 2007;22:1131–5.
26. Osterholm AM, He B, Pitkaniemi J, et al. Genome-wide scan for type 1 diabetic nephropathy in the Finnish population reveals suggestive linkage to a single locus on chromosome 3q. Kidney Int 2007;71:140–5.
27. Moczulski DK, Rogus JJ, Antonellis A, et al. Major susceptibility locus for nephropathy in type 1 diabetes on chromosome 3q: results of novel discordant sib-pair analysis. Diabetes 1998;47:1164–9.
28. He B, Osterholm AM, Hoverfalt A, et al. Association of genetic variants at 3q22 with nephropathy in patients with type 1 diabetes mellitus. Am J Hum Genet 2009;84:5–13.
29. Singh N, Nainani N, Arora P, et al. CKD in MYH9-related disorders. Am J Kidney Dis 2009;54:732–40.
30. Arrondel C, Vodovar N, Knebelmann B, et al. Expression of the nonmuscle myosin heavy chain IIA in the human kidney and screening for MYH9 mutations in Epstein and Fechtner syndromes. J Am Soc Nephrol 2002;13:65–74.

31. Kopp JB, Smith MW, Nelson GW, et al. MYH9 is a major-effect risk gene for focal segmental glomerulosclerosis. Nat Genet 2008;40:1175–84.

32. Kao WH, Klag MJ, Meoni LA, et al. MYH9 is associated with nondiabetic end-stage renal disease in African Americans. Nat Genet 2008;40:1185–92.

33. Freedman BI, Hicks PJ, Bostrom MA, et al. Non-muscle myosin heavy chain 9 gene MYH9 associations in African Americans with clinically diagnosed type 2 diabetes mellitus-associated ESRD. Nephrol Dial Transplant 2009;24:3366–71.

34. Cooke JN, Bostrom MA, Hicks PJ, et al. Polymorphisms in MYH9 are associated with diabetic nephropathy in European Americans. Nephrol Dial Transplant 2012; 27:1505–11.

35. McKnight AJ, Duffy S, Fogarty DG, et al. Association of MYH9/APOL1 with chronic kidney disease in a UK population. Nephrol Dial Transplant 2012;27: 3660.

36. Pearson TA, Manolio TA. How to interpret a genome-wide association study. JAMA 2008;299:1335–44.

37. McDonough CW, Palmer ND, Hicks PJ, et al. A genome-wide association study for diabetic nephropathy genes in African Americans. Kidney Int 2011;79:563–72.

38. Hanson RL, Craig DW, Millis MP, et al. Identification of PVT1 as a candidate gene for end-stage renal disease in type 2 diabetes using a pooling-based genome-wide single nucleotide polymorphism association study. Diabetes 2007;56: 975–83.

39. Shimazaki A, Kawamura Y, Kanazawa A, et al. Genetic variations in the gene encoding ELMO1 are associated with susceptibility to diabetic nephropathy. Diabetes 2005;54:1171–8.

40. Shimazaki A, Tanaka Y, Shinosaki T, et al. ELMO1 increases expression of extracellular matrix proteins and inhibits cell adhesion to ECMs. Kidney Int 2006;70: 1769–76.

41. Hanson RL, Millis MP, Young NJ, et al. ELMO1 variants and susceptibility to diabetic nephropathy in American Indians. Mol Genet Metab 2010;101:383–90.

42. Pezzolesi MG, Katavetin P, Kure M, et al. Confirmation of genetic associations at ELMO1 in the GoKinD collection supports its role as a susceptibility gene in diabetic nephropathy. Diabetes 2009;58:2698–702.

43. Leak TS, Perlegas PS, Smith SG, et al. Variants in intron 13 of the ELMO1 gene are associated with diabetic nephropathy in African Americans. Ann Hum Genet 2009;73:152–9.

44. Millis MP, Bowen D, Kingsley C, et al. Variants in the plasmacytoma variant translocation gene (PVT1) are associated with end-stage renal disease attributed to type 1 diabetes. Diabetes 2007;56:3027–32.

45. Manolio TA, Collins FS, Cox NJ, et al. Finding the missing heritability of complex diseases. Nature 2009;461:747–53.

46. Kaplan JM, Kim SH, North KN, et al. Mutations in ACTN4, encoding alpha-actinin-4, cause familial focal segmental glomerulosclerosis. Nat Genet 2000;24:251–6.

47. Kestila M, Lenkkeri U, Mannikko M, et al. Positionally cloned gene for a novel glomerular protein–nephrin–is mutated in congenital nephrotic syndrome. Mol Cell 1998;1:575–82.

48. Boute N, Gribouval O, Roselli S, et al. NPHS2, encoding the glomerular protein podocin, is mutated in autosomal recessive steroid-resistant nephrotic syndrome. Nat Genet 2000;24:349–54.

49. Hinkes B, Wiggins RC, Gbadegesin R, et al. Positional cloning uncovers mutations in PLCE1 responsible for a nephrotic syndrome variant that may be reversible. Nat Genet 2006;38:1397–405.

50. Winn MP, Conlon PJ, Lynn KL, et al. A mutation in the TRPC6 cation channel causes familial focal segmental glomerulosclerosis. Science 2005;308:1801–4.
51. Kahn CR, Vicent D, Doria A. Genetics of non-insulin-dependent (type-II) diabetes mellitus. Annu Rev Med 1996;47:509–31.
52. Pezzolesi MG, Jeong J, Smiles AM, et al. Identification of rare genetic variants that contribute to diabetic nephropathy in type 2 diabetes through family-based targeted exome sequencing [abstract]. Presented at the 62nd Annual Meeting of the American Society of Human Genetics. San Francisco, November 7, 2012.
53. Veit G, Kobbe B, Keene DR, et al. Collagen XXVIII, a novel von Willebrand factor A domain-containing protein with many imperfections in the collagenous domain. J Biol Chem 2006;281:3494–504.

Pancreas Transplantation and Reversal of Diabetic Nephropathy Lesions

Michael Mauer, MD[a],*, Paola Fioretto, MD, PhD[b]

KEYWORDS

- Diabetic nephropathy • Pancreas transplantation • Type 1 diabetes
- Diabetic glomerular lesions • Reversal healing

KEY POINTS

- Pancreas transplantation is the only available treatment that has restored long-term (10 or more years) normoglycemia without the risks of severe hypoglycemia.
- Diabetic glomerular lesions were not significantly changed at 5 years but were dramatically improved after 10 years, with most patients' glomerular structure returning to normal at the 10-year follow-up.
- Tubulointerstitial remodeling, including decreased interstitial collagen, was possible.

INTRODUCTION

Diabetic nephropathy (DN) is the most important cause of end-stage renal disease,[1,2] leading to more than 45% of all new cases in the United States. The specific DN lesions leading to renal dysfunction in DN are secondary to the diabetic state. DN in type 1 diabetes (T1D) begins primarily as a glomerular disease.[2,3] At the onset of T1D, the 2 major early glomerular lesions, mesangial expansion and increased thickness of the glomerular basement membrane (GBM), are not present but may be demonstrable over the next 5 to 10 years.[4] DN lesions recur in the renal allograft,

This work was supported by grants from the National Institutes of Health (DK13083), the National Center for Research Resources (MO1-KK00400), and by an endowment from the Kroc Research Foundation. During the initial stages of this work, Dr Fioretto was supported by Research Fellowship and Career Development Awards from the Juvenile Diabetes Foundation International.

[a] Department of Pediatrics, Medical School, University of Minnesota, 2450 Riverside Avenue, East Building, MB681, Minneapolis, MN 55454, USA; [b] Department of Medicine, University of Padova, via Giustiniani, 2, 35128 Padova, Italy
* Corresponding author. Department of Pediatrics, Medical School, University of Minnesota, 2450 Riverside Avenue, East Building, MB681, Minneapolis, MN 55454.
E-mail address: mauer002@umn.edu

Med Clin N Am 97 (2013) 109–114
http://dx.doi.org/10.1016/j.mcna.2012.10.009
0025-7125/13/$ – see front matter © 2013 Elsevier Inc. All rights reserved.

and patients with T1D randomized to maximized glycemic control in the first 5 years following kidney transplantation have less mesangial matrix expansion than patients randomized to standard control.[5] There were also lower incidences of microalbuminuria and proteinuria after 7 to 8 years of follow-up[6] in patients with T1D randomized to strict control in the Diabetes Control and Complications Trial. However, the critical role of glycemia in DN pathogenesis was finally proven by the dramatic demonstration of reversal of DN lesions in patients with T1D following successful pancreas transplantation alone (PTA).[7]

PANCREAS TRANSPLANTATION AND DIABETIC RENAL DISEASE

DN largely results from the accumulation of extracellular matrix (ECM) (basement membrane proteins) in the GBM, tubular basement membrane (TBM), and mesangium.[2,3,8–10] Fibrillar types I and III collagens are absent from the glomerulus throughout most of the evolution of DN lesions, appearing only in advanced Kimmelstiel-Wilson nodules and in the final stages and of glomerular scarring.[11] Moreover, these scar collagens, normally present in modest quantities in the interstitium of the kidney, increase at this site only after the glomerular lesions are well established and interstitial expansion is quite advanced.[2]

In healthy people, the fraction of the volume of the glomerulus occupied by the mesangium (mesangial fractional volume [Vv(Mes/glom)]) and GBM width do not change between 16 and 60 years of age.[12] Thus, there is a remarkable ability for the cells of the kidney, throughout adult life, to maintain a near perfect balance between glomerular ECM production and removal, whereas DN lesions result from a disturbance in this balance caused by increased production, decreased removal, or both.[12]

Pancreas Transplantation and Reversibility of DN Lesions

Animal studies provided a proof of concept that DN lesions may, at least in part, be reversible. Thus, after 7 months of diabetes, the cure of diabetes in rats by islet transplantation resulted (in the next 2 months) in the reversal of mesangial matrix and cell expansion but did not affect the increased GBM width,[13] perhaps because the follow-up time was not long enough. However, the reversal of mesangial expansion did not occur in the first 5 years after pancreas transplantation in humans.[14] Moreover, although mesangial expansion in human DN is mainly the result of mesangial matrix accumulation, mesangial matrix and cellular expansion are equivalent in rats. Thus, animal models of the development and reversal of DN are imperfect models of the human condition.

As alluded to earlier, the authors' initial report on the effects of PTA on DN lesions in the native kidneys of 13 PTA recipients was extremely disappointing. Thus, despite 5 years of normoglycemia and insulin independence, established DN lesions did not improve,[14] increased GBM width was unchanged, and Vv(Mes/glom) actually increased further, this due decreased glomerular volume, whereas the total volume of the mesangium per glomerulus (TM) did not change. On the other hand, control patients with persistent T1D had further increases in both Vv(Mes/glom) and TM.[14]

Eight of these 13 PTA recipients returned for repeat research biopsies 10 years after the cure of T1D by PTA,[7] whereas 2 patients required a kidney transplant 6 and 8 years after PTA, 2 lost pancreatic graft function and became diabetic again, and 1 refused the 10-year biopsy. At PTA, these 8 patients were 33 ± 3 years old, had a T1D duration of 22 ± 5 years, and their hemoglobin A_{1c} was $8.7 \pm 1.5\%$. Renal function was difficult to interpret given that cyclosporine causes substantial reductions in glomerular filtration rate[15] and may also reduce albuminuria. The authors observed a dramatic reversal of diabetic glomerulopathy lesions in all 8 patients returning for their 10-year PTA biopsies.[7] GBM and TBM widths all increased at baseline, remained unchanged at 5 years, and were decreased at 10 years compared with the baseline and 5 years; several of the 10-year values were in the normal range and approached normal in the others (**Fig. 1**A, B). As noted earlier, Vv(Mes/glom) and mesangial matrix fractional volume increased significantly from the baseline to 5 years (see **Fig. 1**C, D) because of a decrease in glomerular volume. Glomerular volume was stable from the 5th to the 10th post-PTA years, and Vv(Mes/glom) and mesangial matrix fractional volume were much lower at 10 years than either the baseline or 5-year values (see **Fig. 1**). Total mesangial and total mesangial matrix volumes per glomerulus (unchanged at 5 years) were also markedly decreased at 10 years. The authors also found remarkable remodeling of glomerular architecture in the 10-year versus the baseline and 5-year biopsies. In several biopsies, there was a total disappearance

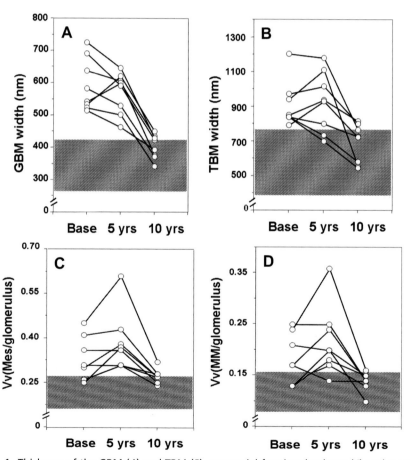

Fig. 1. Thickness of the GBM (*A*) and TBM (*B*), mesangial fractional volume (*C*) and mesangial matrix fractional volume (*D*) at baseline and 5 and 10 years after PTA. The shaded area represents the normal ranges obtained in 66 age- and sex-matched normal controls (mean ± 2 SD). Data for individual patients are connected by lines. (*From* Fioretto P, Steffes MW, Sutherland DE, et al. Reversal of lesions of diabetic nephropathy after pancreas transplantation. N Engl J Med 1998;339:69–75; with permission.)

of Kimmelstiel-Wilson nodules; the authors commonly appreciated open glomerular capillaries, whereas, in previous biopsies in the same patients, glomerular capillaries were greatly compressed by the expansion of the mesangium (**Fig. 2**). Thus, these studies proved that diabetic glomerular and tubular ECM lesions are reversible in humans but not before a delay of at least 5 years.

The basis for this long delay before healing occurred is unknown. One possibility is that, secondary to long exposure to hyperglycemia. ECM molecules are heavily glycosylated and, because glycosylated ECM is more resistant to proteolysis,[16] there is a delay in healing until long-lived ECM is replaced by less glycosylated molecules. A more attractive hypothesis is that renal cells have metabolic memory for the diabetic state[17]; thus, cells behave as if in a diabetic environment for a long time after the establishment of normoglycemia. Both of these hypotheses may be true. Regardless of the mechanisms, at some point after the cure of diabetes, rates of ECM removal begin to exceed rates of ECM production. This situation is active healing, clearly different from a normal situation in adult life where renal ECM production and removal remain in near perfect balance.[12]

All PTA recipients in these studies received cyclosporine, a known nephrotoxic drug.[18,19] In fact, the authors reported that the increase in interstitial expansion and tubular atrophy at 5 years was related to cyclosporine dose and blood levels in the first year after PTA.[15] In the 10-year post-PTA biopsies, the authors observed remodeling of interstitial and tubular lesions. Thus, interstitial fibrosis and tubular atrophy observed at 5 years after PTA significantly improved by 10 years after PTA,[20] demonstrating that the tubulointerstitium can undergo substantial remodeling. There was a decrease in the quantity of renal cortical interstitial fibrillar collagen, which was consistent, once again, with healing characterized by the removal of ECM exceeding its rate of production.[20] The findings in these studies were more consistent with the idea that atrophic tubules underwent reabsorption rather than healing. The nature of these studies did not allow the determination of whether the tubulointerstitial improvements resulted from prolonged normoglycemia, decreased cyclosporine dose, or both. Nevertheless, these PTA studies revealed that these components of the kidney

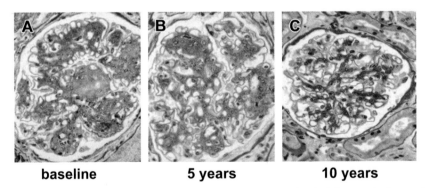

baseline   5 years   10 years

Fig. 2. Glomeruli before and after pancreas transplantation (PTA). (*A*) Typical glomerulus from the baseline biopsy, with diffuse diabetic glomerulopathy and Kimmelstiel-Wilson nodules. (*B*) Typical glomerulus 5 years after PTA shows persistence of diabetic glomerulopathy. (*C*) Typical glomerulus 10 years after PTA, with marked resolution of diabetic glomerulopathy lesions and substantially normal glomerular structure. (*From* Fioretto P, Steffes MW, Sutherland DE, et al. Reversal of lesions of diabetic nephropathy after pancreas transplantation. N Engl J Med 1998;339:69–75; with permission.)

could also undergo changes in the direction of restoration of renal architecture toward normal from the point of substantial injury.

In summary, as previously reviewed these studies have proven that the kidney has intrinsic cellular healing mechanisms for restoring more normal renal structure on removal of the injury stimuli.[21] These processes, in some ways, recapitulate aspects of renal development in that the renal cells seem to know what normal renal structure is and, given the opportunity, will orchestrate the means of getting there. Although there are likely points of no return (ie, severity of structural damage beyond which reestablishment of normal renal architecture is no longer possible), even advanced lesions of diabetic glomerulopathy, including nodular changes, are reversible. A better understanding of the regulation of the cellular mechanisms involved in these healing processes could lead to new approaches to the prevention and treatment of DN as well as other slowly progressive renal diseases.

ACKNOWLEDGMENTS

The authors are indebted to the patients who so generously participated in these studies.

REFERENCES

1. U.S.R.D.S. U.S. renal data system annual report. NIH and NIDDK; 2006.
2. Mauer M, Fioretto P, Woredekal Y, et al. Diabetic nephropathy. In: Schrier RW, editor. Disease of the kidney and urinary tract. Philadelphia: Lippincott Williams and Wilkins; 2001. p. 2083–127.
3. Mauer SM, Steffes MW, Ellis EN, et al. Structural-functional relationships in diabetic nephropathy. J Clin Invest 1984;74:1143–55.
4. Østerby R. Early phases in the development of diabetic glomerulopathy. Acta Med Scand 1975;475:1–84.
5. Barbosa J, Steffes MW, Sutherland DE, et al. The effect of glycemic control on early diabetic renal lesions. A 5-year randomized controlled clinical trial of insulin-dependent diabetic kidney transplant recipients. J Am Med Assoc 1994;272:600–6.
6. Diabetes Complications and Control Trial Research Group. The effect of intensive treatment of diabetes on the development and progression of long-term complications of insulin dependent diabetes mellitus. N Engl J Med 1993;329:977–86.
7. Fioretto P, Steffes MW, Sutherland DE, et al. Reversal of lesions of diabetic nephropathy after pancreas transplantation. N Engl J Med 1998;339:69–75.
8. Fioretto P, Steffes MW, Mauer SM. Glomerular structure in non-proteinuric insulin-dependent diabetic patients with various levels of albuminuria. Diabetes 1994;43:1358–64.
9. Brito PL, Fioretto P, Drummond K, et al. Proximal tubular basement membrane width in insulin-dependent diabetes mellitus. Kidney Int 1998;53:754–61.
10. Steffes MW, Bilous RW, Sutherland DE, et al. Cell and matrix components of the glomerular mesangium in type I diabetes. Diabetes 1992;41:679–84.
11. Falk RJ, Scheinman JI, Mauer SM, et al. Polyantigenic expansion of basement membrane constituents in diabetic nephropathy. Diabetes 1983;32:34–9.
12. Steffes MW, Barbosa J, Basgen JM, et al. Quantitative glomerular morphology of the normal human kidney. Lab Invest 1983;49:82–6.
13. Mauer SM, Sutherland DE, Steffes MW, et al. Pancreatic islet transplantation. Effects on the glomerular lesions of experimental diabetes in the rat. Diabetes 1974;23:748–53.

14. Fioretto P, Mauer SM, Bilous RW, et al. Effects of pancreas transplantation on glomerular structure in insulin-dependent diabetic patients with their own kidneys. Lancet 1993;342:1193–6.
15. Fioretto P, Steffes MW, Mihach MJ, et al. Cyclosporine associated lesions in native kidneys of diabetic pancreas transplant recipients. Kidney Int 1995;48:489–95.
16. Brownlee M, Cerami A, Vlassara H. Advanced glycosylation end products in tissue and the biochemical basis of diabetic complications. N Engl J Med 1988;318:1315–22.
17. Roys S, Sala R, Cagliero E, et al. Overexpression of fibronectin induced by diabetes or high glucose: phenomenon with a memory. Proc Natl Acad Sci U S A 1990;87:404–8.
18. Myers BD, Sibley R, Newton L, et al. The long-term course of cyclosporine-associated chronic nephropathy. Kidney Int 1988;33:590–600.
19. Feutren G, Mihatsch MJ. Risk factors for cyclosporine induced nephropathy in patients with autoimmune diseases. N Engl J Med 1992;326:1654–60.
20. Fioretto P, Sutherland DE, Najafian B, et al. Remodeling of renal interstitial and tubular lesions in pancreas transplant recipients. Kidney Int 2006;69:907–12.
21. Fioretto P, Mauer M. Reversal of diabetic nephropathy: lessons from pancreas transplantation. J Nephrol 2012;25(1):13–8.

Potential New Treatments for Diabetic Kidney Disease

Deanna S. Kania, PharmD, BCPS[a,b], Cory T. Smith, PharmD[a,c],
Christy L. Nash, PharmD, CDE[a,d],
Jasmine D. Gonzalvo, PharmD, BCPS, BC-ADM, CDE[a], Andrea Bittner[a],
Brian M. Shepler, PharmD[a,*]

KEYWORDS

- Pentoxifylline • Bardoxolone • Pirfenidone • Doxycycline • Diabetic kidney disease

KEY POINTS

- Antifibrotic agents, antioxidant agents, ET-a receptor antagonists, and a few other agents with nonspecific or multifaceted mechanisms of action have been evaluated and progressed to small clinical studies in human subjects.
- There is certainly not enough compelling evidence to justify the routine use of any of these products specifically for diabetic kidney disease (DKD) at the moment; however, more well-controlled studies in several hundred patients will help determine which of these may have a place in the DKD treatment armamentarium of the future.
- The effect of diabetes on the progression of kidney disease is a complex process with many mechanisms that may be targetable by new molecular entities and existing drug therapy.

INTRODUCTION

Drug therapy for DKD involves managing hyperglycemia and proteinuria, but there are several new drugs that are being investigated for their ability to interrupt the disease process and delay the progression of DKD. Some of these agents are existing drugs and others are new compounds. As our understanding of the disease process deepens, new targets for drug therapy can be identified and tested. The formation of advanced glycation end products (AGEs), for example, has been studied for 30 years and is one of the processes investigated for potential drug therapy intervention.

AGEs essentially form when a glucose molecule combines with a protein under the right conditions. There are 3 pathways for AGE formation, including the glycation

[a] Purdue University College of Pharmacy, 575 Stadium Mall Drive, West Lafayette, IN 47907-2091, USA; [b] R.L. Roudebush VA Medical Center, 1481 West 10th Street, Indianapolis, IN 46202, USA; [c] Floyd Memorial Hospital, 1850 State Street, New Albany, IN 47150, USA; [d] Mathes Pharmacy, Diabetes Center, and Medical Supplies, 1621 Charlestown Road, New Albany, IN 47150, USA
* Corresponding author.
E-mail address: sheplerb@purdue.edu

Med Clin N Am 97 (2013) 115–134
http://dx.doi.org/10.1016/j.mcna.2012.10.004
0025-7125/13/$ – see front matter Published by Elsevier Inc.

pathway, polyol pathway, and glycoxidation. Once an AGE is formed, it can directly harm the glomerulus specifically by causing glomerulosclerosis and expansion of the extracellular matrix, 2 hallmarks of DKD. AGE receptors have been identified in several structures in the glomerulus including the glomerular basement membrane, mesangium, and endothelial cells and through their activation can cause fibrosis and inflammation.[1] AGEs can cause these deleterious effects in several ways. They can increase gene expression and promote growth factors such as transforming growth factor beta (TGF-b), vascular endothelial growth factor, and connective tissue growth factor (CTGF), as well as induce inflammatory mediators such as interleukin-1 (IL-1), IL-6, and tumor necrosis factor alpha (TNF-a) in addition to causing oxidative stress.[2] Furthermore, as protein begins to leak through the glomerular filtration membrane and enter into the proximal convoluted tubule, it is taken up by the tubule cells stimulating the release of proinflammatory cytokines that promote fibrosis.[3]

Drug therapy targeting the AGE process has focused on different parts of this complex pathway. Aminoguanidine, for example, was an early compound evaluated for its ability to interrupt the formation of AGEs and slow the progression of kidney disease in several animal models.[4–6] In a clinical study evaluating its effects in humans, however, there was no statistically significant difference detected in the primary end point (time to doubling of serum creatinine), although it reduced proteinuria more than placebo.[7] Some significant side effects including aminoguanidine's damaging effect on DNA has also hindered its rise to routine use.[2,8] Other drugs that have demonstrated the ability to interrupt the formation of AGEs include pyridoxamine and ALT-946.[2] Many other drugs under investigation exhibit their pharmacologic effects further along the AGE-induced disease pathway and affect various receptors and processes. **Fig. 1** offers a simplistic overview of the AGE process and indicates where drug therapy may intervene. In reality, this process is much more complex and involves many more biochemical associations. Antifibrotic agents, for example, can inhibit TGF-b, whereas endothelin antagonists block ET-a receptors responsible for vasoconstriction of the efferent arterioles and extracellular matrix inflammation.[9] Some drugs have been observed to have multiple possible mechanisms of action. Pentoxifylline, for example, has both antiinflammatory and antifibrotic properties that could potentially explain its benefit in delaying kidney disease progression in animals.[10–12]

The following review summarizes other potential drug therapies being studied for the treatment of DKD. Only drugs that have advanced to human studies were selected for this review. The agents have been organized into 4 categories based on their proposed mechanisms of action in interrupting the DKD process: antifibrotic agents, antioxidant agents, endothelin antagonists, and those with nonspecific or multifaceted mechanisms of action. **Table 1** summarizes the medications and their proposed mechanisms of action.

ANTIFIBROTIC AGENTS: PIRFENIDONE, DOXYCYCLINE (ADOXA), FG-3019, AST-120 (KREMEZIN), AND TRANILAST (RIBAZEN)

Antifibrotic agents can inhibit growth factors and interfere with collagen and matrix formation. Ultimately, this may prohibit tissue fibrosis and remodeling of the extracellular matrix, as in the case of doxycycline, the only drug in this category that is already approved by the US Food and Drug Administration (FDA) for other conditions. Pirfenidone, AST-120, and tranilast are available outside the United States for other maladies, whereas FG-3019 is a new compound under investigation.

Pirfenidone is an antifibrotic approved in Europe for the treatment of idiopathic pulmonary fibrosis. The agent has been shown to inhibit TGF-b and reduce the level

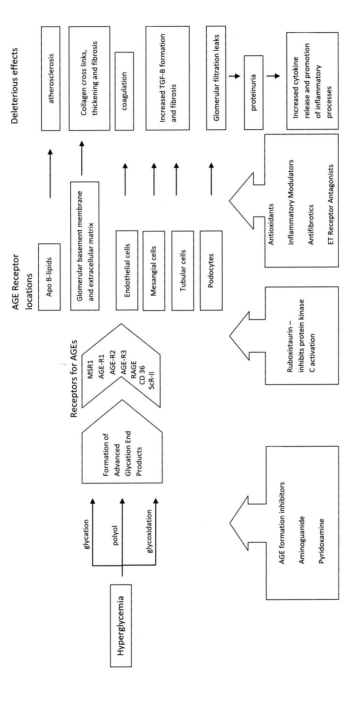

Fig. 1. Overview of AGE formation, development of deleterious effects, and where along the pathway drug therapy may intervene.

Table 1
Drugs and other molecular compounds and their proposed mechanisms of action in effecting the progression of DKD

Drug	Proposed Mechanism of Action
Pirfenidone	Inhibition of growth factors, interfere with collagen and matrix formation, inhibit TGF-b and TNF-a
Doxycycline	Inhibits matrix metalloproteinases
FG-3019	Inhibits connective tissue growth factor and indirectly, TGF-b and IGF-1
AST-120	Adsorption of uremic toxins reduced expression of TGF-b
Tranilast	Inhibits TGF-b release
Bardoxolone	Increased gene expression and transcription factor induction that decreases oxidative stress and pro-inflammatory activity; decreased production of inflammatory cytokines IL-1, IL-6, and TNF-a
Pentoxifylline	Decreased production of pro-inflammatory cytokines
Bosentan	ET-a and ET-b receptor antagonist
Atrasentan	More selective ET-a receptor antagonist
Avosentan	ET-a receptor antagonist
Paricalcitol	Inhibition of TNF-a, IL-2, TGF-b, and fibroblasts
Ruboxistaurin	Inhibits protein kinase C
Palosuran	Urotensin II receptor antagonist
Allopurinol	Xanthine oxidase inhibitor reduces uric acid formation with potential effect on urinary albumin excretion
Fasudil	Inhibits Rho kinase

of TNF-a in animal models.[13,14] These mechanisms can decrease fibrosis in the kidney and may have a renoprotective effect in DKD. Sharma and colleagues[14] performed a randomized, double-blind, placebo-controlled trial of 77 subjects with DKD, with 52 subjects completing the trial. Subjects received pirfenidone 1200 mg/d, pirfenidone 2400 mg/d, or placebo. After 1 year, estimated glomerular filtration rates (eGFR) were significantly increased in the 1200-mg/d pirfenidone group compared with placebo ($+3.3 \pm 8.5$ mL/min/1.73 m^2 vs -2.2 ± 4.8 mL/min/1.73 m^2; $P = .026$). No significant difference in eGFR was seen in the 2400-mg/d pirfenidone group versus placebo (-1.9 ± 6.7 mL/min/1.73 m^2). This result may have been due to the small study size and high dropout rate within the high-dose pirfenidone group. No decrease in albuminuria was seen in the pirfenidone treatment groups. While not specific to diabetic kidney disease, a study currently underway by the National Institute of Diabetes and Digestive and Kidney Diseases (NIDDK) is currently examining the effectiveness of pirfenidone in the treatment of focal segmental glomerulosclerosis, a disease also marked by kidney fibrosis and proteinuria, and may further contribute to the possible role pirfenidone has in therapy.[15]

Doxycycline has been evaluated for its antifibrotic effects, specifically its ability to inhibit matrix metalloproteinases (MMPs). MMPs play an important role in the remodeling of connective tissue. In the context of DKD, an imbalance of MMPs and tissue inhibitors of metalloproteinases leads to an increase in tissue fibrosis.[16] Doxycycline is a nonselective inhibitor of MMPs and may decrease the remodeling of extracellular matrix.[16,17] A study by Naini and colleagues[17] included 35 patients with DKD who were on stable doses of angiotensin-converting enzyme inhibitors (ACEIs) and/or angiotensin II-AT1 receptor blockers (ARBs) and assessed 24-hour urine collections. All patients received doxycycline, 100 mg, once daily for 2 months and were reassessed 4 months after discontinuing the medication. The mean baseline protein-uria of 888 ± 419 mg/d was unchanged at 1 month (884 ± 368 mg/d) but had signifi-cantly declined to 643 ± 386 mg/d (P<.001) at 2 months of therapy. Records of only 12 (34%) patients were obtained for the 4-month washout after discontinuation of doxycycline, which revealed that the amount of proteinuria had increased to 1021 ± 422 mg/d. In an open-label, randomized study by Aggarwal and colleagues,[16] 40 patients with DKD who were on stable doses of ACEIs and/or ARBs with overt protei-nura (defined as >500 mg/d) and antihyperglycemic mediations received either placebo or oral doxycycline, 100 mg, daily for 3 months. Renal parameters were measured at baseline, after 1 and 3 months of therapy, and at 6 months after a 3-month washout period. No significant difference was seen at 1 month; however, although both groups experienced a decrease in proteinuria, the group that received doxycycline had a significantly larger decrease than the group that received placebo (1.22 ± 2.01 vs 1.50 ± 1.50 g/d; P<.05). At 6 months, following the 3-month washout and discontinu-ation of doxycycline, levels of proteinuria returned to nearly pretreatment levels (1.98 ± 2.65 vs 2.17 ± 2.95 g/d at baseline). Neither study observed any significant effects of other renal parameters such as serum blood urea nitrogen, creatinine, or blood pres-sure.[16,17] The effect of doxycycline in DKD is currently continuing to be explored with an ongoing study assessing the possible anti-inflammatory and insulin sensitizing properties via direct measurement of MMP activity and C-reactive protein.[18]

FG-3019 is a recombinant human anti-CTGF monoclonal antibody that has completed a phase I trial for treating microalbuminuria in patients with diabetes. CTGF expression is increased in patients with diabetes and has been shown to increase the fibrogenic activity of TGF-β and insulinlike growth factor 1, as well as inhibit antifi-brotic factors.[19] The open-label dose-escalation trial administered intravenous biweekly infusions of FG-3019 and used a dose of 3 or 10 mg/kg. The urinary albumin-to-creatinine ratios (UACR) were decreased for both the 3- and 10-mg/kg groups, although these data were not statistically significant, likely due to a low study population (n = 9 and n = 10, respectively). However, when both groups were combined, a significant average decline in mean UACR was observed from baseline to day 56 (61 ± 57 and 34 ± 21 mg/g, respectively [P = .027]).[19] Fibrogen, FG-3019's manufacturer, is continuing research into the medication's possible treatment of micro-albuminuria. FG-3019 was recently granted Orphan status by the Food and Drug Administration in July 2012 for the treatment of idiopathic pulmonary fibrosis.[20]

AST-120 (Kremezin) is another agent currently undergoing clinical trial for use in the United States but has been more extensively studied and used in Asian countries, particularly Japan. AST-120 is an oral adsorbent that has been demonstrated to have a protective effect on the progression of both nondiabetic chronic kidney disease (CKD) and DKD by decreasing the amount of uremic toxins.[20] These uremic toxins include biologically harmful substances such as indoxyl sulfate, methylguanidine, and dimethylamine and are thought to contribute either directly or indirectly to toxicity of renal tissues.[21–24] In addition, AST-120 has shown in animal studies to possess anti-fibrotic characteristics via reducing the expression of TGF-b.[24] Of the clinical trials completed in humans, Sanaka and colleagues[22] performed the largest in the popula-tion of patients with DKD, whereby a total of 276 patients were given an average dose of 5 g (5.0 ± 1.4 g) orally daily. After 6 months of therapy, subjects were divided into 3 groups according to changes in serum creatinine (SCr) levels compared with baseline. Subjects with a decrease in SCr levels compared with baseline were grouped as "responders," those with a less than 1.5-fold increase in SCr were grouped as "partial responders," and those with a 1.5-fold or greater increase in SCr were grouped as "nonresponders."[22] About 30% of the subjects were designated as responders

(4.2 ± 1.9 to 3.6 ± 1.8 mg/dL after therapy; P<.001), 52% were designated as partial responders (4.7 ± 1.8 to 5.7 ± 2.3 mg/dL after therapy; P<.001), and 18% were designated as nonresponders (4.4 ± 1.5 to 7.9 ± 2.8 mg/dL after therapy; P<.001).[22] An open-label, randomized controlled study by Konishi and colleagues[21] demonstrated AST-120 to be more effective when initiated in early-stage renal failure by using 6 g once daily in 16 subjects with type 2 diabetes mellitus (T2DM), an SCr level of less than 1.5 mg/dL, and 24-hour urinary protein excretion greater than 0.5 g. Although limited by the small sample size, the study demonstrated that 7 of 10 subjects in the control group had exceeded SCr concentrations of 2 mg/dL at 37 months compared with only 1 of 6 subjects in the AST-120 group at 34 months (P = .039).[21] Research of AST-120 continues with the K-STAR trial (Kremezin Study Against Renal Disease Progression in Korea), which is currently recruiting sugjects. This study will assess AST-120 added to standard-of-care therapy for moderate to sever CKD, although not specifically DKD, overall treatment period of 36 months on a primary composite outcome of initiation of renal replacement therapy, decline of eGFR 50% or more, or doubling of SCr when compared with a standard-of-care group.[25]

Tranilast [N-(3,4-dimethoxycinnamoyl) anthranilic acid] is an antifibrotic agent currently available in Japan and South Korea for the treatment of keloid formation after skin injury and scleroderma. Tranilast exerts its antifibrotic effects through inhibition of TGF-b release, resulting in decreased collagen synthesis by fibroblasts.[26] There is a paucity of trials examining the use of tranilast in patients with DKD. Soma and colleagues[26] randomized 20 subjects with a urinary albumin excretion of 30 to 1000 mg/g creatinine and SCr 1.2 mg/dL or less and taking an ACEI or ARB to either tranilast, 100 mg, orally 3 times per day or placebo. Urinary albumin excretion and urinary type IV collagen excretion were measured at baseline and every 3 months during the 12-month study; values for these assessments were divided by urinary creatinine concentrations to exclude the influence of urine concentration, giving a normal range of less than 10 mg/gCr for urinary albumin excretion and less than 4.9 µg/gCr for urinary type IV collagen excretion. In the tranilast treatment group, both urinary albumin excretion and urinary type IV collagen excretion were significantly decreased compared with the baseline (191 ± 62 vs 279 ± 79 mg/gCr and 4.4 ± 0.90 vs 6.4 ± 0.66 µg/gCr, respectively). In the control group, although both the urinary albumin and urinary type IV collagen excretion rates were higher, no significant changes were observed. The investigators concluded that tranilast seems to decrease urinary albumin and type IV collagen excretion in patients with DKD and may potentially be useful for retarding the progression of early DKD.[26]

ANTIOXIDANT INFLAMMATION MODULATORS: BARDOXOLONE AND PENTOXIFYLLINE (TRENTAL)

Antioxidant inflammation modulators (AIMs) are thought to exert beneficial effects in DKD through increased expression of genes (nuclear factor [NF]-E2-related factor 2 [Nrf1], peroxisome proliferator-activated receptor-γ [PPAR γ], and heme oxygenase 1 [HO-1]), which have been associated with protective effects against acute kidney injury,[27] as well as induction of Nrf2, a transcription factor known to play a key role in decreasing oxidative stress and reducing the proinflammatory activity of the IkappaB kinase-β/NF-κB pathway, resulting in restoration of redox homeostasis in inflamed areas.[28] Furthermore, AIMs decrease the production of inflammatory cytokines, such as IL-1, IL-6, and TNF-α.[2] These mechanisms shed light on a promising future for medications such as bardoxolone and pentoxifylline, although a paucity of literature exists to define the exact role of these medications in the long-term management of DKD.

A phase IIb double-blind, randomized, placebo-controlled trial evaluated the effects of bardoxolone in 227 patients with DKD with a eGFR ranging from 20 to 45 mL/min/1.73 m^2 and T2DM. Participants were assigned to 1 of doses of bardoxolone or placebo (**Table 2**).[29] Although results from this trial reflected increased eGFR values after 24 weeks, concerns have been raised about the mechanism by which bardoxolone increases eGFR. The initial beneficial effects on eGFR were not maintained 4 weeks after discontinuation of bardoxolone. Increases in eGFR by bardoxolone may have resulted from deleterious rather than favorable mechanisms, such as afferent arteriolar dilatation and increased glomerular hydrostatic pressure.[30] Such mechanisms are contrary to the well-established favorable effects of angiotensin blockade seen with ACEI and ARB therapy in patients with diabetic nephropathy.

Bardoxolone therapy in the setting of DKD has been associated with muscle spasms, hypomagnesemia, and nausea. Consequently, adherence to bardoxolone therapy declined to 81%, 42%, and 25%, respectively, in the 25, 75, and 150 mg/d groups at 52 weeks. Long-term studies are needed to further clarify the significance of these adverse effects.[29]

Bardoxolone methyl displays increases in eGFR in individuals with DKD for a time frame of approximately 3 months. However, the long-term safety and efficacy of bardoxolone has not yet been evaluated thoroughly. Furthermore, the mechanism by which bardoxolone increases eGFR warrants further elucidation. Results from the Bardoxolone Methyl Evaluation in Patients with Chronic Kidney Disease and Type 2 Diabetes (BEACON) study have the potential to shed insight on the long-term effects of bardoxolone in slowing the progression to end-stage renal disease (ESRD) and death from cardiovascular causes in patients with advanced CKD and T2DM.[31]

Pentoxifylline is a methylxanthine phosphodiesterase inhibitor that has been studied in individuals with DKD.[32,33] Most pentoxifylline studies are of short duration in a limited number of patients.

An extensive systematic review including 17 studies of pentoxifylline for patients with DKD published between 1986 and 2006 concluded that pentoxifylline treatment results in decreased SCr levels, microalbuminuria, and overt proteinuria when compared with placebo. Furthermore, pentoxifylline decreased proteinuria in a DKD population when compared with routine treatment. In this review, routine treatment was defined as glycemic, blood pressure, and lipid control; anticoagulant or antiplatelet treatment; physical activity and dietary control; or treatment with ACEIs, ARBs, or calcium channel blockers. Pentoxifylline treatment was most commonly associated with headache, dizziness, nausea, and dyspepsia.[32]

A meta-analysis of the effects of pentoxifylline on proteinuria, with or without ACE or ARB treatment, in DKD included 10 studies and a total of 476 subjects. A significant decrease in proteinuria (weighted mean difference −278 mg/d of protein) was demonstrated in these trials when compared with placebo or standard care (95% confidence interval, −398 to −159; $P<.001$), although these results were variable when stratified by overt proteinuria or microalbuminuria. The investigators concluded that a greater decrease in proteinuria was associated with a higher baseline proteinuria ($P = .002$) and shorter study duration ($P<.001$), although the pentoxifylline dose did not have a significant effect on proteinuria ($P = .4$). In a small number of participants, pentoxifylline treatment was associated with dizziness, gastrointestinal symptoms, and headache.[33]

Although pentoxifylline studies demonstrate associated decreases in SCr levels, albuminuria, and overt proteinuria, insufficient evidence exists for pentoxifylline to be recommended as a mainstay of treatment for the management of DKD. Future research should focus on long-term use of pentoxifylline in DKD populations stratified

Table 2
Bardoxolone studies in diabetic kidney disease patients

Trial	Study Population	Treatment Groups	Study Outcomes	Results	Adverse Effects
Pergola et al,[28] BEAM	227 Adults with CKD (eGFR 20–45 mL/min/1.73 m²) and type 2 diabetes	25 mg daily 75 mg daily 150 mg daily	Change from baseline in eGFR at 24 wk and 52 wk	24 wk: 25 mg: 8.2 ± 1.5 mL/min/1.73 m² 75 mg: 11.4 ± 1.5 mL/min/1.73 m² 150 mg: 10.4 ± 1.5 mL/min/1.73 m² (P<.001) 52 wk: 25 mg: 5.8 ± 1.8 mL/min/1.73 m² 75 mg: 10.5 ± 1.8 mL/min/1.73 m² 150 mg: 9.3 ± 1.9 mL/min/1.73 m² (P<.001)	Muscle spasms, hypomagnesemia, mild increases in ALT, and GI side effects
Pergola et al[28]	20 Patients with moderate to severe CKD and type 2 diabetes	25 mg daily × 28 d, then 75 mg daily × 28 d	Change from baseline to day 56 in eGFR Secondary: changes in SCr, CrCl, UACR, BUN, and 24-h creatinine excretion	Increase in eGFR 7.2 mL/min/1.73 m² (P<.001) Secondary: SCr—0.3 mg/dL BUN—4.9 mg/dL CrCl + 14.6 mL/min/1.73 m²	Muscle spasms (n = 7; 35%), chills (n = 3; 15%), cough (n = 3; 15%)

Abbreviations: ALT, alanine aminotransferase; BUN, blood urea nitrogen; GI, gastrointestinal.

by individualized patient characteristics and dosing strategies, such as patient age, duration of DKD, and route of administration.[32] The ongoing Pentoxifylline for Reno-protection in Diabetic Nephropathy (PREDIAN) study will provide additional insight into the potential benefits of pentoxifylline in combination with ACE or ARB treatment compared with ACE or ARB treatment alone in individuals with stage 3 or 4 DKD during a 2-year period.[34]

ENDOTHELIN RECEPTOR ANTAGONISTS: BOSENTAN (TRACLEER), ATRASENTAN, AND AVOSENTAN

Endothelin-1 (ET-1), with its potent vasoactive properties,[35] plays an important role in the development of diabetes-related complications. Plasma and urinary ET-1 levels are elevated in patients with diabetes and have been shown to correlate with decreased renal function, increased blood pressure, and increased albuminuria.[36–41] ET-1 acts on 2 receptors, endothelin A (ET_A) and endothelin B (ET_B). ET_A receptors, located in vascular smooth muscle, arteries, and the glomerulus, cause vasoconstriction, renal sodium retention, cellular proliferation, inflammation, and fibrosis when stimulated.[42] ET_B receptor stimulation has the opposite effect, resulting in vasodilation, sodium excretion, and inhibition of vascular proliferation, inflammation, and fibrosis. These receptors are localized in vascular and glomerular endothelial cells, convoluted tubules, and collecting duct epithelial cells.[41,43] The effect of an endothelin antagonist depends on its selectivity for the ET_A versus ET_B receptors. There are 2 endothelin antagonists approved by the FDA: ambrisentan (Letairis), an agent selective for the ET_A receptor, and bosentan, a nonselective agent. Ambrisentan has not been studied for the treatment of DKD. Other non-FDA approved endothelin antagonists that have been studied for diabetic nephropathy include avosentan and atrasentan.

Bosentan is a dual endothelin receptor antagonist originally approved by the FDA in 2001 for the management of pulmonary artery hypertension. Based on its pharmacologic action, bosentan has recently been studied for its effects on kidney disease in diabetic patients. In a randomized, double-blind, placebo-controlled parallel group study, 46 patients with T2DM for at least 2 years and with microalbuminuria were randomized to bosentan 62.5 mg twice daily titrated to 125 mg twice daily or placebo for 4 weeks. The primary end point was the change in microvascular endothelium-dependent vasodilatation, assessed by the change in digital reactive hyperemia index (RHI). In the bosentan group, the RHI increased from 1.73 ± 0.43 at baseline to 2.08 ± 0.59 at study end ($P<.05$), whereas there was no change in the placebo group (1.84 ± 0.49 to 1.87 ± 0.47). The study was discontinued in three patients in the bosentan group because of adverse events (facial flushing, edema, and respiratory tract infections). There were no changes in the levels of hepatic transaminases during the study period, but there was a significant drop in the hemoglobin level within the bosentan arm, from 13.4 to 12.7 g/dL ($P<.001$).[44] Owing to the vasodilatory and therefore hemodilutional effect of these agents, the drop in hemoglobin level is to be expected. Bosentan's nonselectivity for endothelin receptors may result in more fluid overload or other complications, but data suggest that bosentan may represent a future therapeutic strategy for patients with T2DM and proteinuria.

The efficacy of avosentan, a predominant ET_A receptor antagonist, for the treatment of diabetic nephropathy has been evaluated in 2 human clinical trials.[45,46] The first trial was a randomized, double-blind, placebo-controlled, dosage-range, parallel group study of 286 diabetic patients (either type 1 or type 2) with diabetic nephropathy already on standard therapy with an ACEI and/or an ARB.[45] Patients were randomized to 1 of 5 groups, placebo or avosentan 5, 10, 25, or 50 mg daily for a period of

12 weeks. The primary efficacy parameter was the absolute change in 12-hour urinary albumin excretion rate (UAER) from baseline. Thirty-four patients were withdrawn from the study, leaving 252 patients for final analysis. Mean UAER levels at baseline ranged from 0.79 ± 0.79 to 1.21 ± 1.43 mg/min (see **Table 3**). The mean change in UAER from baseline was significant in all avosentan dosage groups, with the smallest change seen in the 10-mg group and the largest change in the 50-mg group (see **Table 3**). The proportion of patients who experienced 30% or more relative reduction in median UAER was 46.9%, 58.0%, 56.4%, 60.5%, and 23.6% for 5, 10, 25, and 50 mg avosentan and placebo, respectively. Throughout the study period, systolic blood pressure (SBP) and diastolic blood pressure (DBP) did not change significantly in any group. For safety parameters, there was a -0.6 g/dL change in hemoglobin level from baseline across all treatment groups versus 0 g/dL in the placebo group. In addition, 86% of patients who received avosentan versus 95% placebo had a decrease in hemoglobin level of 2 g/dL or less. Overall, the levels of liver enzymes remained stable throughout the treatment period, as increases in enzyme levels were less than 3 times the upper limit of normal for all patients but one (the level of alanine aminotransferase was >8 times the upper limit of normal in 1 patient in the 10-mg avosentan group). During the study, 56.3% ($n = 161$) of patients reported adverse events, with 87% of those being defined as mild or moderate. Serious adverse events were reported in 8% and 5% of patients taking avosentan and placebo, respectively. The most common adverse events were edema, abnormal electrocardiogram (ECG), anemia, and headache, and with the exception of the ECG, they were more common in the avosentan 50 mg group. Edema was the only adverse event that was statistically significantly more prevalent across all treatment groups versus placebo ($P<.01$). There was a dosage-dependent increase in the incidence of fluid-retention episodes in the avosentan arms (11.9%, 21.2%, 15.0%, and 32.1% in the 5-, 10-, 25-, and 50-mg groups) as compared with placebo (3.5%). Five deaths occurred during the study period, with 1 in each of the 5 groups. Causes of death included subdural hematoma, myocardial infarction (2), congestive heart failure, and a gastric bleed, and only 1 was thought to be due to study medication (myocardial infarction). The proportion of patients who withdrew consent or withdrew because of adverse events was dosage dependent (5.1% in the 5-mg group, 18.9% in the 50-mg group, and 3.5% in the placebo group). The investigators concluded that avosentan demonstrated the ability to decrease UAER in patients with diabetic nephropathy and macroalbuminuria, but the optimal dosage in terms of risk-benefit ratio may be defined at 10 mg or less daily.

The second trial with avosentan was a randomized, placebo-controlled, double-blind, parallel group study to assess avosentan's effect on time to doubling of SCr,

Table 3					
Effects of avosentan and placebo on UAER concentrations					
Parameter	Avosentan 5 mg ($n = 49$)	Avosentan 10 mg ($n = 50$)	Avosentan 25 mg ($n = 55$)	Avosentan 50 mg ($n = 43$)	Placebo ($n = 55$)
Baseline UAER (mg/min)	1.11 ± 1.04	0.79 ± 0.79	0.94 ± 0.68	1.21 ± 1.43	1.08 ± 1.20
Week 12 UAER (mg/min)	0.89 ± 1.02	0.68 ± 0.91	0.63 ± 0.64	0.70 ± 0.76	1.25 ± 1.41
Change in UAER (mg/min)	-0.22 ± 0.61	-0.11 ± 0.55	-0.31 ± 0.62	-0.51 ± 1.24	$+0.16 \pm 0.72$
P values vs placebo	$P<.01$	$P<.01$	$P<.001$	$P<.0001$	—

ESRD, or death in patients with T2DM and stage 3 or 4 CKD.[46] Patients were randomized to avosentan 25 mg daily, 50 mg daily, or placebo, and ACEIs and/or ARBs were continued. Almost 1400 patients participated in the trial, and the treatment period was 4 months for both the avosentan arms and 5 months for placebo. There was no statistically significant difference among the 3 groups for the proportion of patients who experienced a doubling of the SCr, ESRD, or death (**Table 4**). At 3 months, the median UACR significantly declined by 40.5% and 38.3% for the avosentan 25- and 50-mg groups, respectively, versus 7.7% placebo ($P<.001$). No statistical difference was found, but fewer patients experienced ESRD when compared with placebo, and more patients died. Death was due to cardiovascular causes in 74% of the 46 cases. In addition to the deaths, more patients experienced serious adverse events in the avosentan group, especially congestive heart failure ($P = .003$ for the avosentan 25-mg group vs placebo) and fluid overload ($P\leq.001$ for both the avosentan groups vs placebo), leading to termination of the trial by the Data Safety and Monitoring Board. Mean hemoglobin levels decreased in patients taking avosentan by approximately 11.0 g/L for both the treatment groups versus 0.1 g/L for placebo ($P<.001$). There was no significant difference in the increase in liver function tests between groups. At the dosages used in this study, avosentan significantly decreased proteinuria in patients with diabetic nephropathy but at the expense of severe consequences in some patients, leading to trial discontinuation. Avosentan may be less selective for the ET_A receptor at the doses of 25 and 50 mg, resulting in the increased fluid overload and incidence of mortality, making these higher dosages inappropriate therapeutic options. Based on both avosentan studies,[45,46] further use and study should be done with avosentan but at dosages of 10 mg or less daily.

As was seen in the A Study of Cardiovascular Events in Diabetes (ASCEND) trial, selectivity at the ET_A receptor may be an important factor for drug selection in the management of DKD. Another endothelin antagonist, atrasentan, has a selectivity of 1800:1 for ET_A and ET_B receptors.[47] In a randomized, double-blind, placebo-controlled, 8-week trial of patients with T2DM already on stable doses of ACEIs or ARBs, 89 subjects were randomly assigned to 4 treatment groups: placebo or atrasentan 0.25, 0.75, or 1.75 mg daily. The primary end point was the change in the UACR, and this was significantly reduced in the 0.75-mg and 1.75-mg atrasentan groups ($P = .001$ and $P = .011$ vs placebo, respectively) (**Table 5**). The UACR reduction in the 0.25-mg arm did not reach statistical significance ($P = .150$). The percentage of subjects who achieved at least a 40% reduction from baseline to the final UACR was statistically significant for only the 0.75-mg group ($P = .029$). The most common adverse event was peripheral edema (9% placebo, 14% 0.25 mg, 18% 0.75 mg, and 46% 1.75 mg). This result was statistically significant for only the 1.75-mg atrasentan group ($P = .007$). Two patients each from the 0.75-mg and 1.75-mg atrasentan groups had

Table 4
Effects of avosentan doses and placebo on doubling of SCr level, ESRD, death, and heart failure

Parameter	Avosentan 25 mg (n = 455)	Avosentan 50 mg (n = 478)	Placebo (n = 459)	Avosentan 25 mg vs Placebo	Avosentan 25 mg vs Placebo
Doubling of SCr	2 (0.4%)	4 (0.8%)	9 (2%)	$P = .405$	$P = .060$
ESRD	20 (4.4%)	24 (5%)	30 (6.5%)	$P = .136$	$P = .405$
Death	21 (4.6%)	17 (3.6%)	12 (2.6%)	$P = .225$	$P = .194$
Heart failure	27 (5.9%)	29 (6.1%)	10 (2.2%)	$P = .008$	$P = .050$

Table 5
Effects of atrasentan doses and placebo on UACR

Parameter	Placebo (n = 23)	Atrasentan 0.25 mg (n = 22)	Atrasentan 0.75 mg (n = 22)	Atrasentan 1.75 mg (n = 22)
Mean change from baseline in UACR (%)	11	21[a]	42[a]	35
Percentage of subjects with ≥40% reduction in UACR	17	30	50[a]	36

[a] Statistically significant when compared to placebo.

to withdraw from the study because of adverse events (congestive heart failure and coronary artery disease in the 0.75-mg group and hypotension and angioedema with peripheral edema in the 1.75-mg group). There were no deaths throughout the study period. There was no significant difference in hepatic enzymes between groups, but as expected, there were changes in hemoglobin concentrations, SBP, and DBP. The mean change in the hemoglobin level was −0.7 g/dL in the 0.25-mg group, −0.4 g/dL in the 0.75-mg group, and −0.9 g/dL in the 1.75-mg group compared with +0.1 g/dL for placebo ($P<.001$, $P = .015$, and $P<.001$, respectively). There was a statistically significant reduction in SBP during the study period for the 0.75-mg group (−8.8 mm Hg, $P = .049$ vs placebo) and in DBP for the 1.75-mg group (−7.4 mm Hg, $P = .042$ vs placebo). Other groups did not achieve statistical significance. This study demonstrated that atrasentan at 0.75 mg or 1.75 mg daily was efficacious in treating albuminuria in patients with T2DM during an 8-week period. The higher selectivity for the ET_A receptor may be an advantage for this agent in decreasing the likelihood of sodium retention from ET_B receptor inhibition. Long-term studies are needed to determine sustainability and safety outcomes.

Endothelin receptor antagonists may offer another therapeutic option to the standard treatment of renin-angiotensin system inhibition for diabetic patients with CKD. They may provide additional cardiovascular and renal protection through reductions in proteinuria, arterial stiffness, and blood pressure. Additional clinical trials with more long-term outcome analyses are needed to determine their true role and establish safety in this patient population.

NONSPECIFIC MECHANISM OF ACTION: PARICALCITOL (ZEMPLAR), RUBOXISTAURIN (ARXXANT), PALOSURAN, ALLOPURINOL (ZYLOPRIM), AND FASUDIL

Paricalcitol, ruboxistaurin, palosuran, allopurinol, and fasudil have either more unique mechanisms of action or multiple mechanisms of action that could explain their effect on kidney disease progression. Paricalcitol, for example, seems to have some antiproteinuric and antiinflammatory properties. Ruboxistaurin is known as a protein kinase C (PKC) inhibitor, which can indirectly exhibit some antifibrotic characteristics through TGF-b inhibition. Similarly, fasudil, a Rho kinase inhibitor also may indirectly retard the formation of renal fibrosis. Palosuran and allopurinol have other mechanisms of proposed action related to their effects on urotensin II and uric acid serum concentrations, respectively.

Paricalcitol is a third-generation synthetic vitamin D analogue approved for the prevention and treatment of secondary hyperparathyroidism in stage 3 to 5 CKD.[48] Paricalcitol directly activates the vitamin D receptors (VDRs) more selectively than first generation vitamin D receptor agonists in the parathyroid glands.[49,50] The activation of the VDRs results in an inhibition of parathyroid hormone (PTH) synthesis and secretion.[49] The natural activator of VDRs, calcitriol (1,25-$(OH)_2$vitamin-D), is produced by the kidney, but plasma concentrations decline as eGFR decreases.[51] As a result, patients with CKD have a deficiency in calcitriol, which causes increased PTH levels and consequently hyperparathyroidism. Lower calcitriol concentrations have also been shown to strongly correlate with a higher risk of diabetes, higher UACRs, and lower eGFRs.[51,52] VDR activators can inhibit renin biosynthesis, have beneficial effects on arterial function and left ventricular hypertrophy, attenuate insulin resistance, and improve immune function.[53,54] Vitamin D analogues such as paricalcitol are preferred VDR activators in patients with CKD because they carry less risk of hypercalcemia and hyperphosphatemia.[53,55,56] Several human studies also suggest that paricalcitol provides renal protection through a reduction in both proteinuria and inflammatory status.[53] The proposed mechanisms for this renoprotection are complex and include among others, inhibition of TNF-a, IL-2, TGF-b, and fibroblast activity.[49]

Agarwal and colleagues,[57] in 3 double-blind, randomized, placebo-controlled trials, compared the suppression of PTH in 220 patients who took either oral paricalcitol or placebo; 195 subjects had tests for dipstick urinalysis at the beginning and the end of study. In 2 trials, subjects received 2 μg of oral paricalcitol (iPTH ≤500 pg/mL), 4 μg of oral paricalcitol (iPTH >500 pg/mL), or placebo, dosed 3 times per week. In the third trial, a once-daily dosing regimen was used and the initial doses were 1 μg (iPTH ≤500 pg/mL) and 2 μg (iPTH >500 pg/mL). The doses were then titrated in 2-μg (3 times weekly) or 1-μg (daily) increments based on PTH, calcium, and phosphorus values. These 24-week studies in patients with CDK stage 3 and 4 found a significant reduction in proteinuria in the patients given paricalcitol compared with the patients given placebo (51% vs 25%, $P = .004$). The reduction observed was independent of the administration of ACEI and/or ARBs.

The VITAL study was a multinational, placebo-controlled, double-blind trial that measured the primary end point of percentage change in geometric mean UACR. This study included patients with T2DM and albuminuria. All subjects were on ACEI or ARB therapy. After 24 weeks of treatment, results showed that the primary end point of reduction in UACR was not significant. In the 1-μg group compared with placebo there was a −11% change from baseline ($P = .23$). In the 2-μg group compared with placebo there was a −18% change from baseline ($P = .053$). A total of 88 patients received placebo, 92 received 1 μg paricalcitol, and 92 received 2 μg paricalcitol, each given one dose daily. However, the proportion of patients who achieved a change in UACR of at least −15% from baseline to the last treatment was significant only in the 2-μg group (55% [51/92], $P = .038$). There was also a reduction in eGFR in the 2-μg paricalcitol group versus placebo, although not significant ($P = .0548$). In this study, no significant changes were seen between the paricalcitol groups and placebo in the measurements of antiinflammatory markers.[51]

In a study of 61 patients, Fishbane and colleagues[58] showed a significant reduction in eGFRs from 15 to 90 mL/min/1.73 m^2 and protein excretion greater than 400 mg per 24 hours in the group that received 1 μg/d paricalcitol compared with the group that received placebo. This 6-month, double-blind randomized study showed changes in protein excretion from baseline to last evaluation of +2.9% in the placebo group and −17.6% in the paricalcitol group ($P<.05$).

In an observational study of 19 patients with proteinuria who received ACEI or ARBs for control of proteinuria, 14 patients responded favorably to paricalcitol treatment. In these 14 patients, there was a 32.9% reduction in proteinuria. In the other 5 patients, no significant change in protein excretion was observed. All subjects were given oral paricalcitol, 1 to 2 μg/d, depending on iPTH levels (1 μg for iPTH ≤500 pg/mL; otherwise dose was 2 μg/d). Dose reduction was required in 2 patients because of increased Ca levels.[49]

A randomized, double-blind, pilot trial of 24 patients (22 completions) found that greater than 50% of the subjects had a significant reduction in the secondary end point of proteinuria. The subjects had stage 2 or 3 CKD and were randomized to placebo, 1 μg, or 2 μg oral paricalcitol for 1 month. Patients were on a stable dose of ACEI or ARB therapy. The treatment/baseline ratio of 24-hour albumin excretion rate was 1.35 in the placebo group ($P = .01$), 0.52 in the 1-μg paricalcitol group ($P<.001$), and 0.54 in the 2-μg paricalcitol group ($P = .01$) ($P<.001$ between group changes). The primary end points were endothelial function and inflammation, of which no changes in vascular smooth muscle function were observed at 1 month. A significant change in the inflammation markers from baseline ($P = .048$) between groups was detected, although the study size was small and limits the generalizability of these results.[59]

None of these paricalcitol studies reported a risk of adverse events in paricalcitol-treated patients that was significantly higher when compared with placebo. In summary, there are data to indicate that vitamin D concentrations are significantly lower in patients with DKD compared with nondiabetic patients with CKD[60] and some preliminary evidence indicating that paricalcitol may have antiproteinuric and antiinflammatory properties in patients with DKD.

Ruboxistaurin is a selective inhibitor of PKC-β, a signal transduction mediator activated by hyperglycemia and associated with diabetic vascular complications.[61–64] In several preclinical studies, PKC-β was linked to the overexpression of TGF-b, leading to the development of glomerulosclerosis and tubulointerstitial fibrosis.[65–68] Tuttle and colleagues[69] performed a randomized, double-blind, placebo-controlled trial in humans evaluating ruboxistaurin 32 mg daily, in addition to renin-angiotensin-aldosterone system (RAAS) inhibitor therapy, for 1 year in 123 patients with T2DM and persistent albuminuria (albumin-to-creatinine ratio 200–2000 mg/g). After 1 year, in patients treated with ruboxistaurin, UACR significantly decreased as compared with placebo ($-24 + 9\%$, $P = .020$ vs $-9 + 11\%$, $P = .430$) and the eGFR in the ruboxistaurin group was maintained ($-2.5 + 1.9$ mL/min/1.73 m^2) in contrast with the placebo group, which lost significant eGFR function ($-4.8 + 1.8$ mL/min/1.73 m^2).[69] Additional studies are needed to determine the efficacy and long term outcomes of ruboxistaurin use in this patient population.

Gilbert and colleagues[62] examined the correlation between the urinary excretion of fibrogenic growth factors, namely, TGF-b, and the extent of tubulointerstitial disease. TGF-b was the prespecified secondary objective in the prospective, double-blind, placebo-controlled study of ruboxistaurin, 32 mg/d, for 1 year in 107 patients with diabetic nephropathy, all receiving an ACEI or an ARB. The study results reflected a significant increase in urinary TGF-b-to-creatinine ratio (TCR) among patients in the placebo group ($+37\%$, $P<.01$) versus no significant TCR increase in patients treated with ruboxistaurin ($+19\%$, $P = NS$). According to this trial, the increased intrarenal production of TGF-b may be an applicable biomarker of renal fibrogenesis and disease progression independent of the RAAS.

Palosuran is a potent, selective, competitive antagonist of the urotensin II receptor. Binding of the urotensin II receptor leads to activation of phospholipase C, increasing the intracellular calcium concentration, and ultimately leading to contraction of vascular smooth muscle. Elevated urotensin II plasma concentrations have been observed in patients with DKD, suggesting a role for urotensin II antagonists in therapy.[70–74] Sidharta and colleagues[75] studied patients with hypertension and type II diabetic nephropathy administered either an ACEI or ARB in an open-label, multi-dose study in patients with normal to mild (CrCl >50 mL/min) and moderate to severe (CrCl ≤50 mL/min) kidney disease. A total of 18 patients completed the trial treatment of oral palosuran 125 mg twice daily for 13.5 days. Results showed a statistically significant decrease in the 24-hour UAER in the group with normal to mildly impaired renal function (26.2%, $P = .027$) but not in the group with moderate to severely impaired renal function (22.3%, $P = .250$). Palosuran was well tolerated and did not lead to any patients' withdrawal from the study.

Comparatively, Vogt and colleagues[76] conducted a multicenter, randomized, double-blind, placebo-controlled study on whether palosuran would reduce urinary albumin excretion and/or systemic blood pressure in patients with hypertension and type 2 diabetic nephropathy already being treated with an ACEI or ARB. A total of 54 patients were randomly treated during 2 treatment phases of 4 weeks each, separated by a 6-week washout period, with palosuran 125 mg twice daily or placebo. At this time, palosuran has not proven to be an effective therapy option to control the progression of renal disease.

Allopurinol is a xanthine oxidase inhibitor that directly reduces the amount of uric acid produced in the body. In the context of DKD, previous studies have revealed that patients with T2DM demonstrate elevated serum concentrations of uric acid that directly correspond to their level of urinary albumin excretion.[77] Furthermore, hyperuricemia may be accompanied by peripheral vascular disease, higher concentration of hemoglobin A1c, more severe albuminuria, lower eGFR, and the early start or rapid progression of diabetic nephropathy.[78–80] Momeni and colleagues[81] evaluated the effect of allopurinol 100 mg daily in decreasing proteinuria through a double-blind, randomized, controlled trial with 40 patients. The study showed that serum concentrations of uric acid (6.44 ± 1.97 vs 5.31 ± 0.79, $P = .02$) and levels of 24-hour urine protein (1011 ± 767 vs 1609 ± 1071, $P = .049$) were both significantly lower after 4 months of treatment with low-dose allopurinol as compared with the control group. The study reported no adverse effects and that the inhibition of uric acid production promotes a significant decrease in proteinuria and, thus, delayed progression of nephropathy.

Fasudil, a specific inhibitor of Rho kinase (ROCK), has been associated with reno-protective effects in the kidney. ROCK inhibition promotes dilation of the afferent and efferent arterioles and reverses angiotensin II-dependent arteriolar vasoconstriction. Renal fibrosis has been linked to the RhoA/ROCK pathway at the cellular level, specifically to epithelial-mesenchymal transdifferentiation during cytoskeletal rearrangements in the podocytes, renal tubule cells, and mesangial cells. Other models of kidney damage have been explored as well; ROCK inhibition reduced structural and functional damage secondary to hypertension and prevented tubulointerstitial fibrosis following unilateral ureteral obstruction.[82,83] Gojo and colleagues[84] reported that administration of fasudil (10 mg/kg) for 30 days had no effect on glycemic control but normalized albuminuria and decreased levels of urinary 8-hydroxyguanosine. Kolavennu and colleagues[85] tested the effects of fasudil (10 mg/kg) for 16 weeks and confirmed that ROCK inhibition was independent of glycemic control and considerably decreased albuminuria, mesangial expansion, accumulation of glomerular type IV collagen, and thickening of the glomerular basement membrane (**Table 4**).[83]

SUMMARY

Antifibrotic agents, antioxidant agents, ET-a receptor antagonists, and a few other agents with nonspecific or multifaceted mechanisms of action have been evaluated and progressed to small clinical studies in human subjects. Although there are limited data at the present time, these early evaluations have produced some favorable results that at least warrant further investigation. There is certainly not enough compelling evidence to justify the routine use of any of these products specifically for DKD at the moment; however, more well-controlled and adequately powered studies in several hundred patients will help determine which of these may have a place in the DKD treatment armamentarium of the future.

REFERENCES

1. Daroux M, Prevost G, Maillard-Lefebvre H, et al. Advanced glycation end-products: implication for the diabetic and non-diabetic nephropathies. Diabetes Metab 2010;36:1–10.
2. Turgut F, Bolton W. Potential new therapeutic agents for diabetic kidney disease. Am J Kidney Dis 2010;55:928–40.
3. Abbate M, Zoja C, Corna D, et al. In progressive nephropathies, overload of tubular cells with filtered proteins translates glomerular permeability dysfunction into cellular signals of interstitial inflammation. J Am Soc Nephrol 1998;9:1213–24.
4. Soulis-Liparota T, Cooper M, Papazoglou D, et al. Retardation by aminoguanidine of development of albuminuria, mesangial expansion, and tissue fluorescence in streptozocin-induced diabetic rat. Diabetes 1991;40(10):1328–34.
5. Friedman E, Distant D, Fleishhacker J, et al. Aminoguanidine prolongs survival in azotemic-induced diabetic rats. Am J Kidney Dis 1997;30(2):253–9.
6. Abdel-Rahman E, Bolton W. Pimagedine: a novel therapy for diabetic nephropathy. Expert Opin Investig Drugs 2002;11(4):565–74.
7. Bolton W, Cattran D, Williams M, et al. Randomized trial of an inhibitor of formation of advanced glycation end products in diabetic nephropathy. Am J Nephrol 2004; 24(1):32–40.
8. Suji G, Sivakami S. DNA damage by free radical production by aminoguanidine. Ann N Y Acad Sci 2006;1067:191–9.
9. Neuhofer W, Pittrow D. Endothelin receptor selectivity in chronic kidney disease: rationale and review of recent evidence. Eur J Clin Invest 2009;39(S2):50–67.
10. Lin S, Chen Y, Chien C, et al. Pentoxifylline attenuated the renal disease progression in rats with remnant kidney. J Am Soc Nephrol 2002;13(12):2916–29.
11. Chen Y, Ng Y, Lin S, et al. Pentoxifylline suppresses renal tubular necrosis factor-alpha and ameliorates experimental crescentic glomerulonephritis in rats. Nephrol Dial Transplant 2004;19(5):1106–15.
12. Tsai T, Lin R, Chang C, et al. Vasodilator agents modulate rat glomerular mesangial cell growth and collagen synthesis. Nephron 1995;70(1):91–9.
13. RamachandraRao S, Zhu Y, Ravasi T, et al. Pirfenidone is renoprotective in diabetic kidney disease. J Am Soc Nephrol 2009;20:1765–75.
14. Sharma K, Ix J, Matthew A, et al. Pirfenidone for diabetic nephropathy. J Am Soc Nephrol 2011;22:1144–51.
15. National Institute of Diabetes and Digestive and Kidney Diseases; Bethesda, MD. Pirfenidone to treat kidney disease (focal segmental glomerulosclerosis). In: Clinicaltrials.gov [Internet]. Bethesda, MD: National Library of Medicine (US). 2000-[cited 2012 Oct 8]. Available from: http://clinicaltrials.gov/ct2/show/NCT00001959 NLM Identifier: NCT00001959.
16. Aggarwal H, Jain D, Talapatra P, et al. Evaluation of role of doxycycline (a matrix metalloproteinase inhibitor) on renal functions in patients of diabetic nephropathy. Ren Fail 2010;32:941–6.
17. Naini A, Harandi A, Moghtaderi J, et al. Doxycycline: a pilot study to reduce diabetic proteinuria. Am J Nephrol 2007;27:269–73.

18. ClinicalTrials.gov. Examination of the anti-inflammatory and insulin sensitizing properties of doxycycline in humans. NLM Identifier: NCT01375491. www. clinicaltrials.gov [Accessed October 8, 2012].

19. Adler S, Schwartz S, Williams M, et al. Phase 1 study of anti-CTGF monoclonal antibody in patients with diabetes and microalbuminuria. Clin J Am Soc Nephrol 2010;5:1420–8.

20. FibroGen Press Release. FibroGen's FG-3019 granted US Orphan drug designation for the treatment of patients with idiopathic pulmonary fibrosis. http://www. fibrogen.com/press/release/pr_1343708794 [Accessed October 8, 2012].

21. Konishi K, Nakano S, Shin-ichi T, et al. AST-120 (Kremezin) initiated in early stage chronic kidney disease stunts the progression of renal dysfunction in type 2 diabetic subjects. Diabetes Res Clin Pract 2008;81:310–5.

22. Sanaka T, Akizawa T, Koide K, et al. Protective effect of an oral adsorbent on renal function in chronic renal failure: determinants of its efficacy in diabetic nephropathy. Ther Apher Dial 2004;8(3):232–40.

23. Ueda H, Shibahara N, Shizuko T, et al. AST-120, an oral adsorbant, delays the initiation of dialysis in patients with chronic kidney disease. Ther Apher Dial 2007;11(3):189–95.

24. Hayashino Y, Fukuhara S, Akizawa T, et al. Cost-effectiveness of administering oral adsorbent AST-120 to patients with diabetes and advance stage chronic kidney disease. Diabetes Res Clin Pract 2010;90:154–9.

25. Clinicaltrials.gov. Kremezin Study Against Renal Disease Progression in Korea (K-STAR). NLM Identifier: NCT 00860431. www.clinicaltrials.gov. [Accessed October 8, 2012].

26. Soma J, Sato K, Saito H, et al. Effect of tranilast in early stage diabetic nephropathy. Nephrol Dial Transplant 2006;21:2795–9.

27. Wu Q, Wang Y, Senitko M, et al. Bardoxolone methyl (BARD) ameliorates ischemic AKI and increases expression of protective genes Nrf2, PPARγ, and HO-1. Am J Physiol Renal Physiol 2011;300:F1180–92.

28. Pergola P, Krauth M, Huff J, et al. Effect of bardoxolone methyl on kidney function in patients with T2D and stage 3b-4 CKD. Am J Nephrol 2011;33:469–76.

29. Pergola P, Raskin P, Toto R, et al. Bardoxolone methyl and kidney function in CKD with type 2 diabetes. N Engl J Med 2011;365:327–36.

30. McMahon G, Foreman J. Bardoxolone methyl, chronic kidney disease, and type 2 diabetes. N Engl J Med 2011;365(18):1746.

31. Bardoxolone methyl evaluation in patients with chronic kidney disease and type 2 diabetes (BEACON). Clinical trial NCT01351675. Available at: www.clinicaltrials. gov. Accessed August 27, 2012.

32. Shan D, Wu H, Yuan Q, et al. Pentoxifylline for diabetic kidney disease [review]. The Cochrane Collaboration. Wiley & Sons, Ltd; 2012.

33. McCormick B, Sydor A, Akbari A, et al. The effect of pentoxifylline on proteinuria in diabetic kidney disease: a meta-analysis. Am J Kidney Dis 2008;52: 454–63.

34. Navarro-Gonzalez J, Muros M, Mora-Fernandez C, et al. Pentoxifylline for renoprotection in diabetic nephropathy: the PREDIAN study. Rationale and basal results. J Diabetes Complications 2011;25:314–9.

35. Yanagisawa M, Kurihara H, Kimura S, et al. A novel potent vasoconstrictor peptide produced by vascular endothelial cells. Nature 1988;332:411–5.

36. De Mattia G, Cassone-Faldetta M, Bellini C, et al. Role of plasma and urinary endothelin-1 in early diabetic and hypertensive nephropathy. Am J Hypertens 1998;11:983–8.

37. Bruno CM, Meli S, Marcinno M, et al. Plasma endothelin-1 levels and albumin excretion rate in normotensive, microalbuminuric type 2 diabetic patients. J Biol Regul Homeost Agents 2002;16:114–7.
38. Haynes WG, Webb DJ. Endothelin as a regulator of cardiovascular function in health and disease. J Hypertens 1998;16:1081–98.
39. Kakizawa H, Itoh M, Itoh Y, et al. The relationship between glycemic control and plasma vascular endothelial growth factor and endothelin-1 concentration in diabetic patients. Metabolism 2004;53:550–5.
40. Peppa-Patrikiou M, Dracopoulou M, Dacou-Voutetakis C. Urinary endothelin in adolescents and young adults with insulin-dependent diabetes mellitus: relation to urinary albumin, blood pressure, and other factors. Metabolism 1998;47:1408–12.
41. Schneider MP, Boesen EI, Pollock DM. Contrasting actions of endothelin ET(A) and ET(B) receptors in cardiovascular disease. Annu Rev Pharmacol Toxicol 2007;47:731–59.
42. Jandeleit-Dahm KA, Watson AM. The endothelin system and endothelin receptor antagonists. Curr Opin Nephrol Hypertens 2012;21:66–71.
43. Ge Y, Bagnall A, Stricklett PK, et al. Collecting duct-specific knockout of the endothelin B receptor causes hypertension and sodium retention. Am J Physiol Renal Physiol 2006;291:F1274–80.
44. Rafnsson A, Bohm F, Settergren M, et al. The endothelin receptor antagonist bosentan improves peripheral endothelial function in patients with type 2 diabetes mellitus and microalbuminuria: a randomized trial. Diabetologia 2012;55:600–7.
45. Wenzel RR, Littke T, Kuranoff S, et al. Avosentan reduces albumin excretion in diabetics with macroalbuminuria. J Am Soc Nephrol 2009;20:655–64.
46. Mann JF, Green D, Jamerson K, et al. Avosentan for overt diabetic nephropathy. J Am Soc Nephrol 2010;21:527–35.
47. Opgenorth TJ, Adler AL, Calzadilla SV, et al. Pharmacological characterization of A-127722: an orally active and highly potent ETA-selective receptor antagonist. J Pharmacol Exp Ther 1996;276:473–81.
48. Zemplar [package insert]. North Chicago: Abbott Laboratories; 2011.
49. Aperis G, Paliouras C, Zervos A, et al. The role of paricalcitol on proteinuria. J Ren Care 2011;37(2):80–4.
50. Sprague S, Llach F, Amdahl M, et al. Paricalcitol versus calcitriol in the treatment of secondary hyperparathyroidism. Kidney Int 2003;63(4):1483–90.
51. De Zeeuw D, Agarwal R, Amdahl M, et al. Selective vitamin D receptor activation with paricalcitol for reduction of albuminuria in patients with type 2 diabetes (VITAL study): a randomized controlled trial. Lancet 2010;376(9752):1543–51.
52. Levin A, Bakris G, Molitch M, et al. Prevalence of abnormal serum vitamin D, PTH, calcium, and phosphorus in patients with chronic kidney disease: results of the study to evaluate early kidney disease. Kidney Int 2007;71:31–8.
53. Gravellone L, Rizzo M, Martina V, et al. Vitamin D receptor activators and clinical outcomes in chronic kidney disease. Int J Nephrol 2011;2011:419524.
54. Vervloet M, Twisk J. Mortality reduction by vitamin D receptor activation in end-stage renal disease: a commentary on the robustness of current data. Nephrol Dial Transplant 2009;24(3):703–6.
55. Lund R, Andress D, Amdahl M, et al. Differential effects of paricalcitol and calcitriol on intestinal calcium absorption in hemodialysis patients. Am J Nephrol 2010;31(2):165–70.
56. Greenbaum L, Benador N, Goldstein S, et al. Intravenous paricalcitol for treatment of secondary hyperparathyroidism in children on hemodialysis. Am J Nephrol 2008;28(1):97–106.

57. Agarwal R, Acharya M, Tian J, et al. Antiproteinuric effect of oral paricalcitol in chronic kidney disease. Kidney Int 2005;68(6):2823–8.
58. Fishbane S, Chittineni H, Packman M, et al. Oral paricalcitrol in the treatment of patients with CKD and proteinuria: a randomized trial. Am J Kidney Dis 2009; 54(4):647–52.
59. Alborzi P, Patel N, Peterson C, et al. Paricalcitol reduces albuminuria and inflammation in chronic kidney disease a randomized double-blind pilot trial. Hypertension 2008;52(2):249–55.
60. Kim M, Frankel A, Donaldson M, et al. Oral cholecalciferol decreases albuminuria and urinary TGF-β1 in patients with type 2 diabetic nephropathy on established renin-angiotensin- aldosterone system inhibition. Kidney Int 2011;80(10):851–60.
61. Way K, Katai N, King GL. Protein kinase C and the development of diabetic vascular complications. Diabet Med 2001;18:945–59.
62. Gilbert R, Kim S, Tuttle K, et al. Effect of ruboxistaurin on urinary transforming growth factor-beta in patients with diabetic nephropathy and type 2 diabetes. Diabetes Care 2007;30:995–6.
63. Ishii H, Jirousek M, Koya D, et al. Amelioration of vascular dysfunctions in diabetic rats by an oral PKC β inhibitor. Science 1996;272:728–31.
64. Koya D, Haneda M, Nakagawa H, et al. Amelioration of accelerated diabetic mesangial expansion by treatment with PKC β inhibitor in diabetic db/db mice, a rodent model for type 2 diabetes. FASEB J 2000;14:439–47.
65. Kelly D, Chanty A, Gow R, et al. Protein kinase C beta inhibition attenuates osteopontin expression, macrophage recruitment, and tubulointerstitial injury in advanced experimental diabetic nephropathy. J Am Soc Nephrol 2005;16: 1654–60.
66. Sharma K, Ziyadeh F. Hyperglycemia and diabetic kidney disease: the care for transforming growth factor-β as a key mediator. Diabetes 1995;44:1139–46.
67. Sharma K, Ziyadeh F, Alzahabi B, et al. Increased renal production of transforming growth factor-β1 in patients with type II diabetes. Diabetes 1997;46:854–9.
68. Houlihan C, Akdeniz A, Tsalamandris C, et al. Urinary transforming growth factor-β excretion in patients with hypertension, type 2 diabetes, and elevated albumin excretion rate: effects angiotensin receptor blockade and sodium restriction. Diabetes Care 2002;25:1072–7.
69. Tuttle K, Bakris G, Toto R, et al. The effect of ruboxistaurin on nephropathy in type 2 diabetes. Diabetes Care 2005;28:2686–90.
70. Matsushita M, Shichiri M, Imai T, et al. Co-expression of urotensin II and its receptor (GPR14) in human cardiovascular and renal tissues. J Hypertens 2001;19:2185–90.
71. Totsune K, Takahashi K, Arihara Z, et al. Role of urotensin II in patients on dialysis. Lancet 2001;358:810–1.
72. Totsune K, Takahashi K, Arihara Z, et al. Increased plasma urotensin II levels in patients with diabetes mellitus. Clin Sci (Lond) 2003;104:1–5.
73. Clozel M, Binkert C, Birker-Robaczewska M, et al. Pharmacology of the urotensin-II receptor antagonist palosuran: first demonstration of a pathophysiological role of the urotensin system. J Pharmacol Exp Ther 2004;311:204–12.
74. Clozel M, Hess P, Qui C, et al. The urotensin-II receptor antagonist palosuran improves pancreatic and renal function in diabetic rats. J Pharmacol Exp Ther 2006;316:1115–21.
75. Sidharta P, Wagner F, Bohnemeier H, et al. Pharmacodynamics and pharmacokinetics of the urotensin II receptor antagonist palosuran in macroalbuminuric, diabetic patients. Clin Pharmacol Ther 2006;80:246–56.

76. Vogt L, Chiurchiu C, Chadha-Boreham H, et al. Effect of the urotensin receptor antagonist palosuran in hypertensive patients with type 2 diabetic nephropathy. Hypertension 2010;55:1206–9.

77. Tseng C. Correlation of uric acid and urinary albumin excretion rate in patients with type 2 diabetes mellitus in Taiwan. Kidney Int 2005;68:196–801.

78. Tseng C. Independent association of uric acid levels with peripheral arterial disease in Taiwanese patients with type 2 diabetes. Diabet Med 2004;21:724–9.

79. Bo S, Cavallo-Perin P, Gentile L, et al. Hypouricemia and hyperuricemia in type 2 diabetes: two different phenotypes. Eur J Clin Invest 2001;31:318–21.

80. Wun Y, Chan C, Lui C. Hyperuricaemia in type 2 diabetes mellitus. Diabetes Nutr Metab 1999;12:286–91.

81. Momeni A, Shadhidi S, Seirafian S, et al. Effect of allopurinol in decreasing proteinuria in type 2 diabetic patients. Iran J Kidney Dis 2010;4(1):28–132.

82. Hayashi K, Wakino S, Kanda T, et al. Molecular mechanisms and therapeutic strategies of chronic renal injury: role of rho-kinase in the development of renal injury. J Pharmacol Sci 2006;100:29–33.

83. Bach L. Rho Kinase inhibition: a new approach for treating diabetic nephropathy? Diabetes 2008;57:532–3.

84. Gojo A, Utsonomiya K, Taniguchi K, et al. The Rho-kinase inhibitor, fasudil, attenuates diabetic nephropathy in streptozotocin-induced diabetic rats. Eur J Pharmacol 2007;192:595–603.

85. Kolavennu V, Zeng L, Peng H, et al. Targeting of RhoA/ROCK signaling ameliorates progression of diabetic nephropathy independent of glucose control. Diabetes 2008;57:714–23.

Diabetes Management in the Kidney Patient

Rajesh Garg, MD[a], Mark E. Williams, MD[b],*

KEYWORDS

- Hyperglycemia • Chronic kidney disease • Diabetes

KEY POINTS

- Multiple mechanisms including altered insulin clearance and changes in insulin resistance contribute to changes in glucose/insulin homeostasis in CKD.
- Hemoglobin A1c may not be an accurate measure of glycemic control in CKD. Glycated albumin may become an alternative to HbA1c in CKD/ESRD.
- Value of tight glycemic control in CKD is not proven. Therefore, goal of treatment should be moderate glycemic control and avoidance of hypoglycemia.
- Pharmacologic therapy for hyperglycemia should be aimed at achieving individualized glycemic goals using agents with lowest risk of hypoglycemia.

Contributing factors to the abnormalities in glucose homeostasis in people with kidney impairment are shown in **Fig. 1**. Multifactorial alterations in glucose homeostasis occur when kidney impairment progresses. Abnormal insulin metabolism involves reduced renal insulin clearance, which is typically present when chronic kidney disease (CKD) reaches stages 4 and 5.[1] Some evidence suggests that a reduction in pancreatic insulin secretion may also contribute.[2,3]

Recent research has explored the mechanisms and clinical significance of another abnormality, insulin resistance, in CKD. A cross-sectional study involving 128 individuals with diabetes showed that homeostasis model assessment–insulin resistance (HOMA-IR) increased significantly with worsening renal disease ($P<.0001$), with no significant difference between the study groups with regard to age, body mass index, duration of diabetes, or glycemic control.[4] Glucose transport mediated by specific transporter proteins is 1 of the major actions of insulin and believed to be rate limiting for glucose uptake in peripheral tissues.[5] In muscle and adipose tissue, insulin stimulates translocation of an intracellular pool of glucose transporters to the plasma membrane and thus promotes glucose entry into the cells. Insulin action starts

[a] Division of Endocrinology, Diabetes and Hypertension, Brigham and Women's Hospital, 221 Longwood Avenue, Boston, MA 02115, USA; [b] Renal Division, Joslin Diabetes Center, 1 Joslin Place, Boston, MA 02215, USA
* Corresponding author.
E-mail address: mark.williams@joslin.harvard.edu

Med Clin N Am 97 (2013) 135–156
http://dx.doi.org/10.1016/j.mcna.2012.11.001
0025-7125/13/$ – see front matter © 2013 Elsevier Inc. All rights reserved.
medical.theclinics.com

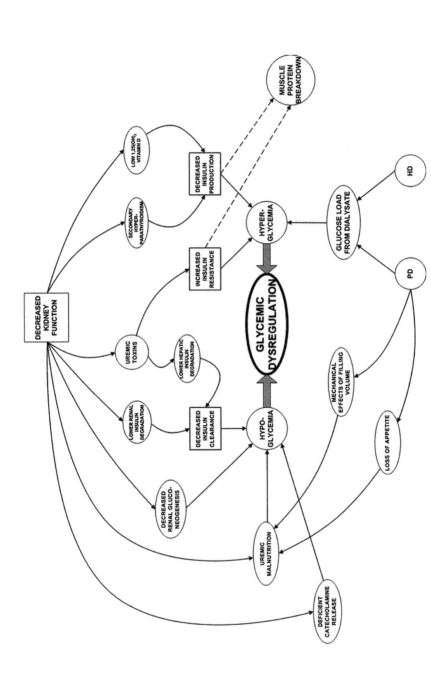

Fig. 1. Overview of glucose/insulin homeostasis in chronic kidney disease/ESRD. Disturbances of glucose metabolism include insulin resistance and glucose intolerance. Several factors contribute to hyperglycemia, which may coexist with hypoglycemia. *Abbreviations:* HD, hemodialysis; PD, peritoneal dialysis.

when the hormone binds to its receptor, which then phosphorylates insulin receptor substrates such as IRS1.[6] Downstream events involve activation of multiple targets such as glycogen synthase, protein kinase C, and endothelial nitric oxide synthase (eNOS), culminating in wide-ranging effects such as enhancement of glucose uptake, glycogenesis, lipogenesis, and cellular proliferation.[7] In CKD, the specific mechanism of insulin resistance involves the insulin receptor-signaling pathway, at sites distal to the insulin receptor, from changes in the generation of intracellular messengers for insulin action,[8] to glucose transport, to effects of insulin on 1 of the intracellular enzymes involved in glucose metabolism itself.[9] Accumulation of uremic toxins, chronic inflammation, excess visceral fat, oxidative stress, metabolic acidosis, and vitamin D deficiency can all affect the insulin signaling mechanisms and induce insulin resistance in CKD. In reality, insulin resistance appears to be somewhat variable among individuals with kidney disease, as it is in other conditions such as type 2 diabetes, obesity, or even in normal subjects.[10]

The improvement in insulin sensitivity associated with dialysis treatment suggests a role for uremic toxins.[11,12] Other data suggest that alterations in body metabolism during CKD could alter adipose tissue secretion patterns. Altered adipokine secretion could then become an important source of proinflammatory molecules capable of creating insulin resistance.[13] Plasma adinopectin levels, for example, are inversely related to kidney function, and decreased adinopectin concentrations may contribute to inflammation and insulin resistance.[14,15] Production of proinflammatory molecules in adipose tissue may also be modulated by oxidative stress, a feature of uremia.[16] Finally, erythropoietin deficiency might contribute to insulin resistance. This possibility was suggested by a recent clinical study indicating that recombinant erythropoietin-treated hemodialysis patients had lower mean insulin levels and HOMA-IR levels than those not treated with erythropoietin.[17]

Clinically, insulin resistance could contribute to protein-energy wasting, atherosclerosis, and cardiovascular complications known to occur in CKD/end-stage renal disease (ESRD) patients. However, the clinical relevance of insulin resistance in the CKD patient is not yet fully understood. Insulin resistance in CKD is a result of known risk factors such as obesity, as well as metabolic abnormalities unique to uremia as already described. Insulin resistance is a common characteristic feature of uremia, regardless of the cause of CKD. The ability of insulin to stimulate peripheral glucose disposal by muscle and adipose tissue is markedly affected in CKD.[18] However, 2 other important actions of insulin, antiproteolytic action and the translocation of potassium ions into cells, may not be affected to the same extent.[18,19] Numerous studies suggest that insulin resistance in uremia appears to be restricted to defects in glucose uptake and muscle protein anabolism. Dialysis patients even without diabetes mellitus or obesity have significant insulin resistance and increased muscle protein breakdown. Protein breakdown in muscle during kidney failure is at least partly mediated through the ubiquitin-proteasome pathway, where it is related to suppression of phosphatidylinositol-3 kinase.[20,21] More attention has recently been focused on the role of insulin resistance in protein-energy wasting.[22] One metabolic report examined the relationship between HOMA-IR and fasting whole-body and skeletal muscle protein turnover, with a goal of determining mean skeletal muscle protein synthesis, breakdown, and net balance in chronic hemodialysis patients without diabetes.[23] HOMA-IR was found to correlate with negative net skeletal muscle protein balance.

Increased attention has been given recently to the contribution of the kidneys to glucose homeostasis through processes that include glucose filtration and reabsorption.[24] Normally, up to 180 g of glucose may be filtered each day by the glomerulus. Nearly all of this filtered glucose is actively reabsorbed in the proximal tubule, mediated through 2 sodium-dependent glucose transporter (SGLT) proteins. The majority of this glucose reabsorption occurs through SGLT2, present in the S1 segment of the proximal tubule.[25] This process has achieved recent therapeutic significance because of the development of SGLT2 inhibitors.[26] Reports indicate that the administration of SGLT2 inhibitors can improve glycemic control through glucosuria in patients with type 2 diabetes, without the risk of inducing severe hypoglycemia.[27] Although SGLT2 mediates 90% of glucose reabsorption in the kidneys, SGLT inhibitors at best appear to inhibit only half that amount. Dapagliflozin is the most advanced SGLT2 inhibitor in clinical trials.[28]

Physiologic studies have also shown that kidney tissues respond to insulin, and activation of targets in the kidney elicits wide-ranging metabolic effects. Of note, insulin resistance in the glomerulus is similar to the insulin resistance found in other vascular tissues. Studies conducted by Mima and colleagues[29] showed dysfunctional insulin signaling in glomeruli and tubules of diabetic and insulin-resistant animals. Based on these data, it has been suggested that glomerular insulin resistance could contribute to the initiation and progression of glomerular lesions in diabetes.[29]

Dysglycemia in diabetes also includes challenges of hypoglycemia, which will be described in more detail. The pathogenesis of hypoglycemia in diabetic CKD patients coexists with other derangements in insulin/glucose metabolism in kidney failure. Altered glucose metabolism, related to insulin resistance and decreased insulin degradation, as well as to effects on metabolism of drugs used to treat hyperglycemia, combine to add further complexity to glycemic management. Reduced renal insulin clearance as the glomerular filtration rate (GFR) falls to 15 to 20 mL/min/1.73 m^2 results in a prolonged action of insulin. The kidneys are the most important extrahepatic organs for degradation of insulin, and renal insulin clearance decreases with declining kidney function. The decline in kidney mass and impaired kidney function simultaneously lead to decreased renal gluconeogenesis, a protective source of glucose production from precursor molecules during starvation.

DETERMINATION OF GLYCEMIC CONTROL IN CKD

Common tests for determining glycemic control in diabetes mellitus are shown in **Fig. 2**. Hemoglobin A1c (HgbA1c) is the standard clinical measure for glucose

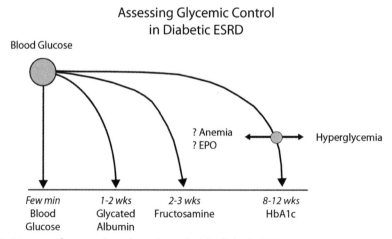

Fig. 2. Measures for assessing glycemic control in diabetic CKD.

monitoring in diabetic patients without kidney impairment. HgbA1c comprises about 4% of total hemoglobin in normal adult erythrocytes. The HgbA1c level reflects average blood glucose concentration over roughly the 3 preceding months.[30] Firm correlation between HgbA1c and blood glucose levels in those with preserved kidney function has been reported in the Diabetes Control and Complications Trial[31] and the A1c-Derived Average Glucose (ADAG) Study.[32] Because the major clinical trials that demonstrated a reduction in microvascular complications with good glycemic control, DCCT for type 1 diabetes[31] and UK Prospective Diabetes Study (UKPDS) for type 2 diabetes,[33] employed HgbA1c levels for predicting their outcomes, the glycohemoglobin level has become the primary basis of diabetes management. A lower HgbA1c in these clinical trials was found to reduce the risk of developing albuminuria, and in those with elevated baseline albumin creatinine ratio (ACR), progression of renal disease was reduced.

However, unreliability of HgbA1c attributed to the analytical, biologic, and clinical variability associated with HgbA1c has been recognized in several clinical conditions.[34] Analytical variability has resolved with introduction of newer assay methods, but the biologic and clinical variability of HgbA1c continue to limit its application to some patients.[35] Many of these factors become relevant when using HgbA1c as a measure of glycemic control in CKD. Analytical biases inherent in the HgbA1c assay that might affect HgbA1c levels in CKD compared with the general population do not appear to be clinically significant anymore with contemporary assays. Unlike the high-performance liquid chromatography assay previously used in routine clinical HgbA1c testing, the contemporary immunoturbidimetric assay is not influenced by high serum urea nitrogen levels. In fact, the most likely causes of HgbA1c discordance from other tests in kidney patients are anemia and the use of erythrocyte stimulating agents (ESAs). In patients with kidney disease, the red blood cell lifespan may be reduced by up to 30% to 70%.[36] Shortened erythrocyte survival in ESRD anemia would be expected to diminish HgbA1c levels by shortening the time for exposure to ambient glucose.[37] In addition, the widespread use of ESAs improves anemia in part by increasing the number of immature red blood cells in the circulation, each with less susceptibility to glycosylation. One case report described a lowering of HgbA1c values with both erythropoietin and darbopoietin analogs.[38]

In spite of that, in the setting of CKD, according to the frequently cited KDOQI (Kidney Dialysis Outcomes Quality Initiative) guidelines of the National Kidney Foundation, the currently recommended HgbA1c targets have not historically differed from those for the general diabetic population (ie, <7%).[39] It is worth noting that the previously referenced seminal glycemic control trials in type 1 and type 2 diabetes (DCCT and UKPDS) excluded patients with significantly impaired kidney function. Furthermore, the strength of the association between glycemic control and clinical outcomes, which hinges on the relationship between hyperglycemia and elevated HgbA1c levels, is now known to be weakened in CKD patients; HgbA1c may overestimate glycemic control in kidney patients. HgbA1c levels appear to be misleadingly lower, resulting in underestimation of hyperglycemia.

Discordance from other metrics of glycemia in clinical research studies[40] have raised concerns about the validity of HgbA1c in predicting outcomes in patients with late stages of CKD. The KDOQI guidelines for diabetic CKD acknowledge a deficiency in data, which would validate the HgbA1c test when kidney function is impaired.[39] This concern has been reinforced by a recent USRDS report indicating that the prevalence of HgbA1c levels over the 7% target was 63% for stages 1 to 2 CKD, but substantially lower (46%) in stages 3 to 4 CKD,[41] an effect unlikely to be attributed to better glycemic management. Similarly, in the authors' large national

ESRD database analysis, the mean HgbA1c value was only 6.77%, and only 35% of patient values were over 7.0%.[42] It is understood that HgbA1c levels tend to be lower in diabetic patients with advanced kidney impairment or in patients who are dialysis-dependent. Peacock and colleagues[43] measured levels of glycated hemoglobin and glycated albumin in 307 patients with diabetes, about 5/6 of whom were undergoing maintenance hemodialysis, and 1/6 were without overt kidney disease. In patients undergoing maintenance hemodialysis, the ratio of glycated albumin to HgbA1c was higher, suggesting that the HgbA1c was relatively reduced, serum glucose levels were significantly underestimated. More recently, Chen and colleagues[44] reported mean glucose levels that were about 10% higher in patients with stages 3 to 4 CKD than an estimated average glucose calculated from the same HgbA1c if applied to patients with normal kidney function, consistent with a reduction in HgbA1c levels in CKD. Poor correlation of HgbA1c and glucose levels were also reported in a recent small study that contrasted 4-day continuous glucose monitoring (CGMS) in type 2 patients undergoing maintenance hemodialysis (N = 19) with a larger group of type 2 diabetic patients without nephropathy (N = 39).[45] The CGMS results and glucose concentrations according to the glucose meter were comparable in patients in both groups. However, glycated hemoglobin and mean glucose concentrations were strongly correlated only in the nondialysis group (r = 0.71); correlation was weaker in those undergoing hemodialysis (r = 0.47). Hemodialysis patients were receiving erythropoiesis stimulating agents, and had lower hemoglobin levels than the comparator group (11.6 vs 13.6 g/dL, $P<.0001$).

Variance in the HgbA1c levels cited previously have raised particular concern with regard to relying on this test as the sole measure of glycemia in the diabetic CKD population. Fructosamine is comprised of those glycated serum proteins that have stable ketoamines (carbonyl group of glucose reacting with the protein's amino group) in their structure. Fructosamine, while increasingly available for the monitoring of diabetes treatment, may not correlate as strongly with fasting serum glucose levels,[34] and the need to correct values for total protein or albumin concentrations remains a potential problem.[46] In a recent report, elevated fructosamine levels were associated with infection and all-cause hospitalization in 100 diabetic CKD patients on hemodialysis.[47] Similar to the HgbA1c findings discussed previously, the study by Chen and colleagues[44] reported that fructosamine levels were also lower than expected for the same glucose concentration in CKD patients, as compared with patients with normal kidney function. Of note, false elevations of fructosamine levels may result from nitroblue tetrazoloium assay interference by serum uric acid.

Relative to the limited use of fructosamine, glycated albumin (GA) is increasingly proposed as a better measure of glycemic control in diabetic patients with CKD/ESRD. Unlike HgbA1c, it has also been suggested that glycated albumin in vivo has biologic properties that could contribute to the pathogenesis of diabetic complications,[48] as an Amadori-modified reaction product capable of inducing oxidative stress and enhancing proinflammatory responses. Albumin undergoes a process of nonenzymatic glycation during glucose exposure, similar to hemoglobin, and accounts for most of the serum glycated proteins. Because the residence time of serum albumin is shorter (a half-life of approximately 20 days),[49] it reflects a shorter glucose exposure, so that the testing interval for monitoring should be monthly. Glycated albumin reflects glycemic control for only the 1 to 2 weeks before obtaining the sample.[50] Glycated albumin can be measured using a bromocresol purple method, and calculated as the percentage relative to total albumin. Using this method, a reference range of about 12% has been determined for nondiabetic individuals with normal renal function.[43] There appears to be a somewhat wider reference interval compared with the more compressed range of measured values for HgbA1c. It has not been validated in dialysis patients. Its precision may be limited in states of abnormal protein turnover, such as from inflammation, hypercatabolic states, peritoneal dialysis, proteinuria, albumin infusions, or gastrointestinal protein losses. In patients with nephrotic range proteinuria, glycated albumin levels may be falsely reduced. However, the case for glycated albumin has been strengthened by an improved assay that is unaffected by changes in serum albumin.

Comparison of glycated albumin to HgbA1c was evaluated in 2 recent studies of kidney patients.[48,50] In a large Japanese study of 538 maintenance hemodialysis patients with type 2 diabetes, 828 patients without diabetes, and 365 diabetic patients without significant kidney impairment, Inaba and colleagues[48] demonstrated significantly lower HgbA1c levels relative to blood glucose or to glycated albumin levels with dialysis, as compared with those without kidney impairment. The ratio of glycated albumin to HgbA1c (with a previously reported ratio of approximately 3.0 in the absence of ESRD) was 2.93 in patients without CKD, and 3.81 in those on dialysis. In a subsequent study from the United States, the glycated albumin/ HgbA1c ratio was again significantly higher in patients who were on dialysis (2.72 vs 2.07).[43] Thus, as an alternative to HgbA1c, evidence linking glycemic control as determined by serum glycated albumin levels to diabetic ESRD outcomes is now emerging. In a recent report, Freedman and colleagues[51] analyzed the association between 3 measures (glycated albumin, HgbA1c, and serum glucose levels) and hospitalization/survival outcomes in diabetic dialysis patients (90% were on hemodialysis). Time-dependent analyses allowed comparisons with available HgbA1c and monthly random serum glucose levels. In the report, mean (standard deviation) serum glycated albumin was 21.5 SDs plus or minus 6%, and HbA1c was 6.9 SDs plus or minus 1.6%. The primary finding was that increased glycated albumin, but not HbA1c or random serum glucose concentrations, was predictive of hospitalization and survival.

VALUE OF GLYCEMIC CONTROL IN CKD PATIENTS

Glycemic management in patients with diabetes and CKD has become increasingly complex, in part reflecting controversies raised in recent studies about safety and efficacy as applied to type 2 diabetes.[52] Challenges cited in improving glycemic control in patients with advanced CKD include therapeutic inertia, monitoring difficulties, and complexity regarding use of a growing list of available treatments in CKD.[53] While HgbA1c combined with home glucose monitoring remains the mainstay for monitoring glycemic control (despite information presented previously), until recently the available evidence regarding the benefit and safety of tight glycemic control in patients with advanced CKD has been limited. There have been no randomized clinical trials to evaluate the effects of glycemic control in patients with late stages of CKD/ ESRD. Recent observational studies have added significantly to available evidence, while providing somewhat contrasting results and significant methodological differences.[42,54,55] Williams and colleagues[42] reported observational findings from a large national ESRD database that mortality risks in diabetic patients did not differ when grouped by Hgb1c levels. There was no overall correlation between glycohemoglobin levels and subsequent 12-month mortality risk, even when adjusted for case-mix and laboratory values. Results in a second study, by Kalantar-Zadeh and colleagues,[54] from a similar-sized retrospective database analysis, differed somewhat, in indicating that higher HgbA1c levels were statistically associated with increased death risk. HgbA1c greater than 10% was associated with a 41% greater risk for all-cause and cardiovascular death. The study used a longer follow-up period, time-dependent survival models, and adjustments for surrogates of malnutrition and inflammation. A subsequent study by Williams and colleagues[55] (**Fig. 3**) modified its analysis to more directly match that of Kalantar-Zadeh, and found that only extremes of glycemia were associated with worsened survival. These studies indicate that the overall relationship between glycemic control and survival outcomes in the presence of ESRD is somewhat weak. A logical conclusion in terms of benefit/risk is to allow somewhat higher HbA1c targets in CKD. The concept that higher HgA1c targets (ie, 7%–8%) may be preferable in those patients with higher levels of comorbidity[56] was also supported by a recent regression analysis involving A1c levels and mortality from the Dialysis Outcomes and Practice Patterns Study (DOPPS).[57] In another observational study, a post-hoc analysis of the 4-D study, a graded relationship between poor glycemic control and mortality caused by sudden cardiac death was reported.[58] Over a median follow-up of 4 years, using patients with an HgbA1c less than 6.0% as the comparator, patients with sudden cardiac death were identified. Patients with an HgbA1c greater than 8% had a greater than 2-fold higher risk of sudden death compared with those with an HgbA1c less than or equal to 6% (hazard ratio [HR] 2.14), with each 1% increase in HgbA1c associated with an 18% increase in the risk of sudden death after statistical adjustments. Sudden death was the single largest cause of mortality (26%). The specific mechanism by which poor glycemic control increases risk of sudden death was not clear. A recent report of 23,296 patients with diabetes and an eGFR between 15 and 60 mL/min/1.73 m^2 evaluated outcomes according to baseline HgbA1c levels (<7, 7–9, >9) over a median follow-up of 3.8 years.[59] For both stage 3 and 4 CKD, higher levels of HgbA1c were associated with an increased risk of death. More recently, an observational report from the

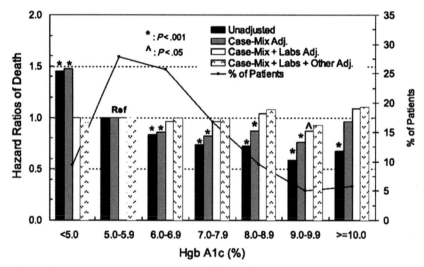

Fig. 3. Relation between glycemic control and hemodialysis survival, among 24,875 hemodialysis patients with follow-up of 3 years, using time-dependent survival models with repeated measures and multiple case-mix adjustments. Data were collected at baseline and every quarter to a maximum of 3 years' follow-up. Extremes of glycemia were weakly associated with survival in the study population. (*Reprinted from* Williams ME, Lacson E Jr, Wang W, et al. Glycemic control and extended hemodialysis survival in patients with diabetes mellitus: comparative results of traditional and time-dependent Cox model analyses. Clin J Am Soc Nephrol 2010;5(9):1595–601; with permission.)

Alberta Kidney Disease Network,[59] in patients with diabetes and more advanced stages of CKD (nondialysis CKD stages 3–5), confirmed that higher HgbA1c levels were associated with markedly worse outcomes, including progression of kidney disease regardless of the baseline eGFR. Confirmation of the renoprotective effect associated with intensive control of hyperglycemia in type 2 diabetes was also suggested by the ADOPT study.[60] Greater durability of glycemic control in those treated with rosiglitizone (compared with metformin and glyburide) was associated with a smaller rise in albuminuria and with preservation of eGFR.

HYPOGLYCEMIA

Patients with diabetes and CKD are at increased risk for hypoglycemia. Diabetes treatment options for patients with advanced CKD are somewhat limited due to safety and tolerability concerns. Increasing attention is being given to the risks of hypoglycemia (<70 mg/dL) in the diabetic CKD population. This is reflected in recent diabetes guidelines, which not express greater concern than in the past about the dangers of hypoglycemia.[52] The American Diabetes Association (ADA) continues to recommend a goal hemoglobin A1c of less than 7.0% or as close to normal and as safely as possible, but without unacceptable hypoglycemia.[61] Increasing pressure to achieve tight glycemic control targets may result in episodes of hypoglycemia, in many cases iatrogenic. Specific factors that might increase the risk of hypoglycemia include use of insulin secretagogues, missed meals, advanced age, duration of diabetes, and unawareness of hypoglycemia.[62] However, published reviews on glycemic control in diabetic CKD patients give little emphasis to risks of hypoglycemia. The greatest risk of harm is in patients with both CKD and diabetes, particularly in the elderly.[63] Partly as a result of mounting concerns about hypoglycemia, the ADA's current Standards of Medical Care in Diabetes recommend less stringent HgbA1c goals, (ie, 7.5–8.0%), as appropriate for those patients with advanced complications, extensive comorbid conditions, or a history of severe hypoglycemia.[52] Adverse consequences of hypoglycemia could partially explain the outcomes from 3 recent clinical trials, ACCORD,[64] ADVANCE,[65] and VADT.[66] The purpose of these landmark studies was to determine whether glycemic management more aggressive than previously recommended (with a goal of achieving HgbA1c levels near 6.0%) would reduce cardiovascular risk in patients with longstanding diabetes. Hypoglycemia occurred more frequently in the intensive therapy arms of all 3 studies. In the ACCORD trial, the rate of hypoglycemic episodes requiring medical assistance was 3 times higher in the intensive group. Likewise, in ADVANCE, severe hypoglycemia was nearly twice as common in the intensive control group, with half of patients in the low HgbA1c group having at least a minor hypoglycemic event during the trial. Notably, these studies failed to demonstrate cardiovascular benefit with the intensive therapy strategy. With regard to the additional risk of CKD, in the ADVANCE trial analysis, higher creatinine levels were an independent risk factor for severe hypoglycemia. Reports on hypoglycemia and advanced kidney disease have generally occurred as case reports, small series, and reviews.[67] However, as many as half of chronic hemodialysis patients with diabetes may suffer hypoglycemia over a 3-month period.[68] Preliminary findings suggest that the risk of hypoglycemia is especially high in diabetic ESRD patients who have greater glycemic variability.[69]

The health consequences of hypoglycemia can be severe, while fear of iatrogenic hypoglycemia may result in poor glycemic control and further risk of diabetic complications. Episodes of cold sweats, agitation, dizziness, disorientation, slurred speech, fatigue, and decreased level of consciousness are typical. However, hypoglycemia unawareness worsens with duration of diabetes. The occurrence of hypoglycemia complicated by central pontine myelinolysis and quadriplegia was recently described.[70] Severe hypoglycemia is known to increase the risk of poor outcomes in patients with diabetes.[71] A powerful stimulant to the sympathetic nervous system, severe hypoglycemia may cause acute secondary adverse cardiovascular outcomes, including chest pain due to coronary vasoconstriction and ischemia, myocardial infarction, serious cardiac arrhythmias, and sudden death.[72] Therefore, 1 of the goals of antihyperglycemic treatment in CKD should be avoidance of hypoglycemia.

STRATEGIES FOR MANAGEMENT OF HYPERGLYCEMIA IN CKD

The management strategy for hyperglycemia in CKD involves a multifaceted approach including dietary changes, an exercise regimen, and drug therapy. Diet and exercise are central components of any therapeutic regimen for all patients with diabetes. Dietary changes and physical activity often improve insulin sensitivity. Meal plans should be individualized to accommodate not only the considerations about renal impairment but also lifestyle and personal preferences of the patient. Most patients with diabetes are overweight, and a dietary plan to promote weight reduction may be appropriate. Protein restriction may be appropriate in some patients, but data on the effect of protein restriction on progression of CKD are controversial. A diet that includes complex carbohydrates from fruits, vegetables, whole grains, legumes, and low-fat milk is encouraged. Similar to diet, the exercise regimen also needs to be individualized. Exercise in diabetic patients with CKD is associated with potential risks as well as benefits. A pre-exercise evaluation should be conducted to determine whether the patient has any contraindications to exercise. Because of the high prevalence of cardiovascular disease in these patients, all patients with typical or atypical cardiac symptoms or an abnormal resting electrocardiogram (ECG) should undergo a cardiac stress test. Patients with severe diabetic retinopathy should avoid exercises that involve valsalva (eg, lifting heavy weights). Patients with severe peripheral neuropathy should avoid repetitive stepping exercise (eg, jogging), which may increase the risk of a foot ulcer. In the absence of contraindications, the exercise program should include both aerobic and resistance exercises. Patients also should be counseled about how to coordinate timing of exercise, meals, medications, and glucose monitoring. Low- to moderate-intensity exercise, such as walking, may have the most significant benefits with minimal risks for most patients. Patients should be encouraged to start with short periods of low-intensity exercise and increase the intensity and duration slowly.

Pharmacologic therapy for hyperglycemia in patients with CKD also needs individualization, because it is affected not only by altered insulin resistance and glucose metabolism and higher risk of hypoglycemia as described previously, but also by altered drug metabolism and concerns about the renal effects of antihyperglycemic drugs. Goals for glycemic control need to be revised and readjusted frequently once renal function starts deteriorating, and pharmacologic management needs frequent changes and/or dose adjustments. Many new noninsulin agents offer a safe and effective option for diabetic patients with CKD.

USE OF NONINSULIN ANTIDIABETIC DRUGS IN THE PRESENCE OF CKD

Many noninsulin agents are currently available for the treatment of type 2 diabetes. Most of these agents have become available within the last 2 decades. While some physicians are skeptical about their use because of a lack of long-term data, the new antidiabetic agents do offer an alternative to insulin therapy and may reduce the risk of hypoglycemia in patients with CKD. There are very few head-to-head comparisons between various noninsulin agents, and data in patients with CKD are scanty. Professional society guidelines on the use of noninsulin agents also leave out patients with CKD.[52,73–76] However, patients with CKD are often eligible for 1 or more of the noninsulin agents and may benefit from them. A brief summary of the available noninsulin agents is given in **Table 1**.

SULFONYLUREAS

Sulfonylureas (SUs) are the oldest and most commonly used noninsulin agents for treatment of type 2 diabetes. They lower blood glucose levels by releasing insulin from the pancreatic β cells via their action on SU receptors that close the adenosine triphosphate (ATP)-sensitive potassium channels. Patients with longer duration of diabetes often have poor β cell reserves and may not respond to SUs. When used in newly diagnosed patients with type 2 diabetes, SUs tend to lose their effectiveness earlier than metformin or thiazolidinediones (TZDs).[77] However, when effective, SUs can cause unregulated insulin release and lead to severe hypoglycemia that can be particularly serious in the presence of CKD.[78] Long-acting SUs like glyburide and chlorpropamide are more notorious for causing hypoglycemia.[79] Shorter-acting drugs, especially those metabolized in the liver like glipizide and glimepiride, are relatively safe and preferred in patients with CKD.[80]

BIGUANIDES

Biguanides are insulin sensitizers, with their main site of action being the liver. They do not cause hypoglycemia when used alone. Metformin is the only biguanide available in the United States. It became available in the United States in 1995, but it has been used in Europe and other parts of the world for the last 3 decades. Therefore, extensive experience is available with this drug. Metformin use was associated with a reduction in incidence of cardiovascular events in the UKPDS trial.[81,82] Metformin use is also associated with a small weight loss. As a result, it is the first-line agent recommended by the ADA and European Association for the Study of Diabetes (EASD) for treatment of type 2 diabetes.[61] However, metformin use in certain patients is associated with a risk of lactic acidosis, a rare but life-threatening condition. Metformin is contraindicated in women with serum creatinine greater than 1.4 mg/dL and in men with serum creatinine greater than 1.5 mg/dL.[83] Other risk factors for lactic acidosis include hypoxemia, sepsis, alcohol abuse, liver failure, myocardial infarction, and shock. It is important to know these contraindications and stop metformin promptly when any of these conditions is present. Studies have shown frequent irrational use of metformin in patients with diabetes and renal failure.[84] Diarrhea and gastrointestinal adverse effects are other common adverse effects of metformin and should lead to a decrease in dose or discontinuation of this drug.

THIAZOLIDINEDIONES

Thiazolidinedione (TZD) drugs are insulin sensitizers and therefore do not cause hypoglycemia if used alone. They act on the PPARγ receptors and improve insulin sensitivity of peripheral tissues like muscle and adipose tissue. Pioglitazone and rosiglitazone are the 2 TZDs currently available in the United States, and both agents are safe in CKD and seem to be effective for glycemic control in patients on hemodialysis.[85–87] However, rosiglitazone is not available in the United States in the open market, because a meta-analysis showed its association with myocardial infarction.[88] Rosiglitazone

Table 1
Noninsulin antidiabetic agents

Drug	Mechanism of Action	Advantages	Disadvantages	Role in Renal Failure
Biguanides: • Metformin	Insulin sensitizer ↓ Hepatic glucose production	Extensive experience No hypoglycemia Weight neutral Likely ↓ CVD Low cost	Gastrointestinal adverse effects Lactic acidosis B-12 deficiency Multiple contraindications, including renal failure, acidosis, hypoxia, infection, dehydration, older age	Cannot be used with serum creatinine >1.5 in men and >1.4 in women
Sulfonylureas: • Glyburide • Glipizide • Glimepiride • Gliclazide	Insulin secretagogue	Extensive experience ↓ Microvascular risk Low cost	Hypoglycemia Weight gain Low durability of effect	Use with caution Glipizide preferred
Meglitinides: • Repaglinide • Nateglinide	Insulin secretagogue	↓ Postprandial glucose excursions Dosing flexibility	Hypoglycemia Weight gain Frequent dosing High cost	Safer than sulfonylureas
Thiazolidinediones: • Pioglitazone • Rosiglitazone	Insulin sensitizer ↑ Insulin sensitivity in muscle and adipose tissue	No hypoglycemia Durability of effect ↓ TGs, ↑ HDL-C ? ↓ CVD (pioglitazone)	Weight gain Edema/heart failure Bone fractures ? ↑ MI (rosiglitazone) ? Bladder ca (pioglitazone) High cost	Safe but concerns about fluid retention
α-glucosidase inhibitors: • Acarbose • Miglitol	Slows carbohydrate digestion/absorption	No hypoglycemia Nonsystemic ↓ Postprandial glucose excursions ? ↓ CVD events	Gastrointestinal adverse effects Dosing frequency Modest ↓ A1c	Contraindicated in renal failure with serum creatinine >2 mg/dL

Drug class	Mechanism	Benefits	Adverse effects / concerns	CKD considerations
DPP-4 Inhibitors: • Sitagliptin • Saxagliptin • Linagliptin	Increased GLP-1, GIP leading to ↑ insulin, ↓ glucagon	No hypoglycemia Well tolerated	Modest ↓ A1c reduction ? Pancreatitis Urticaria High cost	Safe and effective
GLP-1 receptor agonists: • Exenatide • Exenatide- extended release • Liraglutide	Activates GLP-1 receptor leading to ↑ insulin, ↓ glucagon ↓ Gastric emptying ↑ Satiety	Weight loss No hypoglycemia ? Beta cell mass ? CVD protection	Gastrointestinal adverse effects ? Pancreatitis ? Renal failure ? Medullary thyroid ca Injectable High cost	Contraindicated in renal failure due to severe adverse effects and concerns about acute renal failure
Amylin mimetics: • Pramlintide	↓ Glucagon ↓ Gastric emptying ↑ Satiety	Weight loss ↓ Postprandial glucose	Gastrointestinal adverse effects Modest ↓ A1c Injectable Hypoglycemia with insulin Dosing frequency Injection	No data in CKD, should not be used
Bile acid sequestrant: • Colesevelam	Unknown	No hypoglycemia ↓ Low-density lipoprotein	Constipation ↑ Triglycerides Modest ↓ A1c may ↓ absorption of other medications	No data
Dopamine-2 agonists: • Bromocriptine	Modulates hypothalamic control mechanisms ↑ Insulin sensitivity	No hypoglycemia ? ↓ CVD events	Modest ↓ A1c Dizziness/syncope Nausea Fatigue	No data

Abbreviations: ca, carcinoma; CVD, cardiovascular disease.

has also been shown to be associated with increased cardiovascular mortality in hemo-dialysis patients.[89] Pioglitazone, on the other hand, may have some cardiovascular-protective benefits.[90,91] Pioglitazone also has a favorable effect on lipids. Both TZDs cause fluid retention and increase the risk of heart failure, a problem that may be worse in patients with CKD/ESRD. Their use is also associated with increased risk of frac-tures.[92] Recently, concerns have been raised about the increased risk of bladder cancer with pioglitazone.[93] Because of these reasons, TZDs are not a preferred class of drugs for treatment of type 2 diabetes, especially in patients with CKD.

DIPEPTIDYL PEPTIDASE 4 INHIBITORS

Dipeptidyl peptidase 4 (DPP-4) inhibitors are becoming more popular for the treatment of hyperglyecmia in CKD patients because of their better tolerability and low risk of hypoglycemia. By blocking the DPP-4 enzyme, these drugs increase the concentra-tions of endogenous incretins GLP-1 and GIP. Incretins are hormones secreted by the gastrointestinal tract in response to ingestion of food. Incretins stimulate pancre-atic β cells to increase insulin secretion and suppress α cells to decrease glucagon secretion. These effects are dependent on ambient glucose levels, being more potent when glucose levels are high and less potent when glucose levels are low. Thus, incre-tinomimetic drugs are more effective in the postprandial period, when glucose levels are high. However, in a fasting state, their effect is mitigated by low glucose levels, removing the risk of hypoglycemia. Both, GLP-1 and GIP are rapidly broken down by the DPP-4 enzyme, leading to a very short half-life (approximately 2 minutes). Therefore, DPP-4 inhibitors increase the bioavailability of GLP-1 and GIP. They lower glucose levels and do not cause hypoglycemia when used by themselves. Sitagliptin, saxagliptin, and linagliptin are the 3 drugs currently available in this class in the United States. Sitagliptin and saxagliptin need dose adjustment for reduced eGFR because of their renal excretion. Linagliptin is metabolized in the liver and can be used at a fixed dose irrespective of the renal function. Randomized controlled trials have demon-strated safety and efficacy of DPP-4 inhibitors in patients with CKD.[94–98] DPP-4 inhib-itors were also found to be weight neutral in their clinical trials. However, long-term data on their safety and efficacy are still lacking.

GLP-1 RECEPTOR AGONISTS

These drugs have a molecular structure similar to endogenous GLP-1, but they are resistant to metabolism by the DPP4 enzyme. They increase insulin secretion and suppress glucagon secretion in a glucose-dependent manner, thus eliminating the risk of hypoglycemia. These drugs slow gastric emptying and suppress appetite through their central effect, and these effects are responsible for weight loss. However, these effects also lead to nausea and vomiting, which can be more severe in patients with ESRD.[99] Exenatide and liraglutide are the 2 drugs currently available in this class. Both are injectable agents. There are also concerns of acute pancreatitis and acute renal failure with both these agents.[100,101] Moreover, there are concerns of medullary thyroid carcinoma with liraglutide due to C-cell hyperplasia seen in mice injected with liraglutide. Due to their potential adverse effects and poor toler-ance, GLP-1 agonists are often not a good choice in patients with CKD.

MEGLITINIDES

Meglitinides are insulin secretagogues acting by mechanisms similar to SUs. However, they are shorter acting, and their effects are dependent on ambient glucose levels. Therefore, their risk of hypoglycemia is lower, and they are more effective for postprandial glycemic control. Repaglinide and nateglinide are the 2 agents available in the United States. Nateglinide may be preferred in CKD because of lower risk of hypoglycemia, and it has been studied in CKD.[102,103] These drugs require frequent dosing, because they need to be taken before each meal.

α-GLUCOSIDASE INHIBITORS

α-glucosidase inhibitors block the enzyme responsible for digestion of carbohydrates. Acarbose and miglitol are the 2 agents in this class, and both have been shown to reduce HgbA1c in patients with type 2 diabetes. A major adverse effect of these drugs is flatulence. They are also contraindicated in patients with serum creatinine greater than 2 mg/dL because of a risk of accumulation that may lead to liver failure.

BILE ACID SEQUESTRANTS

Colesevelam is a bile acid sequestrant that was originally used for hypercholesterolemia. It can also lower glucose levels in patients with type 2 diabetes and is approved by the US Food and Drug Administration (FDA) for this purpose. The mechanism of the glucose-lowering effect of colesevelam is poorly understood. A major adverse effect is constipation. The drug is used infrequently for patients with or without CKD.

DOPAMINE-2 AGONISTS

Bromocriptine, a dopaminergic agent available for several decades, was recently approved for treatment of hyperglycemia in type 2 diabetes. Its mechanism of action is considered to involve resetting of circadian rhythm in the hypothalamus. Studies have suggested disturbed circadian rhythm in patients with type 2 diabetes that is associated with insulin resistance. Specific benefits or harms of the use of dopamine-2 agonists in CKD are unknown.

AMYLIN MIMETICS

Amylin is a hormone synthesized in pancreatic β-cells and cosecreted with insulin. It slows gastric emptying, increases satiety, and also suppresses secretion of glucagon after a meal. Pramlintide is an amylin agonist that can be used along with insulin to lower the postprandial glycemic excursions. The drug has limited use in patients with type 1 or type 2 diabetes and has not been studied in CKD.

INSULIN THERAPY IN PATIENTS WITH RENAL DYSFUNCTION

Insulin therapy in CKD patient is no different from patients without CKD, other than the fact that insulin requirements may be lower, and insulin action may be prolonged.[104] Therefore, the risk of hypoglycemia with insulin therapy is increased in CKD. A study in hospitalized patients suggested that insulin dose may be reduced by approximately 50% in CKD.[105] Effects of dialysis on insulin sensitivity can further complicate insulin therapy in patients with ESRD.[106] Moreover, presence of glucose in dialysis fluid can affect glycemic control, especially in those on peritoneal dialysis. Insulin therapy is often divided into basal insulin coverage and nutritional insulin coverage. Basal insulin coverage is typically provided by using an intermediate- or long-acting insulin, and nutritional insulin coverage is provided by a short- or rapid-acting insulin (**Table 2**). In CKD, insulin detemir or neutral protamine Hagedorn (NPH) insulin used once or twice daily may be appropriate for basal coverage. Rapid-acting insulin analogs are

Table 2
Insulin therapy in patients with CKD

	Insulin Name	Onset of Action	Peak Effect	Duration	Other Remarks
Basal	NPH	1–2 h	4–8 h	12–18 h	1–2 times daily
	Glargine	2 h	No peak	20–24 h	Once daily
	Detemir	2 h	3–9 h	16–24 h	Once daily
Nutritional	Lispro, Aspart, Glulisine	5–15 min	1–2 h	4–6 h	Can be taken after meals if food intake is unreliable
	Regular	30 min	2–4 h	6–8 h	Less commonly used

appropriate for nutritional coverage in CKD.[107–109] These insulins may even be prescribed after meals in patients with unreliable food intake. It is important to individualize the insulin regimen according to patient's lifestyle, food intake, and dialysis regimen. A regimen consisting of noninsulin agents and basal insulin may be appropriate in many patients with type 2 diabetes. Continuous insulin infusion via an insulin pump may improve quality of life in patients requiring multiple insulin injections, but no studies are available to show a lower risk of hypoglycemia or better glycemic control in patients with CKD.

EFFECT OF TREATMENT CHOICES ON RENAL FUNCTION

A renoprotective effect of glycemic control was demonstrated in early clinical trials of diabetes and confirmed in recent clinical trials. However, an effect of 1 antidiabetic agent over another has not been demonstrated. As mentioned previously, there are few head-to-head clinical trials comparing various antidiabetic agents, and none of these trials was conducted in patients with CKD. A retrospective study suggested that metformin may be associated with lower decline in renal function over time as compared with the use of SUs.[110] However, a possibility of selection bias cannot be ruled out in this study. Some noninsulin agents need to be avoided in patients with CKD, and the doses of others need to be adjusted to avoid their adverse effects. However, at this point of time, no 1 agent can be preferred over another for renoprotective effect.

REFERENCES

1. Mak RH. Impact of end-stage renal disease and dialysis on glycemic control. Semin Dial 2000;13(1):4–8.
2. Akmal M, Massry SG, Goldstein DA, et al. Role of parathyroid hormone in the glucose intolerance of chronic renal failure. J Clin Invest 1985;75(3):1037–44.
3. Mak RH. Intravenous 1,25 dihydroxycholecalciferol corrects glucose intolerance in hemodialysis patients. Kidney Int 1992;41(4):1049–54.
4. Viswanathan V, Tilak P, Meerza R, et al. Insulin resistance at different stages of diabetic kidney disease in India. J Assoc Physicians India 2010;58:612–5.
5. Alvestrand A. Carbohydrate and insulin metabolism in renal failure. Kidney Int Suppl 1997;62:S48–52.
6. Goldstein BJ, Mahadev K, Wu X. Redox paradox: insulin action is facilitated by insulin-stimulated reactive oxygen species with multiple potential signaling targets. Diabetes 2005;54(2):311–21.

7. Chang GY, Park AS, Susztak K. Tracing the footsteps of glomerular insulin signaling in diabetic kidney disease. Kidney Int 2011;79(8):802–4.
8. Hager SR. Insulin resistance of uremia. Am J Kidney Dis 1989;14(4):272–6.
9. Smith D, DeFronzo RA. Insulin resistance in uremia mediated by postbinding defects. Kidney Int 1982;22(1):54–62.
10. Fliser D, Pacini G, Engelleiter R, et al. Insulin resistance and hyperinsulinemia are already present in patients with incipient renal disease. Kidney Int 1998; 53(5):1343–7.
11. DeFronzo RA, Tobin JD, Rowe JW, et al. Glucose intolerance in uremia. Quantification of pancreatic beta cell sensitivity to glucose and tissue sensitivity to insulin. J Clin Invest 1978;62(2):425–35.
12. Schmitz O. Insulin-mediated glucose uptake in nondialyzed and dialyzed uremic insulin-dependent diabetic subjects. Diabetes 1985;34(11):1152–9.
13. Manolescu B, Stoian I, Atanasiu V, et al. Review article: the role of adipose tissue in uraemia-related insulin resistance. Nephrology (Carlton) 2008;13(7):622–8.
14. Lim PS, Chen SL, Wu MY, et al. Association of plasma adiponectin levels with oxidative stress in hemodialysis patients. Blood Purif 2007;25(4):362–9.
15. Guo LL, Pan Y, Jin HM. Adiponectin is positively associated with insulin resistance in subjects with type 2 diabetic nephropathy and effects of angiotensin II type 1 receptor blocker losartan. Nephrol Dial Transplant 2009;24(6):1876–83.
16. Zanetti M, Barazzoni R, Guarnieri G. Inflammation and insulin resistance in uremia. J Ren Nutr 2008;18(1):70–5.
17. Khedr E, El-Sharkawy M, Abdulwahab S, et al. Effect of recombinant human erythropoietin on insulin resistance in hemodialysis patients. Hemodial Int 2009;13(3):340–6.
18. Adrogue HJ. Glucose homeostasis and the kidney. Kidney Int 1992;42(5): 1266–82.
19. Goecke IA, Bonilla S, Marusic ET, et al. Enhanced insulin sensitivity in extrarenal potassium handling in uremic rats. Kidney Int 1991;39(1):39–43.
20. Ikizler TA. Effects of glucose homeostasis on protein metabolism in patients with advanced chronic kidney disease. J Ren Nutr 2007;17(1):13–6.
21. Cusi K, Maezono K, Osman A, et al. Insulin resistance differentially affects the PI 3-kinase- and MAP kinase-mediated signaling in human muscle. J Clin Invest 2000;105(3):311–20.
22. Siew ED, Ikizler TA. Insulin resistance and protein energy metabolism in patients with advanced chronic kidney disease. Semin Dial 2010;23(4):378–82.
23. Siew ED, Pupim LB, Majchrzak KM, et al. Insulin resistance is associated with skeletal muscle protein breakdown in non-diabetic chronic hemodialysis patients. Kidney Int 2007;71(2):146–52.
24. Mather A, Pollock C. Glucose handling by the kidney. Kidney Int Suppl 2011;(120):S1–6.
25. List JF, Whaley JM. Glucose dynamics and mechanistic implications of SGLT2 inhibitors in animals and humans. Kidney Int Suppl 2011;(120):S20–7.
26. Jurczak MJ, Lee HY, Birkenfeld AL, et al. SGLT2 deletion improves glucose homeostasis and preserves pancreatic beta-cell function. Diabetes 2011; 60(3):890–8.
27. Ahmed MH. The kidneys as an emerging target for the treatment of diabetes mellitus: what we know, thought we knew and hope to gain. Int J Diabetes Mellit 2010;2(2):125–6.
28. Liu JJ, Lee T, Defronzo RA. Why do SGLT2 inhibitors inhibit only 30-50% of renal glucose reabsorption in humans? Diabetes 2012;61(9):2199–204.

29. Mima A, Ohshiro Y, Kitada M, et al. Glomerular-specific protein kinase C-beta-induced insulin receptor substrate-1 dysfunction and insulin resistance in rat models of diabetes and obesity. Kidney Int 2011;79(8):883–96.

30. Dunn PJ, Cole RA, Soeldner JS, et al. Reproducibility of hemoglobin Alc and sensitivity to various degrees of glucose intolerance. Ann Intern Med 1979; 91(3):390–6.

31. Rohlfing CL, Wiedmeyer HM, Little RR, et al. Defining the relationship between plasma glucose and HbA(1c): analysis of glucose profiles and HbA(1c) in the Diabetes Control and Complications Trial. Diabetes Care 2002;25(2):275–8.

32. Nathan DM, Kuenen J, Borg R, et al. Translating the A1C assay into estimated average glucose values. Diabetes Care 2008;31(8):1473–8.

33. Stratton IM, Adler AI, Neil HA, et al. Association of glycaemia with macrovascular and microvascular complications of type 2 diabetes (UKPDS 35): prospective observational study. BMJ 2000;321(7258):405–12.

34. Rubinow KB, Hirsch IB. Reexamining metrics for glucose control. JAMA 2011; 305(11):1132–3.

35. Holt RI, Gallen I. Time to move beyond glycosylated haemoglobin. Diabet Med 2004;21(7):655–6.

36. Ly J, Marticorena R, Donnelly S. Red blood cell survival in chronic renal failure. Am J Kidney Dis 2004;44(4):715–9.

37. Little RR, Tennill AL, Rohlfing C, et al. Can glycohemoglobin be used to assess glycemic control in patients with chronic renal failure? Clin Chem 2002;48(5): 784–6.

38. Brown JN, Kemp DW, Brice KR. Class effect of erythropoietin therapy on hemoglobin A(1c) in a patient with diabetes mellitus and chronic kidney disease not undergoing hemodialysis. Pharmacotherapy 2009;29(4):468–72.

39. KDOQI. KDOQI clinical practice guidelines and clinical practice recommendations for diabetes and chronic kidney disease. Am J Kidney Dis 2007;49(2): S12–154.

40. Cohen RM, Smith EP. Frequency of HbA1c discordance in estimating blood glucose control. Curr Opin Clin Nutr Metab Care 2008;11(4):512–7.

41. U S Renal Data System. USRDS 2008 annual data report: atlas of end-stage renal disease in the United States. Bethesda (MD): National Institutes of Health, National Institute of Diabetes and Digestive and Kidney Diseases; 2008.

42. Williams ME, Lacson E Jr, Teng M, et al. Hemodialyzed type I and type II diabetic patients in the US: characteristics, glycemic control, and survival. Kidney Int 2006;70(8):1503–9.

43. Peacock TP, Shihabi ZK, Bleyer AJ, et al. Comparison of glycated albumin and hemoglobin A(1c) levels in diabetic subjects on hemodialysis. Kidney Int 2008; 73(9):1062–8.

44. Chen HS, Wu TE, Lin HD, et al. Hemoglobin A(1c) and fructosamine for assessing glycemic control in diabetic patients with CKD stages 3 and 4. Am J Kidney Dis 2010;55(5):867–74.

45. Riveline JP, Teynie J, Belmouaz S, et al. Glycaemic control in type 2 diabetic patients on chronic haemodialysis: use of a continuous glucose monitoring system. Nephrol Dial Transplant 2009;24(9):2866–71.

46. Ansari A, Thomas S, Goldsmith D. Assessing glycemic control in patients with diabetes and end-stage renal failure. Am J Kidney Dis 2003;41(3):523–31.

47. Mittman N, Desiraju B, Fazil I, et al. Serum fructosamine versus glycosylated hemoglobin as an index of glycemic control, hospitalization, and infection in diabetic hemodialysis patients. Kidney Int Suppl 2010;(117):S41–5.

48. Inaba M, Okuno S, Kumeda Y, et al. Glycated albumin is a better glycemic indicator than glycated hemoglobin values in hemodialysis patients with diabetes: effect of anemia and erythropoietin injection. J Am Soc Nephrol 2007;18(3): 896–903.
49. Alskar O, Korell J, Duffull SB. A pharmacokinetic model for the glycation of albumin. J Pharmacokinet Pharmacodyn 2012;39(3):273–82.
50. Abe M, Matsumoto K. Glycated hemoglobin or glycated albumin for assessment of glycemic control in hemodialysis patients with diabetes? Nat Clin Pract Nephrol 2008;4(9):482–3.
51. Freedman BI, Andries L, Shihabi ZK, et al. Glycated albumin and risk of death and hospitalizations in diabetic dialysis patients. Clin J Am Soc Nephrol 2011; 6(7):1635–43.
52. Inzucchi SE, Bergenstal RM, Buse JB, et al. Management of hyperglycemia in type 2 diabetes: a patient-centered approach: position statement of the American Diabetes Association (ADA) and the European Association for the Study of Diabetes (EASD). Diabetes Care 2012;35(6):1364–79.
53. O'Toole SM, Fan SL, Yaqoob MM, et al. Managing diabetes in dialysis patients. Postgrad Med J 2012;88(1037):160–6.
54. Kalantar-Zadeh K, Kopple JD, Regidor DL, et al. A1C and survival in maintenance hemodialysis patients. Diabetes Care 2007;30(5):1049–55.
55. Williams ME, Lacson E Jr, Wang W, et al. Glycemic control and extended hemodialysis survival in patients with diabetes mellitus: comparative results of traditional and time-dependent Cox model analyses. Clin J Am Soc Nephrol 2010; 5(9):1595–601.
56. Ix JH. Hemoglobin A1c in hemodialysis patients: should one size fit all? Clin J Am Soc Nephrol 2010;5(9):1539–41.
57. Ramirez SP, McCullough KP, Thumma JR, et al. Hemoglobin A1c levels and mortality in the diabetic hemodialysis population: findings from the Dialysis Outcomes and Practice Patterns Study (DOPPS). Diabetes Care 2012.
58. Drechsler C, Krane V, Ritz E, et al. Glycemic control and cardiovascular events in diabetic hemodialysis patients. Circulation 2009;120(24):2421–8.
59. Shurraw S, Hemmelgarn B, Lin M, et al. Association between glycemic control and adverse outcomes in people with diabetes mellitus and chronic kidney disease: a population-based cohort study. Arch Intern Med 2011;171(21): 1920–7.
60. Lachin JM, Viberti G, Zinman B, et al. Renal function in type 2 diabetes with rosiglitazone, metformin, and glyburide monotherapy. Clin J Am Soc Nephrol 2011;6(5):1032–40.
61. American Diabetes Association. Standards of medical care in diabetes—2012. Diabetes Care 2012;35(Suppl 1):S11–63.
62. Amiel SA, Dixon T, Mann R, et al. Hypoglycaemia in type 2 diabetes. Diabet Med 2008;25(3):245–54.
63. Munshi MN, Segal AR, Suhl E, et al. Frequent hypoglycemia among elderly patients with poor glycemic control. Arch Intern Med 2011;171(4):362–4.
64. Gerstein HC, Miller ME, Byington RP, et al. Effects of intensive glucose lowering in type 2 diabetes. N Engl J Med 2008;358(24):2545–59.
65. Patel A, MacMahon S, Chalmers J, et al. Intensive blood glucose control and vascular outcomes in patients with type 2 diabetes. N Engl J Med 2008; 358(24):2560–72.
66. Duckworth W, Abraira C, Moritz T, et al. Glucose control and vascular complications in veterans with type 2 diabetes. N Engl J Med 2009;360(2):129–39.

67. Haviv YS, Sharkia M, Safadi R. Hypoglycemia in patients with renal failure. Ren Fail 2000;22(2):219–23.
68. Sun CY, Lee CC, Wu MS. Hypoglycemia in diabetic patients undergoing chronic hemodialysis. Ther Apher Dial 2009;13(2):95–102.
69. Williams ME, Lacson E Jr, Wang W. High glucose variability increases risk of all-cause and hypoglycemia-related hospitalization in diabetic chronic hemodialysis patients (abstract). J Am Soc Nephrol 2009;20:193A.
70. Vallurupalli S, Huesmann G, Gregory J, et al. Levofloxacin-associated hypoglycaemia complicated by pontine myelinolysis and quadriplegia. Diabet Med 2008;25(7):856–9.
71. Zoungas S, Chalmers J, Ninomiya T, et al. Association of HbA1c levels with vascular complications and death in patients with type 2 diabetes: evidence of glycaemic thresholds. Diabetologia 2012;55(3):636–43.
72. O'Keefe JH, Abuannadi M, Lavie CJ, et al. Strategies for optimizing glycemic control and cardiovascular prognosis in patients with type 2 diabetes mellitus. Mayo Clin Proc 2011;86(2):128–38.
73. Nathan DM, Buse JB, Davidson MB, et al. Medical management of hyperglycemia in type 2 diabetes: a consensus algorithm for the initiation and adjustment of therapy: a consensus statement of the American Diabetes Association and the European Association for the Study of Diabetes. Diabetes Care 2009;32(1):193–203.
74. Rodbard HW, Jellinger PS, Davidson JA, et al. Statement by an American Association of Clinical Endocrinologists/American College of Endocrinology consensus panel on type 2 diabetes mellitus: an algorithm for glycemic control. Endocr Pract 2009;15(6):540–59.
75. Qaseem A, Humphrey LL, Sweet DE, et al. Oral pharmacologic treatment of type 2 diabetes mellitus: a clinical practice guideline from the American College of Physicians. Ann Intern Med 2012;156(3):218–31.
76. Bennett WL, Odelola OA, Wilson LM, et al. Evaluation of guideline recommendations on oral medications for type 2 diabetes mellitus: a systematic review. Ann Intern Med 2012;156(1 Pt 1):27–36.
77. Kahn SE, Haffner SM, Heise MA, et al. Glycemic durability of rosiglitazone, metformin, or glyburide monotherapy. N Engl J Med 2006;355(23):2427–43.
78. Schejter YD, Turvall E, Ackerman Z. Characteristics of patients with sulphonurea-induced hypoglycemia. J Am Med Dir Assoc 2012;13(3):234–8.
79. Holstein A, Plaschke A, Hammer C, et al. Characteristics and time course of severe glimepiride- versus glibenclamide-induced hypoglycaemia. Eur J Clin Pharmacol 2003;59(2):91–7.
80. Rosenkranz B, Profozic V, Metelko Z, et al. Pharmacokinetics and safety of glimepiride at clinically effective doses in diabetic patients with renal impairment. Diabetologia 1996;39(12):1617–24.
81. UK Prospective Diabetes Study (UKPDS) Group. Effect of intensive blood-glucose control with metformin on complications in overweight patients with type 2 diabetes (UKPDS 34). Lancet 1998;352(9131):854–65.
82. Holman RR, Paul SK, Bethel MA, et al. 10-year follow-up of intensive glucose control in type 2 diabetes. N Engl J Med 2008;359(15):1577–89.
83. Runge S, Mayerle J, Warnke C, et al. Metformin-associated lactic acidosis in patients with renal impairment solely due to drug accumulation? Diabetes Obes Metab 2008;10(1):91–3.
84. Pongwecharak J, Tengmeesri N, Malanusorn N, et al. Prescribing metformin in type 2 diabetes with a contraindication: prevalence and outcome. Pharm World Sci 2009;31(4):481–6.

85. Abe M, Okada K, Maruyama T, et al. Clinical effectiveness and safety evaluation of long-term pioglitazone treatment for erythropoietin responsiveness and insulin resistance in type 2 diabetic patients on hemodialysis. Expert Opin Pharmacother 2010;11(10):1611–20.

86. Agrawal A, Sautter MC, Jones NP. Effects of rosiglitazone maleate when added to a sulfonylurea regimen in patients with type 2 diabetes mellitus and mild to moderate renal impairment: a post hoc analysis. Clin Ther 2003;25(11):2754–64.

87. Chiang CK, Ho TI, Peng YS, et al. Rosiglitazone in diabetes control in hemodialysis patients with and without viral hepatitis infection: effectiveness and side effects. Diabetes Care 2007;30(1):3–7.

88. Nissen SE, Wolski K. Effect of rosiglitazone on the risk of myocardial infarction and death from cardiovascular causes. N Engl J Med 2007;356(24):2457–71.

89. Ramirez SP, Albert JM, Blayney MJ, et al. Rosiglitazone is associated with mortality in chronic hemodialysis patients. J Am Soc Nephrol 2009;20(5):1094–101.

90. Dormandy JA, Charbonnel B, Eckland DJ, et al. Secondary prevention of macrovascular events in patients with type 2 diabetes in the PROactive Study (PROspective pioglitAzone Clinical Trial In macroVascular Events): a randomised controlled trial. Lancet 2005;366(9493):1279–89.

91. Schneider CA, Ferrannini E, Defronzo R, et al. Effect of pioglitazone on cardiovascular outcome in diabetes and chronic kidney disease. J Am Soc Nephrol 2008;19(1):182–7.

92. Habib ZA, Havstad SL, Wells K, et al. Thiazolidinedione use and the longitudinal risk of fractures in patients with type 2 diabetes mellitus. J Clin Endocrinol Metab 2010;95(2):592–600.

93. Lewis JD, Ferrara A, Peng T, et al. Risk of bladder cancer among diabetic patients treated with pioglitazone: interim report of a longitudinal cohort study. Diabetes Care 2011;34(4):916–22.

94. Chan JC, Scott R, Arjona Ferreira JC, et al. Safety and efficacy of sitagliptin in patients with type 2 diabetes and chronic renal insufficiency. Diabetes Obes Metab 2008;10(7):545–55.

95. Graefe-Mody U, Friedrich C, Port A, et al. Effect of renal impairment on the pharmacokinetics of the dipeptidyl peptidase-4 inhibitor linagliptin(*). Diabetes Obes Metab 2011;13(10):939–46.

96. Lukashevich V, Schweizer A, Shao Q, et al. Safety and efficacy of vildagliptin versus placebo in patients with type 2 diabetes and moderate or severe renal impairment: a prospective 24-week randomized placebo-controlled trial. Diabetes Obes Metab 2011;13(10):947–54.

97. Nowicki M, Rychlik I, Haller H, et al. Long-term treatment with the dipeptidyl peptidase-4 inhibitor saxagliptin in patients with type 2 diabetes mellitus and renal impairment: a randomised controlled 52-week efficacy and safety study. Int J Clin Pract 2011;65(12):1230–9.

98. Nowicki M, Rychlik I, Haller H, et al. Saxagliptin improves glycaemic control and is well tolerated in patients with type 2 diabetes mellitus and renal impairment. Diabetes Obes Metab 2011;13(6):523–32.

99. Linnebjerg H, Kothare PA, Park S, et al. Effect of renal impairment on the pharmacokinetics of exenatide. Br J Clin Pharmacol 2007;64(3):317–27.

100. Kaakeh Y, Kanjee S, Boone K, et al. Liraglutide-induced acute kidney injury. Pharmacotherapy 2012;32(1):e7–11.

101. Lopez-Ruiz A, del Peso-Gilsanz C, Meoro-Aviles A, et al. Acute renal failure when exenatide is co-administered with diuretics and angiotensin II blockers. Pharm World Sci 2010;32(5):559–61.

102. Devineni D, Walter YH, Smith HT, et al. Pharmacokinetics of nateglinide in renally impaired diabetic patients. J Clin Pharmacol 2003;43(2):163–70.
103. Inoue T, Shibahara N, Miyagawa K, et al. Pharmacokinetics of nateglinide and its metabolites in subjects with type 2 diabetes mellitus and renal failure. Clin Nephrol 2003;60(2):90–5.
104. Rave K, Heise T, Pfutzner A, et al. Impact of diabetic nephropathy on pharmacodynamic and Pharmacokinetic properties of insulin in type 1 diabetic patients. Diabetes Care 2001;24(5):886–90.
105. Baldwin D, Zander J, Munoz C, et al. A randomized trial of two weight-based doses of insulin glargine and glulisine in hospitalized subjects with type 2 diabetes and renal insufficiency. Diabetes Care 2012;35(10):1970–4.
106. Sobngwi E, Enoru S, Ashuntantang G, et al. Day-to-day variation of insulin requirements of patients with type 2 diabetes and end-stage renal disease undergoing maintenance hemodialysis. Diabetes Care 2010;33(7):1409–12.
107. Aisenpreis U, Pfutzner A, Giehl M, et al. Pharmacokinetics and pharmacodynamics of insulin Lispro compared with regular insulin in haemodialysis patients with diabetes mellitus. Nephrol Dial Transplant 1999;14(Suppl 4):5–6.
108. Czock D, Aisenpreis U, Rasche FM, et al. Pharmacokinetics and pharmacodynamics of lispro-insulin in hemodialysis patients with diabetes mellitus. Int J Clin Pharmacol Ther 2003;41(10):492–7.
109. Holmes G, Galitz L, Hu P, et al. Pharmacokinetics of insulin aspart in obesity, renal impairment, or hepatic impairment. Br J Clin Pharmacol 2005;60(5):469–76.
110. Hung AM, Roumie CL, Greevy RA, et al. Comparative effectiveness of incident oral antidiabetic drugs on kidney function. Kidney Int 2012;81(7):698–706.

Comanagement of Diabetic Kidney Disease by the Primary Care Provider and Nephrologist

Brendan T. Bowman, MD[a], Amanda Kleiner, MD[b],
W. Kline Bolton, MD[a],*

KEYWORDS

- Comanagement • Internist • Collaborative care • Diabetic kidney disease

KEY POINTS

- Diabetic kidney disease (DKD) is a common but complex and multifaceted disorder, and few patients achieve current therapeutic targets described in clinical guidelines.
- A coordinated approach to the care of these patients offers the opportunity to improve patient outcomes.
- Guidelines outlining the specifics of coordinating care for patients with DKD do not currently exist.
- Careful collaboration between all health care providers, particularly primary care physicians, nephrologists, and endocrinologists, and the creation of disorder-specific health care systems, offer the best opportunity for improving the management and clinical outcomes of these patients.

INTRODUCTION

Estimates of chronic kidney disease (CKD) prevalence in the United States vary but suggest upwards of 26 million affected individuals, inclusive of all stages of CKD.[1] Within this population, diabetes mellitus (DM) is both a comorbid condition and a cause of kidney disease.[2–4] True prevalence remains difficult to estimate because a definitive diagnosis of diabetic kidney disease (DKD) requires biopsy[5]; however, of the 26 million Americans diagnosed with some form of DM, 20% to 40% will develop renal involvement according to the American Diabetes Association (ADA).[6] Diabetes remains the most common cause of incident end stage renal disease (ESRD) according to the United States Renal Data System's (USRDS) Annual Report.[3] For most clinicians,

[a] Division of Nephrology, Department of Medicine, University of Virginia "Health System", Box 800133, Charlottesville, VA 22908, USA; [b] Division of Endocrinology, Department of Medicine, University of Virginia "Health System", Box 801406, Charlottesville, VA 22908, USA
* Corresponding author.
E-mail address: wkb5s@virginia.edu

Med Clin N Am 97 (2013) 157–173
http://dx.doi.org/10.1016/j.mcna.2012.10.012
0025-7125/13/$ – see front matter © 2013 Elsevier Inc. All rights reserved.

DKD is generally encountered as proteinuria with or without impaired glomerular filtration rate (GFR) in the appropriate clinical setting,[2] although pathologic changes of DM may be present years before clinical signs.[7] Large randomized controlled trials have shown that glycemic control reduces microvascular complications and delays progression of proteinuria[8,9] - important as the risk of ESRD and cardiovascular disease (CVD) increase with progression of proteinuria.[10,11]

Given the significant morbidity and mortality associated with DM, CKD, and ESRD,[3,11] guidelines to assist in diagnosing, stabilizing, and managing DKD have been proposed by various government agencies and professional societies.[2,6,12] CKD alone has been shown to increase mortality but the presence of DM more than doubles mortality, primarily because of CVD.[3]

Although the risks of DKD are better appreciated, evidence suggests that care for CKD and DKD has significant room for improvement.[3,6,13,14] Unfortunately, primary care physicians (PCPs) and nephrologists face increased patient loads and projected workforce shortages, making dedicated time for DKD care difficult to provide.[15,16] These increased demands require PCPs and nephrologists to find more efficient and effective ways to work together.

Proposed primary care delivery models such as accountable care organizations (ACO) and the patient-centered medical home (PCMH) have sought to improve outcomes and reduce costs by integrating the major health care entities (PCPs, hospitals, and specialists) into a single functional entity emphasizing primary care and care coordination.[17–19] Within these models, clear roles and responsibilities of the PCP and specialist have not been assigned. Current practice patterns in DKD management vary widely from the PCP who performs comprehensive care to the physician who refers to the nephrologist for preventive care in any diabetic patient. Regardless of practice styles, evidence exists for the benefits of nephrology involvement in the management of DKD and CKD that persists even after initiation of dialysis.[20–22]

However, barriers to effective collaboration between health care providers exist both in DKD and CKD management. These barriers include low rates of screening, poor recognition of renal disease, late referral for nephrology care, and perceptions of poor communication following referral.[3,23,24] Interventions to address these barriers have been evaluated, but few of these studies take the form of large-scale randomized controlled trials, which is a common problem in renal literature.[25] Most interventions related to collaborative care take the form of improved referral communication, educational interventions, and quality improvement (QI) projects.[26–28] There is no large body of data regarding DKD-specific interventions to improve outcomes, but evaluating the larger body of CKD literature can help inform the topic.

This article discusses areas of weakness in the PCP-nephrology interface, attitudes and perceptions of comanagement, options for attaining euglycemia in DKD, and lastly, proposes a model for DKD care delivery.

SCREENING AND DIAGNOSIS IN DKD

Benefits of early screening and detection in diabetic renal disease derive primarily from early interventions to retard progression of proteinuria and preserve GFR.[8,9,29] In the United States, patients with CKD and diabetes are most often seen by the PCP,[3] making the primary care clinic the logical target of screening and early detection.

Several organizations provide resources for PCPs regarding screening and interpretation of test results. The National Kidney Foundation (NKF) publishes the Kidney Disease Outcomes Quality Initiative (KDOQI) set of clinical practice guidelines, whereas the ADA separately publishes guidelines for diabetes, including renal disease.[2,6] The NKF also operates the Kidney Early Evaluation Program, which promotes screening for at-risk groups, algorithms for confirmatory testing, and results interpretation.[12] The National Institute of Diabetes and Digestive and Kidney Disease promotes screening and management via the National Kidney Disease Education Program. In addition, annual screening targets have been set for DKD as a Healthy People 2020 goal at a modest 37% of the diabetic Medicare population.[3]

The NKF and ADA both recommend annual screening for GFR and proteinuria with follow-up confirmatory testing.[2,6] Recently, the US Preventive Services Task Force concluded there were insufficient data to support routine screening for CKD but, that recommendation did not address DKD.[30] A 2010 Canadian study by Manns and colleagues[31] evaluated cost-effectiveness of screening for CKD and found benefit specifically in diabetic patients, with an acceptable cost per quality-adjusted life year (QALY) of $C22,600. For reference, an intervention less than $50,000 per QALY is considered reasonable from a public health perspective. A summary of screening recommendations for DKD is presented in **Table 1**.

Despite these recommendations, USRDS data show low rates of annual testing for proteinuria, with creatinine testing performed 3 times more frequently.[3] Given the specificity of urine microalbumin testing to the investigation of renal disease, this may be a better indicator of low DKD screening rates. The USRDS Medicare data set also shows low rates of annual microalbuminuria screening at 37.3%.[3] The likelihood of diabetics receiving the recommended combination of urine protein, creatinine, lipid, and eye screening in a given year is a low 25%.[3]

Although screening rates for DKD remain too low, other studies suggest that, even in the presence of diagnostic laboratory values, DKD may simply be underdiagnosed. In a study by Meyers and colleagues,[23] the investigators reviewed a large electronic medical record (EMR) clinical data base, and approximately 35% of diabetic patients showed renal impairment by estimated GFR (eGFR) criteria (eGFR<60 mL/min/1.73 m^2). Despite this, only 20% of the DKD group was documented as having any stage of CKD. Ryan and colleagues[32] found similar results for patients with CKD in reviewing standardized laboratory data and EMRs from 13 primary care clinics. In the study by Ryan and colleagues,[32] these low rates of diagnosis were reported despite the addition of automated eGFR reporting.

Both studies are limited by their retrospective nature and reliance on diagnosis codes or characteristic actions (ie, nephrology referral) to interpret PCP awareness of renal impairment. A more direct method of assessing PCP recognition of DKD was used by Boulware and colleagues[24] using a national survey of family physicians, internists, and nephrologists. In their study, 304 physicians were presented with a clinical vignette and laboratory data including a progressively worsening creatinine (2.1 mg/dL to 2.3 mg/dL) at the time of initial office visit. The investigators purposely did not provide eGFR but did provide all variables necessary to calculate it. Participants were asked to identify the presence and stage of CKD and to assess the need for referral. Responses showed that 59% of family physicians and 78% of internists were able to accurately categorize the patient as having CKD and to stage appropriately (stage 4) versus 97% of nephrologists. KDOQI guidelines recommend referral to a nephrologist at Stage 4; however, fewer PCPs recommended referral (76% family medicine and 81% internal medicine) compared with 99% of nephrologists. These studies suggest an element of decreased awareness of renal disease in primary care.

Recognizing this problem, others have successfully improved renal disease awareness through a variety of interventions. In the CKD literature, Humphreys and colleagues[33] reported a 31% improvement in CKD identification and 40% improvement in blood pressure target achievement with implementation of a QI project using the

Table 1
Screening guidelines for DKD from major professional societies

Organization	Year Reviewed	Target Populations	Acceptable Tests	Frequency of Screening
NKF/KDOQI	2007	All patients with type 1 diabetes of at least 5 y duration. All type 2 diabetics at diagnosis	Serum creatinine with eGFR by MDRD, Cockroft-Gault methods Measurement of albumin/creatinine ratio in a spot urine sample	Annually. Increased albumin/creatinine ratio confirmed twice within following 3–6 mo
ADA	2012	All patients with type 1 diabetes of at least 5 y duration. All type 2 diabetics at diagnosis	Serum creatinine Test of urine albumin excretion	Annually. Increased albumin/creatinine ratio confirmed twice within following 3–6 mo

Abbreviations: eGFR, estimated GFR; MDRD, modification of diet in renal disease.
Data from Klahr S, Levey AS, Beck GJ, et al. The effects of dietary protein restriction and blood-pressure control on the progression of chronic renal disease. N Engl J Med 1994;330:877–84.

Plan-Do-Study-Act methodology. Similar findings were reported by Fox and colleagues[34] implementing a QI and education plan in 2 family practice clinics. In the latter study, a mixed intervention of education and process improvements facilitated by specially trained CKD nurses led to improvements in both diagnosis and medication adjustments. Neither study specifically required a nephrologist.

Kaiser Permanente of Southern California published results from a CKD identification initiative that resulted in a 79% usage rate of CKD diagnosis codes in their prevalent CKD population.[35] This contrasts with the low CKD diagnosis code rate ($\sim$20%) noted in the retrospective chart reviews discussed earlier.[23,32] Here again, most of these patients were never seen by nephrologists, with PCPs performing CKD diagnosis and early stage care.

In the aggregate, these studies suggest that current screening methods may suffer from lack of implementation and, when blood tests alone are used, under-recognition of DKD. Although nephrologists may diagnose DKD more reliably, screening remains most opportunistic in the PCP's office. The United Kingdom and Southern California Kaiser Permanente experiences suggest that dedicated renal disease identification interventions in the primary care office can markedly improve diagnosis.

REFERRAL: OPENING THE DOOR TO COLLABORATION

The benefits of nephrology referral as well as the harms of late referral have previously been described in CKD and DKD literature. A brief list of reported benefits includes reduction in rate of GFR decline, increased use of renin-angiotensin-aldosterone system (RAAS) blockers, and improved mortality.[20–22,36,37] Potential harms of late referral include suboptimal management of mineral bone disorders and anemia, higher rates of dialysis catheter use versus fistulas when initiating renal replacement therapy (RRT), and increased mortality both overall and in the first year of dialysis.[21,38] The KDOQI and ADA recommendations for referral[2,6] are listed in **Table 2**.

Definitions of late referral vary among studies but generally imply a rapid initiation of RRT following referral (<1–4 months) without adequate time to counsel patients on options for ESRD care (including transplantation) or to obtain a fistula if possible, or otherwise a graft. The prevalence of late referrals varies by study and definition, but is commonly reported to be between 20% and 40% in the CKD population.[38,39]

Table 2
Summary of indications for nephrology referral related to DKD from KDOQI and ADA guidelines

Organization	Year Published	Excerpts of Referral Guidelines/Recommendations in DKD/CKD
NKF/KDOQI	2007	Patients with CKD should be referred to a specialist for consultation and comanagement if the clinical action plan cannot be prepared, the prescribed evaluation of the patient cannot be carried out, or the recommended treatment cannot be carried out. In general, patients with GFR <30 mL/min/1.73 m^2 should be referred to a nephrologist
ADA	2012	GFR 45–60 mL/min/1.73 m^2: referral to nephrology if possibility for non-DKD exists (duration type 1 diabetes <10 y, heavy proteinuria, abnormal findings on renal ultrasound, resistant hypertension, rapid decrease in GFR, or active urinary sediment on ultrasound) GFR <30 mL/min/1.73 m^2: referral to nephrologist

Perhaps the largest study of referral patterns and outcomes of patients with diabetes and CKD was performed by Tseng and colleagues,[22] and involved a retrospective review of more than 39,000 Veterans Administration (VA) patients. In that study, the investigators found a mortality benefit proportional to the frequency of nephrology follow-up in patients with stage 3 and 4 kidney disease. In another study, Martinez-Ramirez and colleagues[20] performed one of the few prospective evaluations of referral benefit in patients with CKD and DM. The investigators assigned patients with DM and proteinuria to early nephrology referral, and compared outcomes with a cohort of patients remaining under their family physician's care. Within cohorts, patients were categorized by degree of proteinuria and followed for 1 year. At the conclusion, nephrology care was associated with stable GFR in the study group versus loss in controls, better blood pressure control, increased use of RAAS blocking agents, and decreased nonsteroidal antiinflammatory medication use.

In addition to GFR preservation, the study group also saw decreased progression of proteinuria, with the microalbuminuric group showing the greatest benefit.

Causes of late referral vary, from the patient with rapid decline in GFR making timely referral impossible, to those with insidious disease recognized late in their course. Fischer and colleagues[40] proposed 3 broad causative categories for late referral: patient factors, PCP factors, and health care system factors. PCP-related factors include poor renal disease recognition and lack of screening. Health care system–related factors include fragmented care organizations (part VA, part Medicare, for example) and lack of access to nephrology care. Patient-related factors include older age (>75 years), lack of health insurance, undiagnosed rapid progression of CKD, and poor compliance. A systematic review of late referral causes by Naveneethan and colleagues[41] used a similar system and added poor communication between PCPs and nephrologists to this list.

Boulware and colleagues[24] further explored PCP-nephrologist referral perceptions, surveying both groups regarding comfort with general KDOQI guidelines, ideal referral timing, and desired information from referral. Forty-seven percent of family practitioners and 31% of internists reported difficulty in referring patients at least "a little of the time", and 52% and 29%, respectively, of family practice and internal medicine physicians cited difficulty referring because of lack of local nephrologists. Only a small percentage (<10% in both groups) noted concern that a nephrologist may want to completely take over the patient's care. The investigators found that PCPs electing to refer were more likely to be recent graduates (in practice <10 years) and to self-identify as being familiar with CKD guidelines.

Age may also play a factor as referral rates in CKD are generally lower in the elderly, although not all studies have found this.[39,41,42] Campbell and colleagues[42] reviewed referral decision making by PCPs in the elderly using a clinical vignette and survey. PCP referral decisions were influenced not only by CKD stage but also comorbidities and cognitive abilities, suggesting nuanced referral decisions. This finding suggests the lower rates of elderly CKD referral may be appropriate.

Few studies have evaluated interventions to improve referral in DKD specifically. One study by Stoves and colleagues[26] in the United Kingdom used an e-consult to increase access to and facilitate communication with nephrologists. This study involved electronic review of referrals and patient records by nephrologists followed by electronically communicated recommendations to general practitioners (GPs) through an automated e-consult. This e-consult allowed GPs and nephrologists to determine the necessity of a full clinic visit referral versus providing focused guidance to the GP. Although this intervention reduced total referrals, the appropriateness of referrals was improved in a collaborative manner.

Despite evidence of improved outcomes in DKD with early referral, 20% to 40% of patients initiating dialysis are referred late, with subsequently increased mortality that persists into the period of RRT. Factors specific to patients, health care systems, and providers contribute to this problem. Difficulties in providing access to nephrology care, both real and perceived, are a barrier to referral. Interventions allowing virtual access to nephrology care and educating PCPs on recognition may improve the quality and timeliness of DKD referrals. Allowing PCPs and nephrologists to communicate before referral to determine appropriate referrals may be helpful in reducing rates of unnecessary referrals.

ATTITUDES TOWARD COLLABORATIVE CARE

To our knowledge, the attitudes and expectations of PCPs and nephrologists regarding comanagement of DKD have not been studied. There is no body of literature describing how PCPs and nephrologists divide clinical responsibilities (dietary counseling, prescriptions, lipid management, glycemic control) in day-to-day practice. These matters remain at the discretion of individual providers and are functions of practice patterns and interrelationships. Although there are few DKD-specific data, there are survey data regarding referral in general and CKD comanagement between PCPs and specialists.

In 2000, Gandhi and colleagues[43] performed an electronic survey of PCPs and specialists to determine satisfaction with their current referral and information sharing. Large percentages of both groups were dissatisfied with the information received from the other (28% of PCPs and 43% of specialists). Nearly half of both groups were dissatisfied with the timeliness of communication, suggesting a need for improvement in communication between colleagues.

Specific to CKD, Boulware and colleagues[24] and Diamantidis and colleagues[44] both reported attitudes toward collaboration between PCPs and nephrologists using a stage 4 CKD vignette. The investigators surveyed both groups' preferences in referral communication, frequency of specialist input, transition of primary care activities, and types of information sought. PCPs most often preferred periodic input (every 4–6 months). Most clinicians in both the PCP and nephrology groups agreed on communication regarding confirmation of diagnosis and evaluation, performance of additional testing and evaluation, nutritional advice, and medication regimen advice. Nephrologists were more likely than PCPs to prioritize information related to preparation for RRT and electrolyte disorders.

Regarding longitudinal care, PCPs and nephrologists overwhelmingly preferred the PCP to remain the primary caregiver, which suggests that neither group desires nephrology to "take over" the CKD patients primary care.

In summary, it seems that PCPs and specialists both note problematic communication, with lack of timely reporting and necessary content missing. When PCPs and nephrologists are surveyed, both groups prefer collaboration in which the PCP remains the main caregiver. However, the groups diverge on the timing and importance of CKD complications such as mineral bone disorders, anemia, and preparation for RRT.

DKD CARE DELIVERY MODEL

DKD is a multifaceted entity affecting many organ systems with increased risk for CVD and subsequent mortality, particularly in patients with advanced GFR loss and macroalbuminuria.[10,11] Because of the number of health care professionals involved, and also because the multiple areas of management overlap, there is no definitive model of comanagement in general use. The ADA officially endorses use of the 6-component

Chronic Disease Model (CDM) for DM care; however, the data for use of this model are unproven in kidney disease care.[45] Although further studies of structured interventions are needed, based on current published literature, surveys, and data from CKD and DM, a model of DKD care should consist of at least the following elements:

- Clearly delineated areas of clinical practice agreed on between all providers in advance
- An effective outcomes measurement system and QI strategy
- Integration of multidisciplinary teams with multifactorial interventions
- Effective communication strategy using a shared EMR with access to a fully functional patient chart

In primary care, 2 recent models of care have been promoted heavily: the ACO and PCMH. Both seek to improve patient outcome through emphasizing primary care, improved coordination, and quality metric tracking.[17,18] Both also provide an emphasis on integrated care to maximize the benefits of the PCP-specialist management of comorbidities. The elements of a DKD care model listed earlier can be integrated into these frameworks and differ from the traditional model of 2 to 3 providers that is common at present. **Fig. 1** depicts a traditional 3-provider model with PCP, nephrologist, and endocrinologist. **Fig. 2** depicts the elements of an idealized DKD care delivery model. As shown in the figure, providers, patient, and multidisciplinary team are able to interact through an EMR, and the primacy of the patient-PCP relationship remains intact through an entity such as the PCMH. An integrated QI methodology such as the Plan-Do-Study-Act cycle is embraced by all providers.

ELEMENTS OF THE DKD CARE DELIVERY MODEL

Clear definitions of clinical areas and responsibilities are essential to eliminate overlap and avoid duplicate effort in DKD care. Although all providers have different practice patterns and preferences, the previously discussed survey data suggest that most PCPs and nephrologists have broadly similar views on frequency of referral, information of value expected from referral, and the patient's appropriate medical home.[24,44] Reviewing these surveys suggests that most PCPs prefer nephrology input periodically and would prefer that most health care remain with the PCP. These preferences exclude management of those conditions unique to kidney disease, such as mineral

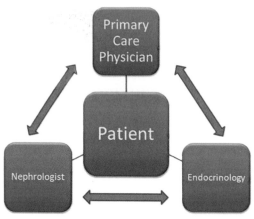

Fig. 1. Traditional model of care for DKD.

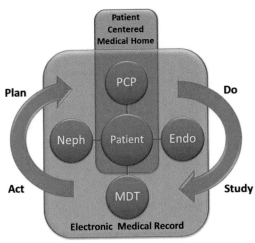

Fig. 2. Proposed model using the PCMH as the primary care entity, with the Plan-Do-Study-Act (PDSA) cycle for QI overlying the EMR as a communication vehicle between providers. The multidisciplinary team (MDT) may be a stand-alone entity, part of a PCMH/ACO or a component of the PCP/specialist practice. The PCMH model is chosen here for example only. ACO structure could be substituted depending on the clinical needs. Many iterative QI programs are acceptable, and the PDSA cycle is selected for example purposes only. Endo, endocrinologist; Neph, nephrologist; PCP, primary care physician.

bone disorders (secondary hyperparathyroidism, hyperphosphatemia, and so forth), anemia of CKD, and preparation for RRT. Using survey data regarding preferred roles by the clinicians, a responsibility matrix can be built to assign areas of management to providers. **Fig. 3** suggests how those roles may transition based on progression of underlying renal disease. These are only suggested role assignments and providers should customize these roles to the individual provider's strengths, weaknesses, and preferences.[46] In short, as long as clinical performance measures (CPMs) are monitored and achieved, it is unimportant which provider assumes a specific role.

Given the overall need for improvement in achieving clinical targets in the care of DKD,[6,13,14] a continuous QI process should be an integral part of a DKD care delivery model. Evaluation and review cycles such as the Plan-Do-Study-Act cycle have been proposed by entities such as the Agency for Healthcare Research and Quality in the care of chronic disease.[47,48] These methods have been used successfully to improve performance in areas as diverse as attainment of blood pressure targets and improvement in quality of referrals.[26,33] The Renal Physicians Association (RPA) provides a CKD toolkit with suggested CPMs that can be applied to DKD to ensure high-quality care delivery.[49] Given the number of health care professionals engaged in DKD management, more potential process flow bottlenecks and breakdowns are possible, necessitating that a QI methodology be integrated into the care model. These concepts are also embraced in the ACO and PCMH models.

A third component of an effective model for DKD would be integration of a multidisciplinary team (MDT). MDTs are groups of care providers, usually physician led, tasked with improving outcomes through multifactorial interventions (diet, lifestyle, social services). Teams typically include a dietician/nutritionist, clinical pharmacist, social worker, nurse practitioners, physician assistant, and specially trained nursing staff.[50–53] MDTs have been studied in diabetes care and are now included specifically in ADA guidelines.[6,54,55] Team-based care was recently the subject of an Institute of

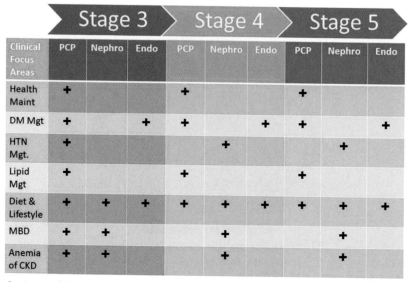

Clinical Focus Areas	Stage 3			Stage 4			Stage 5		
	PCP	Nephro	Endo	PCP	Nephro	Endo	PCP	Nephro	Endo
Health Maint	+			+			+		
DM Mgt	+		+	+		+	+		+
HTN Mgt.	+				+			+	
Lipid Mgt	+			+			+		
Diet & Lifestyle	+	+	+	+	+	+	+	+	+
MBD	+	+			+			+	
Anemia of CKD	+	+			+			+	

Fig. 3. Areas of focus for PCP, nephrologist, and endocrinologist with progression of DKD following development of stage 3 CKD. HTN, hypertension; MBD, mineral bone disorders; Mgt, management; Nephro, nephrologist.

Medicine work group, suggesting the high value of team-based care as a permanent change to the way health care is delivered in the United States.[56]

The effect of MDTs on patients has been best evaluated in CKD, but some studies address DKD specifically. One prospective multicenter 2-year study of a structured care intervention using nurse educators, endocrinologists, and pharmacists in Hong Kong showed improved attainment of glycosylated hemoglobin and blood pressure targets. Patients in the structured care group were also more likely to meet treatment targets, which conveyed a 60% relative risk reduction in reaching ESRD compared with the usual care group.[57] Studies in CKD, on balance, favor the MDT approach.[58–60] For example, a study by Thanamayooran and colleagues[61] showed improved adherence to clinical targets such as blood pressure goals and glycosylated hemoglobin. Wu and colleagues[60] in Taiwan prospectively studied 2 cohorts, 1 assigned to usual care, the other to a structured MDT intervention, and were able to show decreased progression to dialysis and decreased mortality in the intervention group. Hemmelgarn and colleagues[58] retrospectively evaluated elderly patients exposed to MDT and also showed mortality benefit compared with matched controls.

The driver for the effect of MDTs on CKD outcomes is difficult to assess. By nature, these are multifactorial interventions and controlling for each individual intervention is difficult. Nonetheless, the existing data from CKD and DM studies generally show improved achievement of clinical targets, decreased incidence of ESRD, and improved mortality.

The final component of a DKD care delivery model is effective communication between PCPs and specialists. However, both groups perceive important shortfalls in timely, complete, and accurate communication, as shown in provider surveys.[43] Many studies have used EMR systems to improve communication between specialists and PCPs. Stoves and colleagues[26] showed the value of the e-consultation in improving appropriate referrals and reducing total volume of referrals overall using an EMR. Kim-Hwang and colleagues[62] similarly described implementation of an e-referral system resulting in improved clarity of referral reason, reduction of inappropriate referrals, and reduced unnecessary follow-up visits.

Other elements of EMRs suggest promise for improved outcomes but study data are limited or mixed. Chang and colleagues[63] recently reviewed available literature on the use of computerized provider order entry (CPOE) and clinical decision support systems (CDSS) in acute kidney injury and CKD care but this mostly excluded office-based chronic care. A small randomized trial of CDSS for CKD care in a primary clinic noted no clear benefit but was limited in size and duration.[64] A larger 2008 study using a multifactorial intervention of education, practice enhancement assistants, and CDSS to manage CKD in a primary care setting showed improved diagnosis of CKD, but the driver of the improvements was unclear.[34] To our knowledge, data specific to DKD outcomes related to use of CPOE or CDSS have not been separately studied. Supporting data for diabetes care alone using EMRs and CDSSs is more robust but also mixed.[65] We think that, although CPOE and CDSS hold promise, more studies are needed to support the inclusion of these technologies in routine DKD care.

SPECIAL CONSIDERATIONS IN DKD: THE ROLE OF GLYCEMIC CONTROL

Hyperglycemia is the principal metabolic defect occurring in both type 1 and type 2 DM, and euglycemia remains the central management goal.[6] Multiple large, multi-center, randomized controlled trials consistently show the role of glycemic control in reducing the risk of DKD.[8,66,67] It remains controversial whether tight glycemic control prevents the progression of existing microalbuminuria to macroalbuminuria in diabetic patients, with the Kumamoto Study[68] showing a protective effect of tight glycemic control in type 2 DM, whereas the Diabetes Control and Complication Trial (DCCT) was underpowered to show a similar effect in type 1 DM.[8] However, prolonged eugly-cemia can slow the rate of progression in renal injury, even in the presence of known DKD,[69] and guidelines support tight glycemic targets in this group.[6,70,71]

Glycemic control should be a focus in the prevention and management of DKD,[71] but achieving this remains an elusive goal.[72] Most glycemic management for diabetic patients is provided by PCPs working independently, yet few have the resources and support necessary to achieve the glycemic control required to prevent complications of diabetes.[73]

There are several challenges to achieving glycemic control and only a minority of patients achieve these targets.[74] The reasons for this are multifactorial and include patient factors, such as medication nonadherence, health care costs, poor attention to diet, and difficulty with blood glucose self-monitoring,[75,76] and physician factors, such as lack of time for counseling, inadequate education and experience, and clinical inertia.[77,78] Compounding these challenges is the complexity of modifying medication regimens in the presence of underlying renal disease.

Given the complexity of glycemic management in patients with DKD, the ADA recommends all such patients be referred to an endocrinologist.[6] There is evidence showing the benefits of the role of the endocrinologist on glycemic control, either directly, through a traditional referral program, or indirectly, though creation of treatment protocols, supervision and education of other providers, or the creation of specialist diabetes clinics[79-82] Hardy and colleagues[83] showed improvement in DKD-specific end points, such as decline in the rate of decrease in GFR, in an endocrinologist-supervised diabetes nephropathy clinic. The investigators used protocols for the monitoring and management of DKD care, including glycosylated hemoglobin, lipid, and blood pressure targets, patient education, and dietary counseling. All protocols were created in conjunction with an affiliated nephrologist, with whom the care of all patients with advanced DKD was collaboratively managed. Fundamental to the success of this model was the delineation of clinical responsibility, as well as the communication of clear guidelines for the ongoing management of patients by PCPs.

SPECIAL CONSIDERATIONS IN DKD: RENAL DISEASE AND EUGLYCEMIA

The achievement of glycemic control in patients with CKD in general, and DKD in particular, is made more challenging by the pathologic impairments in the production and handling of carbohydrates and insulin that accompany these diseases.

The kidney is a major site of intrinsic glucose production in the fasting state, accounting for approximately 25% of gluconeogenesis.[84] This capacity of the kidney to accomplish gluconeogenesis is impaired with progression of CKD, at a rate that varies between individuals. In addition, the kidneys are the major site of removal and inactivation of circulating insulin, via glomerular filtration, and the intracellular degradation of insulin through a variety of intracellular processes and the action of insulinase.[85,86] The ability of the kidney to remove and inactivate insulin is impaired in CKD, and the resulting reduction in insulin metabolism and clearance induces a prolonged duration of insulin action.

Countering this process is evidence that tissue resistance to insulin is present at all stages of renal impairment, even before a measurable decrease in GFR.[87] This increase in insulin resistance is further compounded by the effect of hyperparathyroidism, low levels of calcitriol, and anemia on pancreatic islet cells and glucose tolerance in CKD.[88,89]

It has long been reported that severe DKD can result in cures of diabetes, or even episodes of spontaneous hypoglycemia.[90] These findings reflect the complex interaction of reduced caloric intake, progressive weight loss, intermittent acidosis, impaired gluconeogenesis, and reduced drug and insulin metabolism that can occur in ESRD. The balance between these processes is variable among individuals, and can translate into a challenging clinical scenario for any single provider. The complexity of disease in DKD alone suggests a need for close collaboration between the PCP, endocrinologist, and nephrologist.

SUMMARY

DKD is a complex and multifaceted disease. A substantial portion of patients remain unable to attain clinical targets for glycosylated hemoglobin, lipids, and blood pressure.[3,14] Improving outcomes requires multifactorial interventions that are best delivered through collaborative care.

Targets for improvement should include screening, diagnosis, and early referral. Following referral, the patient should be cared for in an integrated framework using the 4 elements of an effective DKD care delivery model: clear roles and responsibilities, integrated QI programs, MDT approach, and effective communication facilitated through access to a shared EMR.

Given the differences in the pathophysiology of DM in the renal population, a nephrologist and endocrinologist can be invaluable in improving care for this population. Large-scale trials are needed to validate the cost and usefulness of collaborative care as current data are insufficient. Based on available data, models such as the one proposed here should serve to maximize the strengths of individual providers and provide improved quality of care to patients.

REFERENCES

1. Castro AF, Coresh J. CKD surveillance using laboratory data from the population-based National Health and Nutrition Examination Survey (NHANES). Am J Kidney Dis 2009;53(3 Suppl 3):S46–55.
2. KDOQI clinical practice guidelines and clinical practice recommendations for diabetes and chronic kidney disease. Am J Kidney Dis 2007;49(2 Suppl 2): S12–154.
3. Collins AJ, Foley RN, Chavers B, et al. United States Renal Data System 2011 Annual Data Report: atlas of chronic kidney disease & end-stage renal disease in the United States. Am J Kidney Dis 2012;59(1 Suppl 1):A7, e1–420.
4. Lou Arnal LM, Campos GB, Cuberes IM, et al. Prevalence of chronic kidney disease in patients with type 2 diabetes mellitus treated in primary care. Nefrologia 2010;30(5):552–6 [in Spanish].
5. Olsen S, Mogensen CE. How often is NIDDM complicated with non-diabetic renal disease? An analysis of renal biopsies and the literature. Diabetologia 1996; 39(12):1638–45.
6. American Diabetes Association. Standards of medical care in diabetes - 2012. Diabetes Care 2012;35(Suppl 1):S11–63.
7. Najafian B, Mauer M. Progression of diabetic nephropathy in type 1 diabetic patients. Diabetes Res Clin Pract 2009;83:1–8.
8. The Diabetes Control and Complications Trial Research Group. The effect of intensive treatment of diabetes on the development and progression of long-term complications in insulin-dependent diabetes mellitus. N Engl J Med 1993; 329:977–86.
9. Effect of intensive blood-glucose control with metformin on complications in overweight patients with type 2 diabetes (UKPDS 34). UK Prospective Diabetes Study (UKPDS) Group. Lancet 1998;352(9131):854–65.
10. Yokoyama H, Araki S, Haneda M, et al. Chronic kidney disease categories and renal-cardiovascular outcomes in type 2 diabetes without prevalent cardiovascular disease: a prospective cohort study (JDDM25). Diabetologia 2012;55(7):1911–8.
11. Go A, Chertow GM, Fan D, et al. Chronic kidney disease and the risks of death, cardiovascular events, and hospitalization. N Engl J Med 2004;351:1296–305.
12. Evaluate Patients with CKD. National Institutes of Health 2012. Available at: http://nkdep.nih.gov/identify-manage/evaluate-patients.shtml. Accessed on September 13th, 2012.
13. Owen WF Jr. Patterns of care for patients with chronic kidney disease in the United States: dying for improvement. J Am Soc Nephrol 2003;14(7 Suppl 2): S76–80.
14. Snyder JJ, Collins AJ. KDOQI hypertension, dyslipidemia, and diabetes care guidelines and current care patterns in the United States CKD population: National Health and Nutrition Examination Survey 1999-2004. Am J Nephrol 2009;30(1):44–54.
15. Kohan DE, Rosenberg ME. The chronic kidney disease epidemic: a challenge for nephrology training programs. Semin Nephrol 2009;29(5):539–47.
16. The impact of health care reform on the future supply and demand for physicians updated projections through 2025. 2012. Ref Type: Online Source.
17. Accountable Care Organizations (ACO). 4-5-0012. Centers for Medicare & Medicaid Services. Ref Type: Online Source.
18. Understanding the patient-centered medical home. 2012. American College of Physicians. Ref Type: Online Source.

19. DuBose TD Jr, Behrens MT, Berns A, et al. The patient-centered medical home and nephrology. J Am Soc Nephrol 2009;20(4):681–2.

20. Martinez-Ramirez HR, Jalomo-Martinez B, Cortes-Sanabria L, et al. Renal function preservation in type 2 diabetes mellitus patients with early nephropathy: a comparative prospective cohort study between primary health care doctors and a nephrologist. Am J Kidney Dis 2006;47(1):78–87.

21. Khan SS, Xue JL, Kazmi WH, et al. Does predialysis nephrology care influence patient survival after the initiation of dialysis? Kidney Int 2005;67(3):1038–46.

22. Tseng CL, Kern EF, Miller DR, et al. Survival benefit of nephrologic care in patients with diabetes mellitus and chronic kidney disease. Arch Intern Med 2008;168(1): 55–62.

23. Meyers JL, Candrilli SD, Kovacs B. Type 2 diabetes mellitus and renal impairment in a large outpatient electronic medical records database: rates of diagnosis and antihyperglycemic medication dose adjustment. Postgrad Med 2011;123(3): 133–43.

24. Boulware L, Troll M, Jaar B, et al. Identification and referral of patients with progressive CKD: a national study. Am J Kidney Dis 2006;48(2):192–204.

25. Strippoli GF, Craig JC, Schena FP. The number, quality, and coverage of randomized controlled trials in nephrology. J Am Soc Nephrol 2004;15(2):411–9.

26. Stoves J, Connolly J, Cheung CK, et al. Electronic consultation as an alternative to hospital referral for patients with chronic kidney disease: a novel application for networked electronic health records to improve the accessibility and efficiency of healthcare. Qual Saf Health Care 2010;19(5):e54.

27. Cortes-Sanabria L, Cabrera-Pivaral CE, Cueto-Manzano AM, et al. Improving care of patients with diabetes and CKD: a pilot study for a cluster-randomized trial. Am J Kidney Dis 2008;51(5):777–88.

28. Rayner HC, Hollingworth L, Higgins R, et al. Systematic kidney disease management in a population with diabetes mellitus: turning the tide of kidney failure. BMJ Qual Saf 2011;20(10):903–10.

29. de Boer IH, Sun W, Cleary PA, et al. Intensive diabetes therapy and glomerular filtration rate in type 1 diabetes. N Engl J Med 2011;365(25):2366–76.

30. Moyer VA. Screening for chronic kidney disease: U.S. Preventive Services Task Force Recommendation Statement. Ann Intern Med 2012;157(8):567–70.

31. Manns B, Hemmelgarn B, Tonelli M, et al. Population based screening for chronic kidney disease: cost effectiveness study. BMJ 2010;341:c5869.

32. Ryan TP, Sloand JA, Winters PC, et al. Chronic kidney disease prevalence and rate of diagnosis. Am J Med 2007;120(11):981–6.

33. Humphreys J, Harvey G, Coleiro M, et al. A collaborative project to improve identification and management of patients with chronic kidney disease in a primary care setting in Greater Manchester. BMJ Qual Saf 2012;21(8):700–8.

34. Fox CH, Swanson A, Kahn LS, et al. Improving chronic kidney disease care in primary care practices: an Upstate New York Practice-based Research Network (UNYNET) study. J Am Board Fam Med 2008;21(6):522–30.

35. Rutkowski M, Mann W, Derose S, et al. Implementing KDOQI CKD definition and staging guidelines in Southern California Kaiser Permanente. Am J Kidney Dis 2009;53(3 Suppl 3):S86–99.

36. Campbell GA, Bolton WK. Referral and comanagement of the patient with CKD. Adv Chronic Kidney Dis 2011;18(6):420–7.

37. Herget-Rosenthal S, Quellmann T, Linden C, et al. How does late nephrological co-management impact chronic kidney disease? - an observational study. Int J Clin Pract 2010;64(13):1784–92.

38. Ritz E. Consequences of late referral in diabetic renal disease. Acta Diabetol 2002;39(Suppl 1):S3–8.
39. Arora P, Obrador GT, Ruthazer R, et al. Prevalence, predictors, and consequences of late nephrology referral at a tertiary care center. J Am Soc Nephrol 1999;10:1281–6.
40. Fisher M, Ahya S, Gordon E. Interventions to reduce late referrals to nephrologists. Am J Nephrol 2011;33:60–9.
41. Navaneethan SD, Aloudate S, Singh S. A systematic review of patient and health system characteristics associated with late referral in CKD. BMC Nephrol 2009;9:3.
42. Campbell KH, Smith SG, Hemmerich J, et al. Patient and provider determinants of nephrology referral in older adults with severe chronic kidney disease: a survey of provider decision making. BMC Nephrol 2011;12:47.
43. Gandhi TK, Sittig DF, Franklin M, et al. Communication breakdown in the outpatient referral process. J Gen Intern Med 2000;15(9):626–31.
44. Diamantidis CJ, Powe NR, Jaar BG, et al. Primary care-specialist collaboration in the care of patients with chronic kidney disease. Clin J Am Soc Nephrol 2011;6(2):334–43.
45. Ronksley PE, Hemmelgarn BR. Optimizing care for patients with CKD. Am J Kidney Dis 2012;60(1):133–8.
46. Bolton WK, Owen WF Jr. Preparing the kidney failure patient for renal replacement therapy. Teamwork optimizes outcomes. Postgrad Med 2002;111(6):97–108.
47. Clancy CM. Kidney-related diseases and quality improvement: AHRQ's role. Clin J Am Soc Nephrol 2011;6(10):2531–3.
48. Diabetes care quality improvement: resource guide. 9-14-2012. Ref Type: Online Source. Available at: http://www.ahrq.gov/qual/diabqual/diabqguidemod5.htm.
49. Bolton WK. Renal Physicians Association. Clinical practice guideline: appropriate patient preparation for renal replacement therapy. Guideline Number 3. Renal Physicians Association Guideline. J Am Soc Nephrol 2003;14(5):1406–10.
50. Bolton WK. The role of the nephrologist in ESRD/pre-ESRD care: a collaborative approach. J Am Soc Nephrol 1998;9:S90–5.
51. Bolton WK. Nephrology nurse practitioners in a collaborative care model. Am J Kidney Dis 1998;31:786–93.
52. Holley JL, McGuirl K. Advanced practice nurses in ESRD: varied roles and a cost analysis. Nephrol News Issues 2000;14(3):18–20.
53. Bolton WK, Kliger AS. Chronic renal insufficiency: current understandings and their implications. Am J Kidney Dis 2000;36(6):S4–12.
54. Renders CM, Valk GD, Griffin S, et al. Interventions to improve the management of diabetes mellitus in primary care, outpatient and community settings. Cochrane Database Syst Rev 2001;(1):CD001481.
55. Pimouguet C, Le GM, Thiebaut R, et al. Effectiveness of disease-management programs for improving diabetes care: a meta-analysis. CMAJ 2011;183(2):E115–27.
56. Wynia MK, Von KI, Mitchell PH. Challenges at the intersection of team-based and patient-centered health care: insights from an IOM working group. JAMA 2012;308(13):1327–8.
57. Saxena R, Bygren P, Butkowski RJ, et al. Specificity of kidney-bound antibodies in Goodpasture's syndrome. Clin Exp Immunol 1989;78:31–6.
58. Hemmelgarn BR, Manns BJ, Zhang J, et al. Association between multidisciplinary care and survival for elderly patients with chronic kidney disease. J Am Soc Nephrol 2007;18:993–9.

59. Richards N, Whitfield M, O'Donoghue D, et al. Primary care-based disease management of chronic kidney disease (CKD), based on estimated glomerular filtration rate (eGFR) reporting, improves patient outcomes. Nephrol Dial Transplant 2008;23(2):549–55.

60. Wu IW, Wang SY, Hsu KH, et al. Multidisciplinary predialysis education decreased the incidence of dialysis and reduces mortality-a controlled cohort study based on the NKF/DOQI guidelines. Nephrol Dial Transplant 2009;24:3426–33.

61. Thanamayooran S, Rose C, Hirsch DJ. Effectiveness of a multidisciplinary kidney disease clinic in achieving treatment guideline targets. Nephrol Dial Transplant 2005;20:2385–93.

62. Kim-Hwang JE, Chen AH, Bell DS, et al. Evaluating electronic referrals for specialty care at a public hospital. J Gen Intern Med 2010;25(10):1123–8.

63. Chang J, Ronco C, Rosner MH. Computerized decision support systems: improving patient safety in nephrology. Nat Rev Nephrol 2011;7(6):348–55.

64. Abdel-Kader K, Fischer GS, Li J, et al. Automated clinical reminders for primary care providers in the care of CKD: a small cluster-randomized controlled trial. Am J Kidney Dis 2011;58(6):894–902.

65. O'Reilly D, Holbrook A, Blackhouse G, et al. Cost-effectiveness of a shared computerized decision support system for diabetes linked to electronic medical records. J Am Med Inform Assoc 2012;19(3):341–5.

66. UKPDS 3. Intensive blood-glucose control with sulphonylureas or insulin compared with conventional treatment and risk of complications in patients with type 2 diabetes. Lancet 1998;352(9131):837–53.

67. Ohkubo Y, Kishikawa H, Araki E, et al. Intensive insulin therapy prevents the progression of diabetic microvascular complications in Japanese patients with non-insulin-dependent diabetes mellitus: a randomized prospective 6-year study [see comments]. Diabetes Res Clin Pract 1901;28(2):103–17.

68. Shichiri M, Kishikawa H, Ohkubo Y, et al. Long-term results of the Kumamoto Study on optimal diabetes control in type 2 diabetic patients. Diabetes Care 2000;23(Suppl 2):B21–9.

69. Coppelli A, Giannarelli R, Vistoli F, et al. The beneficial effects of pancreas transplant alone on diabetic nephropathy. Diabetes Care 2005;28(6):1366–70.

70. Gross JL, de Azevedo MJ, Silveiro SP, et al. Diabetic nephropathy: diagnosis, prevention, and treatment. Diabetes Care 2005;28(1):164–76.

71. American Diabetes Association. Nephropathy in Diabetes. Position Statement. Diab Care 2004;27:S79–83.

72. Grant RW, Buse JB, Meigs JB. Quality of diabetes care in U.S. academic medical centers: low rates of medical regimen change. Diabetes Care 2005;28(2):337–442.

73. Quinn DC, Graber AL, Elasy TA, et al. Overcoming turf battles: developing a pragmatic, collaborative model to improve glycemic control in patients with diabetes. Jt Comm J Qual Improv 2001;27(5):255–64.

74. Del PS, Felton AM, Munro N, et al. Improving glucose management: ten steps to get more patients with type 2 diabetes to glycaemic goal. Recommendations from the Global Partnership for Effective Diabetes Management. Int J Clin Pract Suppl 2007;157:47–57.

75. Cramer JA. A systematic review of adherence with medications for diabetes. Diabetes Care 2004;27(5):1218–24.

76. Odegard PS, Gray SL. Barriers to medication adherence in poorly controlled diabetes mellitus. Diabetes Educ 2008;34(4):692–7.

77. Phillips LS, Branch WT, Cook CB, et al. Clinical inertia. Ann Intern Med 2001; 135(9):825–34.
78. Shah BR, Hux JE, Laupacis A, et al. Clinical inertia in response to inadequate glycemic control: do specialists differ from primary care physicians? Diabetes Care 2005;28(3):600–6.
79. Phillips LS, Ziemer DC, Doyle JP, et al. An endocrinologist-supported intervention aimed at providers improves diabetes management in a primary care site: improving primary care of African Americans with diabetes (IPCAAD) 7. Diabetes Care 2005;28(10):2352–60.
80. de Sonnaville JJ, Bouma M, Colly LP, et al. Sustained good glycaemic control in NIDDM patients by implementation of structured care in general practice: 2-year follow-up study. Diabetologia 1997;40(11):1334–40.
81. Verlato G, Muggeo M, Bonora E, et al. Attending the diabetes center is associated with increased 5-year survival probability of diabetic patients: the Verona Diabetes Study. Diabetes Care 1996;19(3):211–3.
82. Graber AL, Elasy TA, Quinn D, et al. Improving glycemic control in adults with diabetes mellitus: shared responsibility in primary care practices. South Med J 2002; 95(7):684–90.
83. Hardy K, Furlong N, Hulme S, et al. Delivering improved management and outcomes in diabetic kidney disease in routine clinical care. Br J Diabetes Vasc Dis 2007;7:172–82.
84. Gerich JE, Meyer C, Woerle HJ, et al. Renal gluconeogenesis: its importance in human glucose homeostasis. Diabetes Care 2001;24(2):382–91.
85. Valera Mora ME, Scarfone A, Calvani M, et al. Insulin clearance in obesity. J Am Coll Nutr 2003;22(6):487–93.
86. Mak RH, DeFronzo RA. Glucose and insulin metabolism in uremia. Nephron 1992; 61(4):377–82.
87. Becker B, Kronenberg F, Kielstein JT, et al. Renal insulin resistance syndrome, adiponectin and cardiovascular events in patients with kidney disease: the mild and moderate kidney disease study. J Am Soc Nephrol 2005;16(4):1091–8.
88. Hajjar SM, Fadda GZ, Thanakitcharu P, et al. Reduced activity of Na(+)-K+ ATPase of pancreatic islets in chronic renal failure: role of secondary hyperparathyroidism. J Am Soc Nephrol 1992;2(8):1355–9.
89. Chagnac A, Weinstein T, Zevin D, et al. Effects of erythropoietin on glucose tolerance in hemodialysis patients. Clin Nephrol 1994;42(6):398–400.
90. Runyan JW Jr, Hurwitz D, Robbins SL. Effect of Kimmelstiel-Wilson syndrome on insulin requirements in diabetes. N Engl J Med 1955;252(10):388–91.

Index

Note: Page numbers of article titles are in **boldface** type.

A

A Study of Cardiovascular Events in Diabetes (ASCEND) trial, 3, 10–11, 125–126
Acarbose, 146, 149
ACCORD (Action to Control Cardiovascular Risk in Diabetes) trial, 45, 82, 143
Accountable care organizations, 164–165
A1c-Derived Average Glucose Study, 139
Actinin, genes for, 101
Action in Diabetes and Vascular Disease: Preterax and Diamicron-MR Controlled Evaluation study, 10
Action to Control Cardiovascular Risk in Diabetes (ACCORD) trial, 45, 82, 143
Acute kidney injury, in type 2 diabetes, 20
Adiponectin, in obesity, 67
ADVANCE study, 82, 143
Advanced glycation end products
    as drug targets, **115–134**
    formation of, 77, 116–117
AGTR1 gene, 94
Albuminuria, 1–2. *See also* Microalbuminuria.
    in type 2 diabetes, 8–11
    incidence of, 9–10
    obesity and, 65–66
    prevalence of, 8
    progression of, 9–10
    renal impairment without, 6–7
Aliskiren, 24, 41–42
Aliskiren Trial in Type 2 Diabetes Using Cardiovascular and Renal Disease Endpoints (ALTITUDE) trial, 42
Allopurinol, 25, 129
Alpha-glucosidase inhibitors, 146, 149
ALTITUDE (Aliskiren Trial in Type 2 Diabetes Using Cardiovascular and Renal Disease Endpoints) trial, 42
Amylin mimetics, 147, 149
Angiotensin II type I receptor gene, 94
Angiotensin receptor blockers, 23–24, 38–42, 83–85
Angiotensin-converting enzyme inhibitors, 23–24, 38–42, 83–85
Angiotensin-converting enzymes, in hypertension, 34
Antifibrotic agents, 116–120
Antioxidant inflammation modulators, 120–123
ASCEND (A Study of Cardiovascular Events in Diabetes) trial, 3, 10–11, 125–126
AST-120, 119–120
Asymmetric dimethylarginine, in hypertension, 36
Atrasentan, 43–44, 125–126

Med Clin N Am 97 (2013) 175–183
http://dx.doi.org/10.1016/S0025-7125(12)00231-3
0025-7125/13/$ – see front matter © 2013 Elsevier Inc. All rights reserved.

medical.theclinics.com

AUH gene, 99–100
Australian Diabetes, Obesity, and Lifestyle study, 8
Avosentan, 25, 43–44, 123–126

B

Bardoxolone, 25, 120–123
BEACON (Bardoxolone Methyl Evaluation in Patients with Chronic Kidney Disease and Type Diabetes 2) study, 121
Benazepril, for hypertension, 40
BENEDICT (Bergamo Nephrologic Diabetes Complications Trial), 23
Bergamo Nephrologic Diabetes Complications Trial (BENEDICT), 23
Biguanides, 145–146
Bile acid sequestrants, 147, 149
Bosentan, 43, 123
Bromocriptine, 147, 149

C

Candesartan, for hypertension, 40
Captopril, for hypertension, 38
Carnosinase 1 gene defects, 94
Casale Monferrato study, 8–10
China National Survey of Chronic Kidney Disease, 2–3
Chronic Disease Model, 164
Chronic Kidney Disease Epidemiology Collaboration formula, 1
Chronic Kidney Disease Prognosis Consortium, 9–10
Clinical decision support systems, 167
Clorpropamide, 145
CNCP1 gene defects, 94
Cohen diabetic rats, 54
COL28A1 gene, 102–103
Colesevelam, 147, 149
Collaborative care, for diabetic kidney disease, **157–173**
    attitudes toward, 163
    barriers to, 158
    care delivery model for, 163–167
    diagnosis of, 158–161
    euglycemia and, 168
    glycemic control in, 167–168
    referral in, 161–163
    screening in, 158–161
Combination Angiotensin Receptor Blocker and Angiotensin Converting Enzyme Inhibitor for Treatment of Diabetic Nephropathy study, 39
Communication, in collaborative care, 166–167
Computerized provider order entry, 167
Cystatin C, 12–13
Cytokines, in obesity, 67

D

DCCT (Diabetes Control and Complications Trial), 5, 24, 139
DEMAND (Developing Education on MA for Awareness of renal and cardiovascular risk iN Diabetes) study, 2–3, 11, 55

Diabetes Control and Complications Trial (DCCT), 5, 24, 139
Diabetes mellitus, in kidney disease, **135–156**
Diabetes Mellitus Treatment for Renal Insufficiency Consortium, 20
Diabetic kidney disease
    definition of, 1
    economic burden of, 3
    end-stage. *See* End-stage renal disease.
    epidemiology of, **1–18,** 19–21, 75–76
    genetic factors in, **91–107**
    hypertension in. *See* Hypertension.
    in elderly persons, **75–89**
    in prediabetes, 12
    in type 1 diabetes, 3–8
    in type 2 diabetes, 8–12
    natural history of, 5–8, 78–79
    nonproteinuric, 20–21, **53–58**
    obesity and, **59–74**
    pancreas transplantation for, **109–114**
    pathophysiology of, 76–80
    subclinical, 12–13
    treatment of, 21–25
        cooperative approach to, **157–173**
        in elderly individuals, 80–86
        multifactorial, 24–25
        new, **115–134**
    worldwide burden of, 2–3
Dialysis Outcomes and Practice Patterns Study (DOPPS), 142
DIAMETRIC database, 9
Diet, for diabetes mellitus, 144
Dimethylarginine dimethylaminohydrolase, in hypertension, 36
Dipeptidyl peptidase 4 inhibitors, 147–148
Direct renin inhibitors, for hypertension, 42
DNA sequencing, in diabetic kidney disease, 101–104
Dopamine-2 agonists, 147, 149
DOPPS (Dialysis Outcomes and Practice Patterns Study), 142
Doxycycline, 118–119

E

EDIC (Epidemiology of Diabetes Interventions and Complications) study, 5–7, 24
Elderly individuals, diabetic kidney disease in, **75–89**
    diagnosis of, 80
    epidemiology of, 75–76
    natural history of, 78–79
    pathophysiology of, 76–80
    treatment of, 80–86
ELMO1 gene, 98–100
Enalapril, for hypertension, 36
Endothelial cells, dysfunction of, in hypertension, 34, 36, 42–44
Endothelin, in hypertension, 36
Endothelin receptor blockers, 25, 123–126

End-stage renal disease
    causes of, 60
    epidemiology of, 3
    genetic factors in, 91–107
    in elderly individuals, 76
    in type 1 diabetes, 4, 6–7
    incidence of, 4, 6–7, 20
    mortality in, 6–7
    obesity and, 59–62
Engulfment and cell motility gene, 98–100
Epidemiology of Diabetes Interventions and Complications (EDIC) study, 5–7, 24
Estimated glomerular filtration rate, heritability of, 92–97
Ethnic factors, in diabetic kidney disease, 10–11, 91–107
Euglycemia, in collaborative care, 168
Exenatide, 147–148
Exercise, for diabetes mellitus, 144

        F

Familial clustering, in diabetic kidney disease, 92–93
Family Investigation of Nephropathy and Diabetes (FIND) collection, 94
Fasidil, 129
FG-3019, 119
Fibrosis, inhibitors of, 116–120
FIND (Family Investigation of Nephropathy and Diabetes) collection, 94
Finnish Diabetes Register, 6–7
Free oxygen radicals, in hypertension, 36–37
Fructosamine, for glycemic control assessment, 140

        G

Genetic factors, in diabetic kidney disease, **91–107**
    familial clustering in, 92–93
    genome-wide association scans in, 98–101
    genome-wide linkage analysis in, 93–98
    next-generation sequencing in, 101–104
Genetics of Kidneys in Diabetes collections, 100
Genome-wide association scans, in diabetic kidney disease, 98–101
Genome-wide linkage analysis, in diabetic kidney disease, 93–98
Gliclazide, 146
Glimepiride, 145–146
Glipizide, 145–146
Glomerular filtration rate
    in early diabetes, 12–13
    in obesity, 63–64
    in prediabetes, 12
Glomerulonephritis, postinfectious, 21
Glomerulopathy
    age-related, 77
    in obesity, 63–64, 66–68
GLP-1 receptor agonists, 147–148

Gluconeogenesis, in kidney, 168
Glucose abnormalities, in kidney disease, **135–156**
    glycemic control in, 138–150
    hypoglycemia, 143–144
    overview of, 136–138
Glyburide, 145–146
Glycated albumin, for glycemic control assessment, 140–141
Glycemic control, in kidney disease, 24, 81–82, 138–150
    challenges in, 144
    choices for, 150
    hypoglycemia in, 143–144
    in collaborative care, 167–168
    insulin for, 149–150
    noninsulin drugs for, 144–149
    testing for, 141–143
    value of, 138–141

H

Hemodialysis, glycemic control in, 139–141
Hemoglobin A1c measurement, 138–143
Heritability, of diabetic kidney disease, 92–93
Hyperfiltration
    in hypertension, 33–34
    in obesity, 63–64
Hypertension, **31–51**
    clinical context of, 32–33
    incidence of, 32–33
    obesity and, 64–65
    pathophysiology of, 33–37
    prevalence of, 32–33
    target treatment for, 32
    treatment of, 22–23, 38–45, 82–83
Hypertension Optimal Treatment trial, 45
Hypoglycemia, in diabetes mellitus treatment, 143–144

I

IDNT (Irbesartan Diabetic Nephropathy Trial), 22, 45
Inflammatory markers, in obesity, 67
Insulin, for diabetes mellitus, 149–150
Insulin resistance, in kidney disease, 135, 137
Interleukin-6, in obesity, 67
International Diabetes Federation Diabetes Atlas, on worldwide burden, 2
Irbesartan, for hypertension, 41
Irbesartan Diabetic Nephropathy Trial (IDNT), 22, 45

J

Joslin Study of the Natural History of Microalbuminuria, 5, 7
Joslin Study on the Genetics of type 2 Diabetes collection, 92–93

K

Kaiser Permanente Northwest, cost statistics in, 3
Kaiser Permanente of Southern California, 161
KEEP (Kidney Early Evaluation Program), 76
Kidney Dialysis Outcomes Quality Initiative, 139–140, 158–159
Kidney disease
    diabetic. *See* Diabetic kidney disease.
    glucose abnormalities in, **135–156**
Kidney Disease Outcomes Quality Initiative, 45
Kidney Early Evaluation Program (KEEP), 76, 159
Kimmelstiel-Wilson disease, 20
Kremezin Study Against Renal Diseases Progression in Korea (K-STAR), 120

L

Leptin, elevated, in obesity in, 67
Lifestyle changes, for diabetes mellitus, 144
Linagliptin, 147–148
Linkage analysis, in diabetic kidney disease, 93–98
Liraglutide, 147–148
Lisinopril, for hypertension, 40
Losartan, for hypertension, 41, 43

M

Matrix metalloproteinase inhibitors, 118–119
Meglitinides, 148–149
Metabolic syndrome, 21
Metformin, 145–146
Microalbuminuria, 1–2
    in nonproteinuric diabetic kidney disease, 53–58
    in type 1 diabetes, 3–8
    in type 2 diabetes, 8–11
    incidence of, 6
    obesity and, 65–66
    prevalence of, 5
    progression of, 5, 7–8
Miglitol, 146, 149
Mineralocorticoid receptor antagonists, for hypertension, 39
Modification of Diet in Renal Disease Study equation, 1
Mortality
    in end-stage renal disease, 6–7
    in type 2 diabetes, 9
Multidisciplinary team, 165–166
MYH9 gene, 98
Myosin heavy chain 9 gene, 98

N

Nateglinide, 146, 149
National Health and Nutrition Examination Survey (NHANES), 55, 76

National Institute of Diabetes and Digestive and Kidney Diseases study, 118
Nephrin
    genes for, 101
    in obesity, 67
Nephrologists, in collaborative care, **157–173**
Nephropathy, diabetic. *See* Diabetic kidney disease.
Next-generation sequencing, in diabetic kidney disease, 101–104
NHANES (National Health and Nutrition Examination Survey), 55, 76
Nicorandil, for hypertension, 43
Nitric oxide, in hypertension, 36
Nonproteinuric diabetic kidney disease, 20–21, **53–58**

O

Obesity, diabetic kidney disease and, **59–74**
    epidemiology of, 60–62
    pathophysiology of, 62–68
    prevalence of, 59
ONTARGET (Ongoing Telmisartan Alone and in Combination with Ramipril Global Endpoint
    Trial), 23, 39
Oxidative stress, in hypertension, 36–37

P

Palosuran, 128–129
Pancreas, transplantation of, **109–114**
Paricalcitol, 126–128
Patient-centered medical home, 164–165
Pediatric patients, end-stage renal disease in, 20
Pentoxifylline, 120–121, 123
Phospholipase C, epsilon 1 gene, 101
Pioglitazone, 145–146, 148
Pirfenidone, 116, 118
Pittsburgh Epidemiology of Diabetes Complications Study, 6
Plasmacytoma variant translocation gene, 99–100
Podocin
    genes for, 101
    in obesity, 67
Pramlintide, 147, 149
Prediabetes, kidney function in, 12
PREDIAN (Pentoxifylline for Renoprotection in Diabetic Nephropathy) study, 123
PREVEND (Prevention of Renal and Vascular End state Disease), 65–66
Prevention of Renal and Vascular End state Disease (PREVEND), 65–66
Primary care providers, in collaborative care, **157–173**
Proteinuria. *See also* Albuminuria; Microalbuminuria.
    diabetic kidney disease without, 20–21, **53–58**
    in type 1 diabetes, 4–7
    incidence of, 4, 6
    natural history of, 5–8
    prevalence of, 5
PVT1 gene, 99–100

R

Ramipril Efficacy in Nephropathy (REIN) study, 42
Randomized Olmesartan And Diabetes MicroAlbuminuria Prevention (ROADMAP) study, 22–23
Receptor for AGE, 77
Referral, in collaborative care, 161–163
REIN (Ramipril Efficacy in Nephropathy) study, 42
RENAAL trial, 43
Renal Data System, 3
Renal Insufficiency and Cardiovascular Events study, 11–12
Renin inhibitors, for hypertension, 42
Renin-angiotensin system
    blockade of, 23–24, 38–42
    in hypertension, 34–35
    in obesity, 67–68
Repaglinide, 146, 149
Rho kinase inhibitors, 129
ROADMAP (Randomized Olmesartan And DiabetesMicroAlbuminuria Prevention) study, 22–23
Rosiglitazone, 145–146, 148
Rubosistaurin, 128

S

Saxagliptin, 147–148
Shanghai Diabetic Complications Study, 8
Single nucleotide polymorphisms, in diabetic kidney disease, 93–104
Sitagliptin, 147–148
Sodium
    reabsorption of, in hypertension, 33–34
    restriction of, for hypertension, 42
Spironolactone, for hypertension, 41
Steno Memorial Hospital study, 4–5, 7, 9
Sulfonylureas, 145–146
Sulodexide, 56
Swedish Linköping study, 6
Swedish National Diabetes Register, 11
Sympathetic nervous system, increased activity of, in hypertension, 36
Systolic Hypertension in the Elderly Population, 82–83

T

Telmisartan, for hypertension, 23, 39
Thiazolidinediones, 145–146, 148
Trandolapril, 23
Tranilast, 120
Transforming growth factor-β, 68, 94
Transient receptor potential cation channel subfamily C genes, 101
Transplantation, pancreas, for diabetic kidney disease, **109–114**
Tubuloglomerular feedback, 63
Tumor necrosis factor-α, in obesity, 67

U

United Kingdom Prospective Diabetes Study (UKPDS), 9, 22, 24, 81–82, 95, 139
United States Renal Data System, 20
Uric acid control, 25

V

VA NEPHRON study, 39
Valsartan, for hypertension, 40
Veterans Affairs Diabetes Trial, 82, 143
VITAL study, 127
Vitamin D, for hypertension, 42

W

Wisconsin Epidemiologic Study of Diabetic Retinopathy, 8

Moving?

Make sure your subscription moves with you!

To notify us of your new address, find your **Clinics Account Number** (located on your mailing label above your name), and contact customer service at:

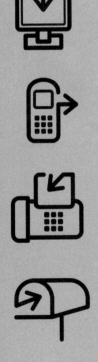

Email: **journalscustomerservice-usa@elsevier.com**

800-654-2452 (subscribers in the U.S. & Canada)
314-447-8871 (subscribers outside of the U.S. & Canada)

Fax number: **314-447-8029**

Elsevier Health Sciences Division
Subscription Customer Service
3251 Riverport Lane
Maryland Heights, MO 63043

ELSEVIER